MW01515834

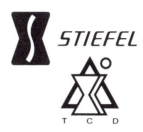

STIEFEL

T C D

Compliments of / Gracieuseté de Stiefel Canada Inc.

For Dr Sandy Skotnicki
with thanks and best wishes

Robert Jackson
August 1998

Morphological Diagnosis of Skin Disease

MORPHOLOGICAL DIAGNOSIS OF SKIN DISEASE

A Study of the Living Gross Pathology of the Skin

ROBERT JACKSON, MD, FRCPC

DERMATOLOGIST, OTTAWA CIVIC HOSPITAL
EMERITUS PROFESSOR OF MEDICINE (DERMATOLOGY)
UNIVERSITY OF OTTAWA

With a Foreword by
Thomas B. Fitzpatrick, MD

1998 MANTICORE PUBLISHERS

© Copyright Robert Jackson under the International Copyright Union.

All rights reserved. No part of this publication, in the original language or any translated language, may be reused, republished, reproduced, stored in a retrieval system, or transmitted in any form without prior written permission from the publisher. Requests for permissions or further information should be sent to the publisher, Manticore Publishers, Grimsby, Ontario, Canada.

NOTICE

This book is sold on the understanding that the publisher is not engaged in rendering medical or other professional services. The authors and publishers have done all they can to ensure that the care which may be recommended in this book reflects the best current practices and standards (this includes choice of medication and dosage). However, as research, regulations and clinical practices are constantly changing, you are encouraged to check all product information sheets from all medical packages. If in doubt about anything in this book or on the product information sheets, contact your personal physician for advice on proper procedure.

For Manticore Publishers
Design and Production: Bond Creative Communications

Body text is set using the Minion family of types designed by Robert Slimbach. Heading are set using the Myriad family of types designed by Robert Slimbach and Carol Twomby.

Printed in Canada
ISBN 1-896918-02-6

for
Dr. Barney Usher
Dr. Henry E. Michelson
Dr. George S. Williamson

*A student is not a vessel to be filled
but a lamp to be lighted.*

—Russian proverb

The true mystery of the world is the visible, not the invisible.
—Oscar Wilde

*Basic lesions are the alphabet without which
nobody can read the language of the skin.*
Jean Darier 1856-1938, l'hôpital Saint Louis, Paris

*There is an old axiom in Viennese dermatology that if you cannot
make a diagnosis you must make a good description, and the better
the description the more apt one is to arrive at a diagnosis.*
Henry E. Michelson 1888-1972, dermatologist,
University of Minnesota–Arch Dermatol 1966;93:250

*Harvey's law: When what you see does not easily resemble or remind
you of a clinical diagnosis, be sure to ask yourself–has something
been done or applied to the lesion.*
Harvey Finkelstein, dermatology resident 1982-1985,
now dermatologist, Ottawa Civic Hospital

Foreword

With the new emphasis on primary care medicine, there appears to be a notion that the clinical skill of diagnosing skin lesions, the precious possession of the trained dermatologist, can be quite easily learned by general physicians who are now, in fact, doing "punch" biopsies of skin with the hope that this will clinch the diagnosis. Gross pathology of skin is the basic and first aspect of diagnosis in dermatology. Prof H. Haxthausen said that "we often have to call in the aid of the microscopic and other special laboratory examinations, but the fundamental basis of all dermatological diagnoses is, however, always direct macroscopic observations". For the trained dermatologist, a methodical scanning of the clinical lesions leads to the diagnosis. For example, four elements of morphology lead to the clinical diagnosis of the two type of herpes infection (herpes simplex and herpes zoster) 1) type of lesion: vesicle, 2) shape: umbilicated vesicles, 3) arrangement (a "bouquet" of vesicles), 4) distribution: unilateral, in a linear pattern along a dermatome in herpes zoster.

Robert Jackson, MD has been a pioneer in preserving the body of knowledge of morphologic diagnosis in dermatology at a time when morphology is a neglected aspect of residency training. This is regrettable because dermatologic diagnostic skill needs to be revitalized with training program instruction in morphologic diagnosis. With the advent of managed care the clinical domain of dermatology can be extenuated: surgery of tumors and cosmetic procedures can be performed by plastic surgeons; severe acne can be treated with oral isotretinoin, fungous infections by new highly effective oral drugs. Yet the large body of inflammatory disorders (psoriasis, eczema, etc.) requires the morphologic skill of a dermatologist for diagnosis in order to select the proper treatment; these disorders cannot be treated by topical corticosteroids alone. The psoriasis reaction pattern occurs not only in psoriasis, but also in fungous disease of the skin, seborrheic dermatitis, secondary syphilis, mycosis fungoides, drug eruptions. The correct diagnosis will result in effective treatment.

This book should be studied by every resident in training and, furthermore, a copy should be at hand in every dermatologist's office so that he/she can continue to perfect his/her morphologic "eye".

Thomas B. Fitzpatrick, M.D., PhD., D.Sc. (Hon.), D.Sc. (Hon.)
Wigglesworth Professor of Dermatology, Emeritus
Chairman, Emeritus
Department of Dermatology, Harvard Medical School
Chief Emeritus, Dermatology Service
Massachusetts General Hospital
Boston, Massachusetts

What thou seest, write in a book

REV. 1:11

*Frye has observed repeatedly that he repeats himself and that
he wouldn't trust any writer who did not.
He adds that what he hopes for, of course, is an increase in lucidity*

Double Vision–Frye: An Appreciation by Johan Aitkin.
University of Toronto Press, 1991, p. xi

*The most difficult problem is to learn to see.
All else is comparatively simple.*

Alfred Stieglitz, 1911. 1864–1946, American photographer.
Stieglitz A. Letter to John Garo.
Wilson's Photographic Magazine. 1911; October: 437

Preface

The purpose of this handbook is to describe in detail the visible changes in the skin and visible mucosae in various morbid conditions. It is designed primarily for dermatology residents but may also be useful to dermatologists and other physicians interested in increasing their knowledge of the living gross pathology of the skin.

The need for this handbook became obvious when I could not find among the current standard English dermatological texts sufficiently detailed morphological descriptions for use in training dermatology residents. These residents must know not only that a skin condition is keratosis pilaris but be able to detail all the various morphological findings characteristic of this disease. They must also be able to give a detailed differential diagnosis[1] of follicular eruptions which may simulate keratosis pilaris and know the significant diagnostic morphological details.

I believe that the raison d'etre for the speciality of dermatology is that dermatologists can with the naked eye make diagnoses that other physicians cannot. Knowledge in such fields as histopathology, physiology, biochemistry, and immunoelectrophoresis will not help the dermatologist who cannot tell pityriasis rosea from guttate parapsoriasis by clinical examination. This is the nitty gritty of dermatology. It is important that dermatologists do not forget it.

The emphasis is on the morphology of skin diseases with particular reference to differential diagnosis. Diagnosis of diseases and the morphological variations of diseases commonly misdiagnosed by residents and staff physicians are stressed.[2] The minutiae of common diseases such as eczema, psoriasis and acne form a large portion of this book.

The concept implied in the term visual literacy[3] has much to recommend it and perhaps indicates in two words what I am trying to provide with this handbook.

Despite the nonmorphological advances in dermatology, it is amazing how much of day-to-day practice is still based on the intelligent appraisal of the living gross pathology of skin diseases. This book is not based on pathogenetic mechanisms, because for many skin conditions and diseases we have no idea why or how the condition or disease occurs. This is particularly true for some morphological groupings (e.g. the keratoses, the verrucosities, and the atrophies, scleroses, and dystrophies).

The text has been based in part on residents' descriptions of conditions submitted to me as part of their training. Many of the cases were presented and discussed at the weekly dermatology rounds held at the Ottawa Civic Hospital. I am indebted to all the residents who have stimulated me to put this handbook together. Their names are listed below:

Dr. R.N. Richards	1967–68	Dr. S.A. Gardere	1968–69
Dr. R.H. Adams	1969–70	Dr. J.F. Hogan	1969–70
Dr. P.J. Craan	1970–71	Dr. J.D. Amiss	1970–71

Dr. Francois Panaccio 1971–72   Dr. J.M. Grainge 1971–72
Dr. A.J. Williams 1972–73   Dr. Paul Brisson 1972–73
Dr. R.J. Conklin 1973–74   Dr. N.M. Mayer 1973–74
Dr. O. Fournier-Blake 1974–75   Dr. David Gratton 1974–75
Dr. G.A. Wasserman 1975–76   Dr. N.J. Shiffman 1975–76
Dr. B.H. Wolk. 1975–77   Dr. E. O'Brien 1976–77
Dr. M.J. Gulliver 1976–77   Dr. P.F. Horan 1977–78
Dr. J.D. Walker 1977–79   Dr. S.A. Laughlin 1977–80
Dr. K.A. Barber 1978–79   Dr. S.M. Swiggum 1978–79
Dr. M. Davis. 1979–81   Dr. R. Kunynetz 1979–82
Dr. M. Pratt 1980–83   Dr. L. Weatherhead 1980–83
Dr. C. Ruddy 1981–84   Dr. D. Quintal 1982–84
Dr. H. Finkelstein 1982–85   Dr. J. Rivers 1983–85
Dr. J. Martin. 1984–85   Dr. F. Thompson 1984–85
Dr. D. McAuley 1985–86   Dr. E. Minuk 1985–87
Dr. S.M. Swiggum 1985–87   Dr. S. Ryan 1985–87
Dr. S. Murray 1986–87   Dr. R. Tremaine 1987–88
Dr. C. Tsoulis 1987–89   Dr. J. Keddy-Grant 1987–90
Dr. L. Parsons. 1987–90   Dr. S. Sapra 1988–90
Dr. D. Keeling. 1988–91   Dr. K. Holfeld 1989–92
Dr. M. Robern 1990–92   Dr. C. Kelly 1990–93
Dr. L. Hurst 1990–93   Dr. W. Taylor 1991–94
Dr. G. Beaulieu. 1991–94   Dr. K. Edstrom 1993–95
Dr. K. Baxter. 1994–97   Dr. S. Skotnicki 1994–97
Dr. V. Taraska 1995–98

There are only a few photographs, illustrating the basic lesions of each chapter. The handbook is to be used in the outpatient clinic or at the bedside. The patient becomes the photograph. To try and depict all the various and manifold varieties of skin diseases by photographs is not possible–either in black and white or color. Most atlases contain the most extensive and flagrant aspect of a disease that the author has ever seen. To use these as a typical example of morphology seems a gross deception. The difficult diagnoses are those where the disease is undeveloped or developed in a way quite different from that shown in so-called classical photographs. I have included a photograph in each chapter to demonstrate a typical morphological group.

I have been asked why there are not more photographs. The implication is that by showing many photographs of a skin disease, you could teach how to diagnose skin disorders. The belief is dermatologically naive. It illustrates how little the non-expert health professional knows about how dermatological diagnoses are made.

One does not make a sophisticated diagnosis by looking through a series of colored photographs and finding one that seem to agree with what you see. The diagnosis is made by pattern recognition which has been learned by repeated directed and guided exposure to patients with skin disease.

Acne vulgaris has 14 lesions. Would photography enthusiasts suggest that all 14 lesions be documented? Would they suggest that only common variants be shown?

Would mild, moderate and severe examples be shown of each of the 14 lesions? Would photographs of each stage be included? It becomes quite clear that this approach is completely impractical.

Another factor seemingly not understood by those advocating hundreds of photographs is that most authors include only the most severe example in their texts. What about the patient who has mild or moderate disease? Would their case be recognized?

So, a few photographs may help and that I have included.

But, the patient is the photograph.

We have found it instructive to have one resident describe what he/she sees and have another resident make the diagnosis based on this description without looking at the patient. The same technique can be used using 35 mm colour transparencies. Line drawings have been scattered here and there throughout the text.

Two textbooks which have helped me immensely are Darier's Textbook of Dermatology (translated by S. Pollitzer, Lea & Febiger, 1920) and H.W. Siemens' General Diagnosis and Therapy of Skin Diseases (translated by K. Weiner, University of Chicago Press, 1958).* Unfortunately, both are now out of print. The overview portion at the beginning of each chapter is taken largely from either or both of these texts. I have altered, updated, clarified and re-written a considerable amount of this material. Some paragraphs and occasional pages of text have not been changed; quotation marks are used for this material.

Some sketches or diagrams have also been re-drawn from those in Siemens and Darier. They are so indicated in the text.

A glossary is included because of the lack of consistency in the meaning of dermatological terms. I have tried to explain what I mean when I use a certain term, just like Willian[4] did many years ago. My choice is based more on clarity than historiographic principles. I have also included some notes on a method of visual examination and the basic approach to morphological diagnosis in the appendix. The names given to the surface anatomical regions are in the appendix.

Without entertaining the argument as to whether or not one should use eponyms[5,6] I have found it useful to include them in the text. When this has been done, I have added historical footnotes. It seems only fair to identify those who have gone before and contributed so much. The eponyms are listed at the bottom of the page where they are first used in the text. For convenience, there is a complete separate index of the eponyms, with dates, specialty, location, and pagination in the text. In this index of eponyms every page on which a particular eponym is present is listed.

Any comments on the contents or format will be welcomed.

ROBERT JACKSON, MD
Ottawa, Canada
May 1998

---

* Available from University Microfilms in bound photocopy form, P.O. Box 1346, Ann Arbor, MI 48106, Invoice No. 684106, $14.00.

References:
1. Korting GW, Denk R. Differential diagnosis in dermatology. Curth HO, Curth W. trans. Philadelphia: WB Saunders, 1976. A sophisticated text–not for amateurs.
2. Jackson R. True confessions of a dermatologist: Memorable mistakes and misadventures. Int J Dermat 1994;33:68–73.
3. Jackson R. The importance of being visually literate: Observations on the art and science of making a morphological diagnosis in dermatology. Arch Dermatol 1975;111:632–636.
4. Willian R. On cutaneous disease. Philadelphia: Kimber and Conrad, 1809.
5. Wright V. In defence of eponyms. BMJ 1991;303:1600–1602.
6. Eisenberg A. Eponymous science. Sci Am 1993;269:144.

Contents

Chapter One – *Erythemas*

Chapter Two – *Urticarias*

Chapter Three – *Purpuras*

Chapter Four – *Telangiectases*

Chapter Five – *Eczemas*

Chapter Six – *Erythematosquamous Dermatoses*

Chapter Seven – *Erythrodermas*

Chapter Eight – *Vesicles*

Chapter Nine– *Bullous Dermatoses*

Chapter Ten–*Pustules and Pustular Dermatoses*

Chapter Eleven–*Papules*

Chapter Twelve–*Nodules*

Chapter Thirteen– *Nodes or Subcutaneous Nodules*

Chapter Fourteen– *Ulcers and Erosions*

Chapter Fifteen– *Keratoses*

Chapter Sixteen–*Verrucosities*

Chapter Seventeen–*Dyschromias*

Chapter Eighteen–*Cutaneous Atrophies, Scleroses, and Dystophies*

Chapter Nineteen–*Hypertrophies*

Chapter Twenty–*Folliculoses*

Chapter Twenty-One–*Trichoses*

Chapter Twenty-Two–*Onychoses*

Chapter Twenty-Three– *Hidroses*

Chapter Twenty-Four– *Cysts*

Chapter Twenty-Five– *Sinuses and Fistulae*

Chapter Twenty-Six– *Burrows*

Appendices

Indices

Acknowledgements

The photographs were taken by the Audio-Visual Department of the Ottawa Civic Hospital, Mr. Peter Medcalf, Chief. The epidermal line drawings were made by Michael Duguay, medical illustrator, Ottawa Civic Hospital. Many of the drawings were redrawn from Siemens' text. Miss E. Jackson provided the other schematic drawings. Miss Andrea Cross, medical illustrator, Ottawa Civic Hospital, rendered the line drawings of the hair shafts.

Many have helped me in the gestation and birth of this book. I cannot thank them all, but Karen Brownson and Mrs. Jean McNeil have contributed above and beyond the call of duty. I especially acknowledge the assistance of my wife, Nonie, who typed the manuscript and helped in many other ways. Without her, I doubt this book would ever have been written.

The steadfast support of Dr. Donald C. Montgomery of Ottawa and Dr. R. Roy Forsey of Montreal is also acknowledged.

Dr. James D. Walker of Ottawa proofread the final copy and made many corrections and valuable suggestions.

R.J.

Introduction
A Basic Approach to Morphological Diagnosis

This text on the living gross pathology of the various conditions of the skin has been organized on a morphological basis. The diseases have been placed in chapters according to main basic lesions. Syndromes developing from these basic lesions are also included. Other subsidiary basic lesions that may occur as part of the disease are described at that time, for example, basal cell carcinoma is placed in the chapter on tumor nodules (the ulcer often present is part of the total description). Detailed morphological descriptions of conditions that must be considered in the differential diagnosis have been included.[1,2] Each chapter begins with an overview defining and describing the various types and forms of each lesion.

This handbook is not intended to be an encyclopedic review of all morbid diseases of the skin. For example, the seven or more types of Ehlers-Danlos, the six or more types of epidermolysis bullosa and the many varieties of xeroderma pigmentosum are not mentioned. In fact, since emphasis is on diagnosis, when a combination of rare and bizarre cutaneous findings is present and can be defined easily as such, not all of the morphology is described. This is particularly true of some of the congenital malformations. The problem in diagnostic clinical dermatology is not with such conditions, but with variations and atypical lesions of much more common diseases such as eczema and psoriasis.

Tropical skin diseases are not described in great detail.

An important point to remember with regard to many skin diseases is that the characteristic clinical features are often most easily seen (and also histologically shown) in areas where the disease most commonly occurs (e.g. psoriasis on the buttocks and elbows as compared with psoriasis on the face, discoid lupus erythematosus on the face or scalp as compared with the forearm, atopic dermatitis in the antecubital fossa as compared with the midscapular area). This does not apply to infants and children, who tend to have similar lesions in all areas (e.g. scabies lesions on palms and soles).

It is also true that, where there is great difficulty in clinically distinguishing between certain eruptions (e.g. lichen simplex chronicus and psoriasis on the nape of the neck), there will probably also be difficulty in histological distinction.

In almost all diseases, the diagnosis must be made on the basic lesion, not on the location. The location is not of primary importance in making a diagnosis, although it may help in classifying the type of eruption that should be considered in the differential diagnosis. For example, scabies does not occur on the scalp of adults, rosacea does not occur on the legs, and acne does not occur on the palms and soles. However, these examples are surely so ludicrous as to be without value. Only scabies and the photodermatoses can almost always be diagnosed on the location alone. An intermediate group for which location may help make a diagnosis. For example, dermatitis herpetiformis rarely occurs on the hands, and a chronic bullous eruption with oral mucosal lesions is more likely to be pemphigus than dermatitis herpetiformis or bullous pemphigoid. The trouble is that there are always exceptions, and if the diagnosis is based solely or even mainly on the location, it is, dermatologically speaking, an unsound diagnosis.

When examining any skin eruption, be sure to look for a well-developed lesion. In some eruptions (e.g. lichen planus and pityriasis rosea), some of the lesions do not show all characteristics. With eruptions due to poison ivy, the sharply marginated square or linear areas may not be present everywhere. With eczema, only a few areas may show vesiculation or the sequelae thereof. With molluscum contagiosum, only the larger lesions may show delling. Umbilication may not be a feature of all chicken pox lesions. In addition to looking for well-developed lesions, it is important to realize that all lesions of a particular eruption may not, strictly speaking, be those of a basic primary lesion. For example, some morbilliform or roseolar erythemas may have small papules in the centers of some lesions; some lesions of chicken pox may not be visibly blistered, but present as turgid urticarial papules; some drug-induced roseolar erythemas may show central purpura. In deciding what the basic lesion is, a well-developed lesion and one which fairly represents the vast majority of the lesions should be used for characterization. The concept that each lesion has a life has been illustrated in dermatopathology.[3]

The technique of visual examination (search behavior[4,5]) has been studied in considerable detail in relation to radiologists studying radiographs. Apparently only a very small portion of the radiograph is ever examined–large areas are never actually studied. Also, the routine of search behavior varies from one well-trained radiologist to another. One finding is that when the suspected diagnosis was known to the examining radiologist, the chance of an error was greater than when the radiograph was examined "blind", that is with no prior history. The relationship of these (and other) findings to the technique of dermatological search behavior has not been determined. However, experts in morphological dermatology prefer to see the eruption before they take a history. Whether this is always practical is a moot point, but examination and diagnosis before history taking is an excellent teaching technique.

To determine exactly what is meant by the name of certain morbid skin conditions, it is sometimes useful to refer to the original description.[6] It is interesting to see that a term or name given originally no longer, in some cases, means the same thing. For example, the original description of Bowen's disease did not include mucosal lesions; now, however, Bowen's disease of the vulva is a commonly used term. It should be pointed out that the original "classic"* description is often neither original nor classic.[7]

---

* Classic: outstandingly important or authoritative; (Fowler) original.

The best use of this handbook occurs when you have read, marked and inwardly digested the glossary. This is particularly important because I have tried to assign exact meanings to such words as papules, nodules, nodes, plaques, and tumors. Until we agree on the same word for the same lesion, communication and the learning of morphology are not possible.

Because the material in this text is lesionally and not disease oriented, the arrangement of the indices is quite different from the average dermatological text. Before using the indices it is highly recommended that you read the introductory note on the indices on page 483.

I have written this book for the postgraduate student, registrar, or resident in dermatology, and dermatologists as well as the intellectually curious. For the undergraduate student or intern, a similar but simplified approach can be found in Dermatology for the House Officer.[8]

References

1. Jackson R. On a clear day you can see forever. Arch Dermatol 1991;127:1151–1153.
2. Jackson R. Morphology revisited. Int J Dermatol 1993;32:77–81.
3. Ackerman, AB, Ragaz, A. The lives of lesions: Chronology in dermatopathology. New York:Masson, 1984.
4. Thomas, EL, Movements of the eye. Sci Am 1968;219:88–95.
5. Thomas,EL, Search behavior. Radiol Clin North Am 1969;VII:403–417, 485–497.
6. Shelley WB, Crissey JT. Classics in clinical dermatology. Springfield:CC Thomas, 1953.
7. Fowler, HW. A dictionary of modern english usage. 2nd edition. Oxford: Clarenden Press, 1965.
8. Lynch PJ. Dermatology for the house officer. Baltimore:Williams & Wilkins, 1987.

CHAPTER 1
Erythemas

> *A reaction in the skin characterized by an active or passive redness of the skin, more or less sharply marginated, usually temporary, and which disappears upon finger pressure. May be widespread or localized.*

Many of the disseminated varieties of the conditions described in Chapters 1, 2, and 3 have been called toxic erythemas, especially when erythema, urticaria, and purpura are present in one eruption. These are considered to be stages of the same underlying process. Toxic erythemas are symmetrical and usually appear rapidly.

Overview

Erythema is an active or passive redness of the skin. It may be circumscribed, or more or less diffuse, usually temporary and disappears momentarily under pressure from a finger. It may be widespread, localized, or generalized. It is the first and most common skin reaction produced by an external or internal irritant. It is always present in inflammations, and therefore precedes and/or accompanies many other lesions as an erythematous base or halo.[1]

One of the main components of skin color in the white race is the blood within the vessels of the skin (the others are the amount of melanin, the thickness of the horny layer, and the carotene in the fat). When the stratum corneum epidermis is thin or absent, the skin is redder because the red color of the blood is more obvious; examples of this increased redness are abrasions, blister bases, and the mucosae and semimucosae. In inflammation, the redness is caused by the dilatation of the vessels allowing the red color of the blood to show through.

By applying firm, direct pressure to the skin with a glass slide (diascopy), the blood can be extruded from the vessels. The skin then appears quite pale. This simple technique is useful to distinguish between the red color of the blood in vessels in erythema and the extravascular blood pigments of purpura.

Rubor, calor, dolor, and tumor (red, heat, pain, and swelling) are the cardinal signs of inflammation. The temperature of the inflamed skin is raised. There are various shades of red produced by these inflammatory erythemas. These colors are related to the acuteness and intensity of the inflammation and to the color and intensity of the accompanying cellular infiltrations. Table 1 lists a few of these. Erythema may last for months; this residual erythema can be useful in diagnosis as, for example, in healed lesions of impetigo.

The noninflammatory or vasomotor erythemas can be active or passive in nature. Examples of the active erythemas are the emotional erythemas* (erythema fugax, erythema pudoris), the flushed face of the febrile and the hectic flush of the excited.[2] This active erythema is produced by both dilatation of blood vessels and increased blood flow. Passive erythemas are darker and more bluish red, and are produced by congestion or relative

Table 1: Various Red Colors and Their Possible Significance	
Bright Hot Red	*Boil, emotional flush* *Vascular, inflammatory, active congestion*
Deep Red	*End stage of inflammatory red,* *passive congestion*
Brown Red	*Granuloma*
Carmine Red	*Discoid lupus erythematosus*
Flat Purple Red	*Dermatomyositis, systemic lupus*
Papular Purple Red	*Lymphocytic accumulations*
Cooked Ham	*Secondary syphilis on palms and soles*

Portions of the Overview are taken and modified from Siemens[1] (pp. 25–30).

*"With Europeans the whole body tingles when the face flushes intensely; and with races of men who habitually go nearly naked, the blushes extend over a much larger surface than with us."[2] (us = Europeans) There is no reason to flush in areas of skin usually covered by clothes.

stasis in the small veins and capillaries of the skin. Cyanotic skin usually feels cool. The pale spots produced by pressure on cyanotic skin recover color slowly. Passive erythemas may be seen on the extremities as well as the nose and ears.

Some types of erythema are complicated by the presence of other lesions. Deformed erythemas are associated with other findings such as dermal edema (urticarial erythema), cellular infiltration (papular erythema, nodal erythema), hemorrhage (purpuric erythema), pigmentation (pigmented erythema), blisters (bullous erythema), and scale (squamous erythema).

Some types of erythema can be classified by their configuration and extent:

Scarlatiniform erythema is a more or less general, bright, and uniform redness. Late and extensive lamellar desquamation is common. Extensive generalized or persistent scarlatiniform erythemas are erythrodermas. It may start as morbilliform or roseolar erythemas.

Morbilliform erythema consists of numerous disseminated erythematous spots up to 5 mm in diameter, occasionally becoming confluent. These spots are less bright red than the red in scarlatiniform erythemas. Characteristically, they start small and gradually increase in size. They have distinct margins and rarely are slightly elevated in the center. Late desquamation is absent or insignificant.

Roseolar erythema consists of numerous 1 to 2 cm disseminated erythematous spots. Late desquamation is absent or insignificant. These eruptions are the opposite of cutis marmorata, i.e., the spotted erythemas are located in the skin at the points where the arterioles bring blood to the skin.

Erythema in patches or figurate or gyrate erythema are congestive spots, patches, with circinate or arcuate borders (erythema marginatum).

Some erythemas may be distinguished by duration (syphilitic roseola). Another group are the persistent erythemas (erythema perstans, erythema annulare centrifugum), which often are also figurate.

Just as the skin becomes darker and redder by vasodilation, so it becomes lighter and paler by constriction of the blood vessels or reduction of their numbers. Everybody knows this phenomenon from the vasomotor paleness associated with fright and fear. Circumscribed constriction of blood vessels makes pale spots that can be easily confused with depigmented spots. The whitish shade of older scars can be explained by a reduction in the number of blood vessels and depigmentation. Pale spots without other skin changes are encountered in nevus anemicus. In this condition, reduction in the blood supply leads to permanent blanching of the skin. Nevus oligemicus is a persistent fixed area of livid erythema on the trunk.[3] Exaggerated physiologic speckled mottling of limbs is caused by slight vasoconstriction of the small cutaneous blood vessels.[4] Some skin lesions have white colored anemic halos (halo nevus) or depigmented halos (Woronoff ring).

D. L. Woronoff, Moscow

Widespread or Disseminated Erythemas

There are three useful descriptive morphological terms for the disseminated erythemas, viz. scarlatiniform or generalized, morbilliform, and roseolar. These have been defined in the Overview of this chapter.

Unfortunately, from a morphological point of view, many identical varieties of disseminated erythemas are the result of so many different causes (e.g. viral, bacterial, and parasitic diseases; drug-induced erythemas; collagen diseases) that it is difficult to present a diagnosis. Disseminated erythemas that are reasonably diagnostic are described first. Presentations of some of the disseminated erythemas that do not have a diagnostic morphology then follow.

Measles (Rubeola)

The eruption starts as faint red spots around or behind the lobes of the ears, the upper lateral parts of the neck, along the hairline, and on the posterior parts of the cheeks in an episode of measles. The blotchy and mottled erythema becomes more prominent with diffuse edema as the eruption spreads rapidly over the entire face, neck, upper arms, and upper part of the chest within approximately the first 24 hours. During the next 24 hours the eruption spreads over the back, abdomen, entire arms, and upper part of the thighs. As it finally reaches the lower extremities on about the third day, it is already fading slightly in the first afflicted areas, which develop a reddish brown color. The eruption disappears in the same order as it appears. A fine branny desquamation may occur. Fever, a slight hacking cough, coryza, and a diffuse conjunctivitis are almost always present. Red mottling of the hard and soft palates may occur. Koplik's spots are grayish-white dots with a slightly reddish mottled areola. They tend to occur on the buccal mucosae opposite the lower molars.

Variations in the measles erythema include a minor variety with only a scattering of lesions, a confluent erythema with edema especially noticeable on the face and, rarely, few to widespread petechiae, especially in measles post vaccination.

German Measles (Rubella)

The eruption consists of a blotchy and at times pinpoint erythema, which starts on the face and rapidly spreads to the upper torso and extremities. In some cases, the eruption may be confluent. Retroauricular, posterior cervical and postoccipital lymph nodes are enlarged and tender.

DIFFERENTIAL DIAGNOSIS

The eruption of German measles is distinguished from measles by the following findings: (1) the rash is less extensive, (2) browning on fading of the erythema is not present, (3) the degree of edema is less, (4) a purpuric element is extremely rare, and (5) desquamation is rare.

High fever, hacking cough, coryza, conjunctivitis, and Koplik's spots are usually not seen in German measles.

Henry Koplik, 1858-1927, Physician, New York, U.S.

Scarlet Fever

The Scarlet fever eruption is a diffuse, bright red erythema that blanches on pressure. It starts on the base of the neck, axillae, and groins, later spreading to the trunk and extremities. The face is not extensively involved, although the cheeks may be flushed. The perioral area may be pale. Petechiae are not uncommon. After 3 to 7 days, the rash fades and is followed by an extensive branny or lamellar desquamation, especially in the groins, axillae, and fingertips.

There is a high fever. Deeply erythematous and purpuric lesions may be seen in the mouth with a purulent discharge on the tonsils. The cervical lymph nodes are enlarged and tender.

The diagnosis of these three diseases is based not solely on the characteristics of the eruption, but also on the mucosae, lymph node abnormalities, and other findings.

Serum Sickness

Serum sickness, as from the injection of horse serum, has the following characteristics:

1. The exanthemata may be urticarial, scarlatiniform, rubella-like or polymorphous. Facial edema and itching are common. It lasts 2 to 3 days. The rash starts first at the site of injection, then it becomes symmetrical, the urticarial element is itchy and there is a rubella-like pattern of the extensor surfaces of the extremities.
2. The fever is remittent and lasts till the end.
3. Lymphadenopathy is generalized. It begins before the rash and fever and subsides before the end of the reaction.
4. Miscellaneous findings are pitting edema and weight gain, arthralgias, enlarged spleen, leukopenia, and albuminuria.

Serum sickness-type patterns can be seen after injections of foreign proteins, but also after some drugs, notably penicillin.

Miscellaneous

Erythema infectiosum (fifth disease) presents with a fairly characteristic slapped cheek appearance as well as a reticulated erythema of the extremities.

Kawasaki's disease has bilateral conjunctural injection; upper respiratory erythemas (such as red tongue or cracked lips); peripheral extremity edema, erythema, and peeling; and enlarged tender lymph nodes.

The diagnosis of other disseminated erythemas becomes much more difficult after the above three conditions have been excluded, and admittedly, at times even the above conditions cannot be diagnosed with certainty. Also, to compound confusion further, some of the below named conditions are not clearly defined entities.

Exanthem subitum, enterovirus, echovirus, reovirus, rhinovirus, and coxsackievirus infections may present with varying sorts of disseminated erythemas. Some erythemas may be photosensitive. Disseminated erythemas may also occur during the course of

Coxsackie, a Town in the State of New York
T. Kawasaki, Japanese Paediatrician

infectious mononucleosis, with mumps, with some forms of generalized staphylococcal or streptococcal disease, and as a scarlatiniform id from certain types (usually kerion) of trichophytosis. Rarely rickettsial infections and toxoplasmosis may have to be considered as a cause of disseminated erythemas.

DIFFERENTIAL DIAGNOSIS

The easily flushed skin of hyperthyroidism and the disseminated erythema sometimes seen with anaphylaxis may occasionally present problems in diagnosis.

The various erythemas of acute or subacute systemic lupus erythematosus may present a problem in differential diagnosis, although, as with many of the other conditions listed before, other findings will help in the diagnosis. In systemic lupus erythematosus, the erythema is primarily one of the upper half of the body; it is usually more extensive on the face and is often associated with edema. Erosive, necrotic, purpuric lesions are common, and a fixed purplish erythema of the periungual and knuckle areas and thenar and hypothenar eminences may also be seen. Telangiectases in the periungual area are seen. The so-called butterfly erythema on the nose and cheeks may be present. The facial lesions are sharply demarcated and of a dusky red or cyanotic tinge. The erythema is fixed. Mucosal erythemas and erosions may occur.

This eruption of systemis lupus erythematosus should be distinguished from the erythemas of dermatomyositis, which is more purplish, more centered about the eyes, and occurs frequently with circumoral pallor. Other erythemas of dermatomyositis may be located on the elbows, knees, and over the knuckles on the dorsa of the fingers. Periorbital edema and edema over the involved muscles may also be present in the acute phase. With atrophy, whitish and brownish areas, this eruption is called poikiloder-matomyositis. Some areas may assume the picture of *atrophie blanche*. In longstanding cases, calcific deposits may develop, especially about the joints of the extremities. Atrophy of proximal muscles may be marked. These purplish lichenoid papules over the knuckles have been called Gottron's papules.

Many disseminated erythemas have no diagnostic pattern and, in many, no cause is found, especially mild minor forms of a few days' duration.

Syphilitic Roseola

Syphilitic roseola consists of an eruption of peach blossom (very light pink) spots becoming deeper pink after a few days. The spots are rounded or oval in shape and never scaly. Flanks, chest, back, and abdomen are the areas usually affected. It lasts from 3 to 8 weeks. Enlarged lymph nodes, mucous patches, and alopecia may also be present.

DIFFERENTIAL DIAGNOSIS

The eruption is distinguished from pityriasis rosea or scaly eczemas by its lack of scale, from most drug eruptions because of its slow onset and lack of itching or burning.

Heinrich Adolf Gottron, 1890–1974, German Dermatologist, Breslau

Erythema Multiforme

The eruption of erythema multiforme is characterized by nummular congestive spots, the center of which promptly become cyanotic; the spots spread, remaining flat or becoming wheal-like or papular, sometimes discoid or depressed in the centers. This livid color of the spots, their bright red border, and their shape are quite characteristic. The lesions may also be whitish in the middle, appear to be bullous or actually become so, or the center can be purpuric. They extend rapidly and sometimes give rise to marginate spots, or even to rings. The sites of predilection are dorsal surfaces of wrists, hands and forearms, knees, elbows, and feet, and the palms and soles. A subsiding herpes simplex eruption may be seen on the vermilion border of the lower lip and occasionally the sequelae of a severe sunburn are also present, indicating the cause of the herpes simplex.

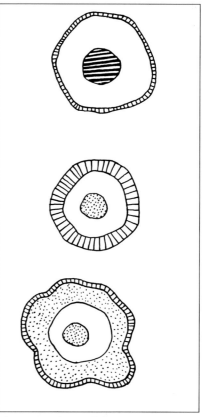

The bullous variant has the same distribution, but in this variant, some or most have a vesicle or tense bulla filled with a lime-yellow fluid. The bullae occupy the entire surface of the papular elevation, the center, or sometimes only the periphery. Target lesions are of three types (Fig. 1.1). One is purely papular and consists of a large (up to 1.0 cm), dark purplish disk surrounded by a lighter ring at the periphery of which there is a 1 mm darker red ring. The second shows a central bulla surrounded by an urticarial wheal, surrounded by an erythematous border. The third has a central bulla or crust with a ring of bright red urticarial erythema, then a bullous circle, and finally a narrow erythematous border. Rarely, this third type displays up to six alternating circles of urticarial wheals and bullous circles. Oral mucosal and lip lesions are common and present as superficial, varying-sized circular erosions covered with a yellowish nonadherent exudate with a bright erythematous halo. They may be confluent on the lips, which present as affected by a diffuse crusted fissured erythema. In some

Figure 1.1 Erythema multiforme, types of target lesions. *Upper,* Dark purplish disc surrounded by a lighter red, in turn surrounded by a small dark red ring at the periphery. *Middle,* Central bulla surrounded by an urticarial weal, which is surrounded by an erythematous border. *Lower,* Central bulla or crust with a ring of bright red urticarial erythema, then a bullous circle, and finally a narrow red border.

cases, these lesions are extensive and may involve the tongue and tonsillar fossa. Occasionally other mucosae are involved (e.g. conjunctiva and glans penis). On the conjunctiva, the bullae may be intact. In the early phases, only the vesiculobullous blistering phase may be obvious, with patches, clumps, and linear lesions without any erythema or iris lesions. Even pox-like lesions may be seen. In these cases the extensive ulcerative mucosal lesions, the distribution, and the passage of time will ascertain the diagnosis. At times, the localization of lesions seems to be related to trauma or to exposure to ultraviolet light. The lesion recurs at the same site.

Erythema multiforme major is the name given to the more severe mucocutaneous variety, which often has systemic involvement. It has been called the Stevens-Johnson syndrome even though Hebra described it in the nineteenth century and others such as Lewin classified erythema multiforme into mild and malignant (i.e. those with systemic effects) types.[5]

DIFFERENTIAL DIAGNOSIS

The differential diagnosis between the bullous variant and other bullous diseases is discussed under bullous eruptions.

Widespread drug-induced erythemas may be present with blistering or bullous lesions and with mouth lesions. Drug-induced erythemas may be difficult to distinguish from classical erythema multiforme. Usually in these multiforme erythemas, the target lesions are not present, the erythema is not in varying-sized circles, but is diffuse. In addition, the hands, elbows, knees, and mouth distribution is not reliable. Also, nodose erythema lesions may occur. In eruptions due to drugs, these lesions tend to be atypical (more lesions, less deep, areas other than the skin involved, nonbruising) when compared with true erythema nodosum.

Erythema Toxicum Neonatorum

This is a blotchy morbilliform erythema with many lesions, most profuse on the trunk (especially the chest); less in the face, arms, thighs; and scanty on the forearms and legs. Small (2 mm) papules or pustules are also present in the more extensive cases. Edema of the eyelids may also be present. This eruption occurs only in the newborn. Transient neonatal pustular melanosis may represent a similar condition in darker skinned races.

Drug-Induced Erythemas

Apart from the childhood erythemas, these drug-induced erythemas are the most common and the most difficult to classify.[6] Shear and Solomon[7] have put some of these erythemas into the acute and delayed hypersensitivity syndromes.

In general, they may be morbilliform, roseolar, scarlatiniform, or erythrodermic. Usually of sudden onset, they are symmetrical, and appear first on the torso and inner surface of the arms although occasionally they may start over friction and pressure areas such as the elbows, knees, and buttocks. Rarely, linear lesions may be present. These

Ferdinand von Hebra, 1816–1880, Austrian Dermatologist
Frank Chambliss Johnson, 1894–1934, U.S. Pediatrician
Lewin
Albert Mason Stevens, 1884–1945, U.S. Pediatrician

presumably represent a type of Koebnerization. The eruption usually disappears without desquamation and without pigmentation except for in the rare disseminated fixed drug type. Purpuric lesions are not uncommon, especially on the legs, ankles, and feet. In general, mucosal involvement (except for the bullous erythema multiforme variety and the occasional mucosal erythema) and lymphadenopathy (except for some types of anticonvulsant drug erythemas) is unusual. Sometimes other varieties of eruptions occur either with or without erythema, as in urticarial erythema, erythema with vesicles or bullae, erythema with various types of folliculitis, erythema with ulcerative and necrotic lesions, erythema with nodose lesions, erythema with fungating ulcerative granulations, erythema with extensive detachment of the upper layers of the epidermis (scalded skin syndrome), and erythema with pustulation.

Certain drugs induce erythema that appears similar to other disease entities (e.g an entity called hydralazine-induced systemic lupus erythematosus). In patients with drug-induced eruptions that simulate other diseases, the drug erythema may have atypical features. For example, in drug-induced erythema multiforme (as compared with post herpes simplex erythema multiforme), the distribution may be more random, for example, sparing the dorsa of the hands and feet, may be without mucosal lesions, and may have nodose lesions on the legs.

Finally, disseminated drug erythemas from a topical application of a drug must be considered. Following the application of mercury to one area, an intense confluent erythema develops, starting in the large body folds (i.e. axillae and groins). This spreads almost all over and is accompanied by exfoliation, giving the impression of an eruption from systemically administered mercury. Topically applied sulfonamides may produce an erythema with fungating ulcerative granulations; topically applied iodoform may produce an erythematous-bullous eruption.

A feature common to many disseminated drug reactions is that they may continue to appear after the causative drug has been discontinued. Apparently, the damage has been done, but is not obvious to the naked eye until a few days have passed. A suggested name for this phenomenon is fallout.

If toxic erythemas become universal and remain persistent, then by definition they become primary erythrodermas (see Chapter 7).

The drug erythema must be distinguished from an id or autosensitization dermatitis occurring as a secondary phenomenon from an acute eczematous process (i.e. varicose eczema). Id reactions mimic the original eruption and are therefore basically a blotchy fine papulovesicular eruption, not an erythema. Id reactions are usually much more pruritic than drug eruptions.

Eczematous (i.e. blistering, weeping, and crusting) dermatoses are rarely caused by the systemic administration of drugs.

Scratching can cause all sorts of lesions on the skin, but does not cause a disseminated erythema with scaling, large erosionsor ulcers, or deep fissures.

Heinrich Koebner, 1823–1904, German Dermatologist

Remember that patients, particularly in the hospital, have a variety of substances applied to the skin. Alcohol, special lotions, and new soaps can easily cause an extensive erythema and irritant eczema, especially in the elderly bed-ridden patient, and particularly in the hot dry air of the hospital during the winter.

Other non-drug causes of sudden widespread erythemas (toxic erythemas) must also be considered, including viral exanthemata or enanthemata, erythemas from pyogenic organisms, and erythemas of collagen vascular disease.

I have included under the erythemas the lesions commonly referred to as erythema from physical causes, despite the fact that at times some of the lesions of eczema are present. However, they do not show spongiosis, precluding classification as eczema.

Erythema Calorica

Burn

The first lesion from a burn is erythema with swelling. The second lesion is a bulla, which forms immediately or within a few hours. The bullae vary in size, may be deep or superficial, and contain a lemon-yellow fluid or gelatinous material. After rupture, the base is a bright red shining surface. If the bullae do not rupture, they shrivel and dry. Secondary pyoderma may occur. The third lesion is a sloughing, coagulation, and necrosis of the cutis (sometimes even deeper). The tissue looks gray and lifeless. Bullae appear at the periphery of these lesions. The course is that of nonprogressive dry gangrene. After healing, hypertrophic scars and keloids are common, especially over moving parts.

Burns may be produced by burning or incandescent bodies, by heated substances (solid, liquid, or gaseous), electricity, by caustic agents.

Frostbite

In frostbite, the region is of a cadaveric pallor, followed, after warming, by intense bluish red congestion. In more severe cases, bleb formation and sloughing occur more on the tips of toes, fingers, pinnas, and other extremities. On healing, there is considerable scarring, but less than might be predicted from the original injury. The course is that of dry gangrene.

Chilblains (pernio) as defined by Rook is an acute itching erythematous swelling of the subcutaneous tissues and dermis which comes up over a few hours and slowly subsides in one to two weeks. It often occurs in patients with acrocyanosis. He states that blistering and ulceration may occur.

Trench or immersion foot, the result of exposure of the feet to an above freezing, damp environment, consists of a purplish and very painful swelling that interferes with walking. The erythema may be accompanied by purpura, bullae, and occasionally sloughing.

Erythema Actinica

Sunburn

A few hours after excessive exposure to sun, the exposed surfaces present an intense congestion with swelling, burning, and itching. Exposed surfaces are usually the face,

Arthur Rook, 1918–1991, English Dermatologist, Cambridge

especially the nose and ears, and the hands. There may be large flaccid bullae, especially on the tops of the shoulders. The symptoms last for a few days, then the epidermis desquamates in large sheets, and only a slight pigmentation remains.

The edema, scaling, and blisters that occur on the face after excessive ultraviolet light therapy may be intense, causing complete closure of the eyelids. In patients with psoriasis receiving ultraviolet therapy, the bullae may be limited to the psoriatic plaques.

Following a severe sunburn of the legs, a persistent erythema with skin tenderness and ankle edema may be present for as along as 1 to 2 months.

Apart from sunburn, it is not an easy task to classify and describe the morphology of the various reaction patterns to sunlight or ultraviolet light.

Other Abnormal Reactions to Sunlight
In Table 2, the morphological changes are reasonably clear and are described elsewhere except for the morphological change which comes from exogenous presence of a photosensitizer, polymorphous light eruption (PLE) including actinic prurigo, and miscellaneous diseases.

In the presence of a photosensitizer (see Table 2), the contact diseases including pollenosis all show an eczematous response except for some of the phytopho-toeruptions that present primarily as linear or blotchy light to medium red-brown to brown patches. The systemic photosensitizers usually present as erythemas with various deformations such as purpura, bullae, and exfoliation.

For polymorphous light eruption(see Table 2) I would include the following varieties: papular, plaque-like (or large papular), erythematous (or erythema multiforme, erythema solare perstans), eczematous actinic prurigo, Hutchinson's summer prurigo, and papular photodermatitis of North American Indians. The last three conditions are closely related and may be the same.

Morphological findings in the miscellaneous diseases (see Table 2) include the following: solar urticaria (hives); hydroa vacciniforme (bullous, scarring); light aggravated atopic dermatitis (lichenification); as well as forms showing eczematous changes, including lichenification, such as actinic reticuloid, persistent light reaction, and photosensitive eczema.

Remember that some of the eruption may spill over into areas not directly exposed to the sun, but the majority and most severe portion will be on sun-exposed areas. The conditions and diseases are discussed under the appropriate basic lesion.

Many chemicals, when taken orally or applied, increase the sensitivity of the skin to sun and ultraviolet light (see Table 2). An eruption on the sun-exposed areas, especially the V of the neck, is also seen in pellagra, where fissures, ecchymoses, bullae, and residual pigmentation are quite common. Phytophotodermatitides are eruptions produced by external contact with plants and their extracts after subsequent exposure to light. A brown residual pigmentation is seen in berloque contact dermatitis on the sides of the neck at the sites of application of perfumes containing aromatic oils.

Jonathan Hutchinson, 1828–1913, English Surgeon, Dermatologist, and Syphilologist, London

Table 2: Classification of Causes of Abnormal Reactions to Sunlight	
Loss or Lack of Protection	*Fair skin* *Albinism* *Xeroderma pigmentosum*
Presence of a Photosensitizer	*Endogenous: Porphyrins* *Exogenous: Contact* *Systemic*
Light Alone (not due to lack of protection or to presence of an identifiable photosensitizer)	*Polymorphous light eruption (PLE) including actinic prurigo* *Autoimmune diseases* *Pellagra (possibly endogenous presence of a photosensitizer)* *Some genodermatoses* *Viral infections* *Certain browning diseases (e.g. melasma)* *Miscellaneous diseases:* *Solar urticaria* *Hydroa vacciniforme* *Light aggravated atopic and seborrheic dermatitis and rosacea* *Actinic reticuloid* *Persistent light reaction* } *Chronic actinic dermatitis* *Photosensitive eczema*

Chronic actinic dermatitis (see Table 2) includes a group of diseases that are persistent and disabling. The actinic reticuloid variety can produce leonine facies with biopsies showing a lymphomatous process. There may also be a persistent and recurrent "dyshidrosiform" eczema pattern on the palms and soles. The persistent light reaction develops into leonine facies less often, and has a quite banal histology. It is often preceded by a proven allergic or photoallergic contact dermatitis. Occasionally, underlying endogenous eczema exists, and in some patients, no underlying cause can be determined.

— Exogenous contact or systemic photodermatitis
— Polymorphous light eruption including actinic prurigo
— Light aggravated atopic and seborrheic dermatitis and rosacea
— Photosensitive eczema
— Persistent light reaction } Chronic actinic dermatitis
— Actinic reticuloid

Acute Radiodermatitis

Acute radiodermatitis presents as a rather dull erythema with some oozing of serum. As the process subsides, a light brownish scaliness ("moist desquamation") occurs (Fig. 1.2) frequently follicular. Follicular pustules may be seen. Light brown pigmentation is a common sequela. If the dose of ionizing radiation is low, or given in fractionated doses over a long period of time, the reaction is minimal or nonexistent.

Bullae, indolent ulcers, and necrosis may appear following huge doses given at a single setting.

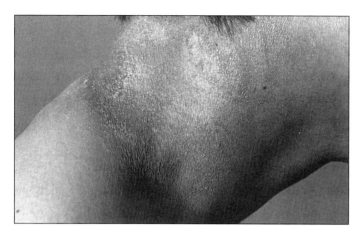

Figure 1.2 Acute radiodermatitis demonstrating a subsiding erythema with scaling and browning following Cobalt [60] irradiation.

Necrolytic Migratory Erythema

The basic lesion of necrolytic migratory erythema is an annular or gyrate erythema with a variable degree of scaling and peripheral flaccid bullae, and erosions with crusting (Fig. 1.3). The central third of the face, lower abdomen, groins, buttocks, thighs, and ankles are sites of predilection. The eruption may change rapidly from time to time. Glossitis, stomatitis, and angular cheilitis are often present. The patient is usually obviously sick, may be diabetic, and may have abdominal pain.

Acute Neutrophilic Febrile Dermatosis (Sweet's Syndrome)

Varying sized, bright red, tender plaques scattered on the arms, neck, and upper torso are found in Sweet's syndrome. They commonly blend one into another, forming figure eights. There may be some scaling behind the elevated active border. The outline is sharp and may be map-like. Lesions are usually several centimeters in diameter; borders are elevated; some central clearing may be seen; the surface is roughened; and there is no crusting, ulceration, or scarring. Sweet's syndrome usually occurs in women and is recurrent. A pre-existing illness may occur 1 to 2 weeks before the first lesion appears.

It could be argued that this condition is more of a plaque than an erythema. It is listed here because it has the color of acute erythema. I regard it as a deformed erythema.

DIFFERENTIAL DIAGNOSIS

The differential diagnosis of disseminated erythemas is summarized in Table 3.

Robert Douglas Sweet, English Dermatologist

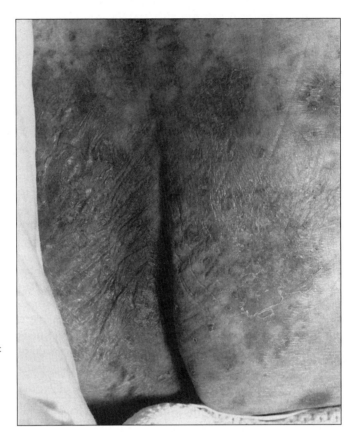

Figure 1.3 Necrolytic migratory erythema on buttocks. Note the erythema and superficial scaling.

Table 3: Differential Diagnosis of Disseminated Erythemas	
Drug	*Sudden onset, symmetrical, purpuric on ankles, not itchy*
Viral	*Many patterns of development, lymphadenopathy*
Bacterial	*Toxic patient, usually localized*
	Primary focus
Systemic Lupus	*Upper half of body, face, edema, elevation of temperature,*
Erythematosus	*purplish erythema and telangiectasia ("butterfly shape")*
Dermatomyositis	*Heliotrope color on eyelids, elbow and knee erythema,*
	muscle weakness
Erythema Multiforme	*Mouth, hands, feet, elbows; target lesions*
Physical	*Heat, cold and sun, localized to areas of contact*
Miscellaneous	

Localized Erythemas

Intertrigos

Intertrigo is the congestive redness of two contiguous surfaces. Verrucous changes are common in intertriginous areas and are often a sign of chronicity.

Intertrigo is ordinarily observed, especially in obese individuals, in the fold between the buttocks and on the crural surface of the thighs. In the obese, it is also seen under the breasts, in the hypogastric fold, in the groin and axillary regions, or in newborn infants on the buttocks, the folds of the neck, and so on. More or less vivid redness bounded by irregular or diffuse margins exist; local heat, pigmentation, and sometimes lichenification develop; and intertrigo is usually symmetrical.

The following differential diagnosis should always be considered in lesions occurring in the intertriginous areas. I have labeled some of them with the adjective intertrigo to emphasize the difficulty commonly encountered in distinguishing one from another and all of them from simple intertrigo.

Erythrasma is a scaly patch in the genitocrural fold (or axillae, submammary area, and between the toes) with distinct, polycyclic, and serrated circumference. The color is uniformly light brown, the surface is level, powdery, finely squamous, and often cross-hatched in very fine folds. There is no vesiculation of the margins. The eruption is relatively stationary.

Inguinal epidermophytosis (eczema marginatum) occurs on the medial aspect of the root of the thighs. Observations include nummular spots of a bright red color, sharply outlined, confluent in patches with red circinate borders, often finely vesiculated or bordered by small papules and occasionally pustules, with white lamellar scales. The center usually fades or remains pigmented light brown, interspersed with scanty scales and excoriations or with small crusts caused by scratching. Secondary scaly patches often originate on the thighs, pubis, and buttocks. The penis and scrotum are not involved; neither is the perianal mucosa or semimucosa.

In *intertriginous pyoderma*, the medial aspect of the thighs, suprapubic area, and the buttocks, especially in the obese, sweaty, hypertrichotic man, commonly have follicular pustules and boils. Resolving lesions may show scarring and/or light brown pigmentation. This may or may not be associated with intertrigo. The creases may be free of lesions. There may be a relationship with hidradenitis.

In *intertriginous moniliasis*, the crease has a deep red moist surface. At the periphery of this large central area, the moistness lessens and more scale of a soft, filmy, superficial, exfoliation type is present with peripheral undermining. There are numerous, satellite, nonfollicular vesiculopustules (1 to 2 mm) decreasing in number and size as one moves farther from the central large lesion. These older satellite lesions have small scaly collarettes. Diffuse brown-black pigmentation may occur at the periphery of intertriginous moniliasis.

Intertriginous lichen simplex chronicus is a basically confluent papular eruption usually forming somewhat asymmetrical lichenified areas reasonably well, but not sharply, demarcated. Excoriations are common. The border is not arcuate and the median raphé of perineum, scrotal sac, and vulva are commonly involved as well as the perianal mucosa and skin. Brown pigmentation is common. Scaliness is uncommon.

Intertriginous psoriasis presents as symmetrical vivid red plaques, denuded of scales, and often oozing with no central clearing. The border shows more typical psoriatic scaling and is sharply demarcated. The border is rather straight, occasionally arcuate, and nonintertriginous lesions are arcuate with no undermining of the periphery. The involvement may be patchy (e.g. on the hairy vulva) with normal skin between involved areas. Penile lesions are common. Fissuring in the creases also may occur. In infancy, psoriasiform napkin dermatitis is centered in the gluteal area with the lesions becoming smaller in size and fewer in number outward from the primary area.

Inguinal tinea versicolor is a spotty, scaly eruption, which in extensive cases, can be present in the groin. The eruption may have a brown color, but is usually patchy and nonconfluent, and does not have a distinct, polycyclic, and serrated border. It is often present on the upper torso.

Infantile gluteal erythema is related to intertrigo and radiates from the intergluteal fold to the thighs, back, and abdomen. The inner crease areas are often spared. It is extremely common and caused not so much by friction as by contact with dejecta. Sometimes the condition is a simple erythema, often of a coppery red color, covering a large area, or in patches; in other cases the erythema is complicated by fissures or vesicles and oozing erosions (eczematous changes), or again, it becomes covered by ulcerations and pyodermal lesions. Other flexural areas such as the axillae, postauricular crease, and neck folds may be involved. The scalp may have a diffuse scaling reminiscent of seborrhea. In the form described as papulo-lenticular erythema or posterosive syphiloid by Sivestre and Jacquet,[8] those erosions appear as raised, moist papules. Other names for this condition are granuloma gluteal infantum and papuloerosive diaper dermatitis.

Intertriginous trichophytosis (nonblistering). This type of tinea cruris is similar to inguinal epidermophytosis, but the lesions are larger, have no vesicles, show more brown pigmentation, and are common on the buttocks. Many of the lesions have incomplete arcuate peripheral borders. It is very rare in women.

In *intertriginous atopic dermatitis*, the eruption may be brightly red, and as it is affected by the same friction, heat, and maceration as in eczema, the pattern may be very similar. Usually, however, there is less weeping and more lichenification. At times also, the eruption has the appearance of a lichen simplex chronicus. This condition is rarely located solely in intertriginous areas.

Intertriginous seborrhea: I do not recognize this as an entity (see "Seborrhea" in Chapter 6).

Leonard Marie Lucien Jacquet, 1860–1914, French Dermatologist
Sivestre

Intertriginous eczema shows the basic lesion of eczema elsewhere with modifications due to the friction, moisture, and heat of the area. The apposing folds show a raw, partially denuded epidermis, frequently with fissuring in the creases. The lesions are poorly demarcated with peripheral, blotchy, irregular papulovesicles. There is no peripheral undermining and the border is not arcuate. Edema and lichenification are frequently seen, especially on the genitalia, and in the median raphé of perineum and the perineum.

DIFFERENTIAL DIAGNOSIS

A summary and differential diagnosis of Intertrigo is provided in Table 4.

Table 4: Differential Diagnosis of Intertrigo	
Simple	
Erythrasma	*Light-brown, distinct, even patches with polycyclic borders*
Epidermophytosis or Trichophytosis	*Arcuate lesions with central brown, cleared areas — penis, scrotum, mucosa, and semimucosa not involved*
Pyoderma	*Follicular pustules and boils*
Candidiasis	*Crease involved, superficial eroded peeling in center, satellite lesions*
Lichen Simplex Chronicus	*Confluent papular (lichenified) eruption with poorly demarcated borders —medial raphé, scrotum, vulva, mucosa, and semimucosae often involved*
Psoriasis	*Vivid red plaques, no scales in center, scales on arcuate border, no underminings, patchy*
Tinea Versicolor	*Spotty, branny scale, brown, other areas*
Infantile Gluteal	*Sparing of deep creases, coppery red color, oozing*
Eczema	*Raw, denuded, oozing, poorly defined, edema, lichenification on mucosa and semimucosa*

Acrocyanosis

This is a chronic congestion of the extremities (usually hands), which are of a purplish red color, habitually cold, and often damp and flaccid. The ischemic spot produced by digital pressure requires a long time, sometimes nearly a minute, to resume its red color by the inflow of blood. Frequently, there is an initial phase of blanching. This condition is brought on by exposure of the extremities to ordinarily tolerable cold. Acrocyanosis is sometimes seen in severe infantile atopic dermatitis. Unless occupational, it is rare in men.

Symmetrical Lividity of the Soles

This is a tender erythema on the plantar surface of the toes, anterior third of the foot, and the heels. The patches of erythema are reasonably well defined, and hyperhidrosis is moderate to extensive. The palmar surfaces are not usually involved.

Raynaud's Phenomenon

Of "local syncope and asphyxia," Raynaud wrote:

> ...without appreciable cause, one or many fingers become pale and cold all at once; in many cases it is the same finger which is always first attacked; the others become dead successively and in the same order.... The determining cause is often the impression of cold...sometimes even a simple mental emotion is enough (to bring on these changes)....In the more pronounced cases,...the pallor of the extremities is replaced by a cyanotic colour...a vermilion colour shows itself at the margin; little by little it gains ground.... Finally, a patch of deep red is formed on the extremities of the fingers. This patch gives place to the normal pink colour, and then the skin is found to have entirely returned to the primitive condition.

Raynaud then described the second type, in which bilateral gangrene was a prominent feature, as follows:

> I hasten now to the symptoms of symmetrical gangrene properly so called.... In the slight cases the ends of the fingers and toes become cold, cyanosed, and livid, and at the same time more or less painful. In grave cases the area affected by cyanosis extends upwards for several centimeters.... Finally, if this state is prolonged for a certain time, we see gangrenous points appear on the extremities; the gangrene is always dry and may occupy the superficial layers of the skin from the extent of a pin's head up to the end of a finger, rarely more.[9]

DIFFERENTIAL DIAGNOSIS

Erythromelalgia is the term given to painful red hot feet. Immersion foot, polycythemia rubra vera, multiple myeloma, systemic lupus erythematosus, and Raynaud's phenomenon must be considered in the differential diagnosis of red feet.

Cutis Marmorata (Marbled Skin) (Livedo Reticularis)

Cutis marmorata[10,11]* is a passive erythema characterized by a usually transient, but occasionally persistent, purplish reddening that appears on the skin as a network of strands of varying size, enclosing round or oval areas. These areas have a normal color and correspond to the territories of direct blood supply, whereas the strands of the network represent the anastomotic zones between these territories. Secondary lesions such as lichenification, ulceration, brown pigmentation (erythema ab igne), and dermal papulation are occasionally seen. It is seen mainly on the arms, thighs, and torso.

Cutis marmorata or livedo reticularis occur in many conditions. Circulatory disorders, exposure to cold, and periarteritis nodosa are some examples. In some patients, it is lifelong and of no significance. "Starburst" livedo reticularis has been reported as occurring as a stage of cutaneous periarteritis nodosa. In cutaneous, periarteritis nodosa, numerous flame–or star-shaped areas of erythema occur, particularly on the lower extremities.

Maurice Raynaud, 1834–1881, Paris, French Surgeon and Medical Historian
*Many of the observations of Lewis[10] are still valid today.

Rosacea

Rosacea[12] is a more or less diffuse active erythema of the face, particularly the central portion. Superficial telangiectases slowly develop, especially on the nose. Later, small undulating venules ramify over the nasolabial folds, the alae nasi, and on the nose. Both the erythema and the multiple telangiectases contribute to the redness. The skin becomes thickened with hypertrophied sebaceous glands. Superficial acneform folliculitis may occur. This passes through stages of papules, pustules, and crusting, resulting in minute scarring. Severe flushing and blushing is common.

Erythema and edema and a minute telangiectasia may extend almost up to the hairline, with a few scattered small purpura in some patients with rosacea treated by long-term topical fluorinated corticosteroids. When the applications are stopped, a very extensive small follicular pustulation may be seen along with edema. (See persistent perioral dermatitis later in this Chapter.)

In some patients with rosacea, in addition to the erythema and telangiectasia, a micropapular eruption may be seen, especially on the chin. These are the apple-jelly papules of Lewandowsky (rosacea-like tuberculid of Lewandowsky). In some cases the papules become confluent and form purplish, firm granulomatous plaques up to 3/4 cm in diameter.

Rhinophyma consists of a thickened skin with dilated and funnel-shaped sebaceous pores. The nose is either uniformly increased in size or covered with firm globular protuberances or pedunculated tumors. The surface of the nose is a purplish red color, lumpy, with large-sized varicose venules, riddled with sebaceous orifices, and often dotted with pustules. The same changes may occur in the skin at the orifice of the external auditory meatus (otophyma). Basal cell carcinomas are usual in rhinophyma.

Rosaceous eye changes can include hyperemia and telangiectases of the lid margins with an erythematous blepharitis, conjunctival hyperemia most marked in the interpalpebral fissure, and phlyctenule-like papules without ulceration, limbal telangiectases, and superficial corneal opacities.

DIFFERENTIAL DIAGNOSIS

Rosacea must be distinguished from the following:

Acne has as its basic lesions comedones, which are rare in rosacea unless they occur as a part of dermatoheliosis. Also, the skin between the acne lesions is not as inflamed or telangiectatic as the intervening skin in rosacea. Oiliness is more a feature of acne than of rosacea. Acne is commonly present on areas beyond the central portion of the face, and often on the neck and upper torso. Dermal inflammatory nodular granulomas are rare in rosacea. Rhinophymatous changes do not occur in classical acne vulgaris.

I give rosaceous acne the following characteristics:

1. Usually female, mid-twenties, with extensive flushing and blushing.

Felix Lewandowsky, 1879–1921, German Dermatologist, Breslau

2. The presence of comedones and inflammatory lesions of acne vulgaris including granulomatous (cystic) lesions, often with scars of previous acne lesions.

3. The presence of enlarged papulous orifices particularly in the infra-orbital area. This area often has a reddish brown color with some seborrheic-type scaling.

4. Patients with rosaceous acne do not have as persistent or intense erythema and telangiectasia.

5. As these patients age, the acne vulgaris seems to decrease in severity and eventually a more characteristic rosacea develops.

6. As a rule, these patients tend to respond much more slowly and not so well to appropriate anti-acne therapy. Even when they have developed mainly "true" rosacea, they do not respond as well as the average rosacea.

Discoid lupus erythematosus has closely adherent carpet-tack scales, areas of atrophy, and forms varying-sized plaques between which the intervening skin is normal. Nonfacial lesions (e.g. ear, scalp) are common. There are no pustules. Now rare, bromodermas, iododermas, and follicular syphilodermas and tuberculids should be considered.

The flushing and telangiectatic blood vessels in the late stages of the carcinoid syndrome may resemble rosacea. There are neither acneform folliculitis lesions nor hypertrophic changes. Polycythemia (primary or secondary) may present as erythema on the face.

Plaque-like solar eczema presents a 2 to 4 cm purplish plaque, which may have excoriations and scaliness on the surface. The border is rather sharp with occasional telangiectatic blood vessels visible. There is no atrophy, no follicular plugging, and the lesions are more violaceous than carmine colored. Pustules are absent as is persistent erythema of the noneczematous skin. Persistent solar erythema on the cheeks (erythema multiforme type of solar dermatitis) shows no scale, no scarring, and no telangiectases; it may be impossible to distinguish from the erythematous type of localized facial lupus erythematosus, and there are no pustules.

Persistent perioral dermatitis is a poorly defined entity consisting of 1 to 2 mm follicular papules, micropustules, erythema, and branny scaliness located on the chin, sides of the mouth, upper lip, and nasolabial folds. Large pustules and telangiectases are rarely present. Although it occurs almost entirely in women, a variety called granulomatous perioral dermatitis is seen in children.

The telangiectases produced on the face in the fair-skinned from habitual exposure to the sun can produce a ruddy background erythema. This at times can resemble the early erythema of rosacea. Both the telangiectases and ruddy erythema due to sun damage and the telangiectases and erythema from rosacea may be present in the same patient.

Table 5 summarizes the differential diagnosis of chronic facial erythemas.

Table 5: Differential Diagnosis of Chronic Facial Erythemas	
Rosacea	*Pustules and telangiectases, scarring*
Discoid Lupus Erythematosus	*Atrophy, carpet tack scale, tumid purple plaques*
Solar Eczema and Erythema	*No atrophy, no pustules, no telangiectasia*

Fixed Drug Eruptions

The basic lesion in fixed drug eruptions is a persistent erythematous brown-purplish patch, situated anywhere, usually one or two in number. They are round or oval in shape, well defined, and initially slightly urticarial. After a few days, the redness subsides and a fine or lamellar desquamation occurs, but the brown (or even black) pigmentation persists to fade only after a long time. The lesion occurs at the same site hours after taking the causative drug. If the drug is taken repeatedly, more patches may occur, but the original one or two spots also become erythematous and urticarial. Rarely, flaccid bullae develop on the patches.

On the tongue or mucosal aspect of the genitals, the lesions are usually briefly erythematous, then bullous, and then erosive. Brown pigmentation is not such a prominent feature on the mucosal lesions.

Figurate Erythemas

Erythema in patches or figurate erythema[13] consists of erythematous spots, patches, or surfaces of irregular shape, discoidal, or variable configuration (e.g. erythema marginatum). The lesions are usually transient or may move around, or may recur (e.g. erythema marginatum of rheumatic fever). A peripheral advancing erythematous border with clearing in the center and exfoliation between (i.e. scaling of inner trailing edge) may occur. Sometimes a residual light brown color is visible in the center. If symptoms persist for several months, they may be called erythema perstans and may represent such conditions as tick bites (erythema chronicum migrans, Lyme disease), subacute systemic lupus erythematosus, spots of macular leprosy, toxic eruptions of underlying carcinomas (erythema gyratum repens), and trichophytids (erythema annulare centrifugum). In the latter condition, the primary lesion is an acute, usually blistering tinea (often a kerion) of the hairy parts, or acute vesiculobullous tinea of the webs and plantar skin. None of the transient, mobile, recurrent, or persistent localized erythemas are clear-cut morphological entities.

Emotional erythema is a transitory redness, arranged in spots or as a network appearing over the chest, neck, and shoulders of certain individuals upon embarrassment of the person, and is identical with the emotional redness of the face.

Lyme (Old Lyme), Town in CT.

Erysipelas

The basic lesion marking erysipelas is a varying sized plaque that is tense, edematous, slightly elevated, and irregular in contour with an abrupt border. The lesion has a rosy or crimson-red color with a smooth, shiny, or glazed surface. The affected part is warm and sometimes tender. Lymphangitis, regional tender lymphadenitis, chills, and fever are often, but not always, present. Larger palm-sized areas may develop. As the lesions subside, a deep purple-brown color may be seen with extensive branny desquamation.

In more severe cases, vesicles or bullae (sometimes hemorrhagic) occur in the erythema with, rarely, dry gangrene and ulceration. In the gangrenous forms, frank pus may be present. Sites predilection are the head and neck, but lesions may occur anywhere. Inflammatory edema and erythema are pronounced on soft elastic tissues (e.g. eyelids, scrotum, and ears). When hairy areas are involved, toxic alopecia develops. Recurrent attacks, especially on the ears (from external otitis), on the legs (from stasis sequelae with superimposed eczema), and on the arms (especially with postmastectomy and postradiation lymphedema) lead to a permanent edema and thickening of the dermal tissues, in some cases resembling elephantiasis. Recurrent erysipelas also occurs in those who have had multiple operations in the lower abdomen with such diagnoses as adhesions, pelvic inflammatory disease, Crohn's disease or bowel cancer. The picture in one of recurrent severe chills and fever with leucocytosis. On the skin the tumid plaques of erysipelas are usually seen on the abdomen, flanks or buttocks. The clinical dermatological differential diagnosis includes acute contact dermatitis, a fixed drug eruption or perhaps a traumatic erythema. Some will get better without penicillin.

Usually, the site of original invasion by the streptococcus is not obvious.

DIFFERENTIAL DIAGNOSIS

Herpes zoster and simplex (recurrent or primary) may present at the beginning of an infection with an acute tender erythema, but if the grouped vesicles are not yet clearly visible, it will be difficult to distinguish these conditions from erysipelas. This is especially true with herpes zoster and primary herpes simplex, where fever and lymphadenitis may also be present.

A patient with acute contact eczema (particularly facial poison ivy eczema) may present with acute edema and erythema and, again, before the oozing or linear blistering streaks are visible, some confusion with erysipelas is possible. There is often some indication of linear, sharply marginated edges. Fever and lymphadenitis are not present.

Rosacea appears as a nonelevated erythema with telangiectasia and follicular pustules.

Erythematous lupus erythematosus is manifested as more purplish, less elevated, erythematous plaques, without regional adenitis.

Carcinoma erysipeloides (inflammatory carcinoma) is basically a bright-red firm plaque occurring on the chest wall. The edges of the infiltration are poorly defined, except where tongue-like, dull red prolongations extend from the margins. Usually other features such as papular or nodular tumors, sclerosis, marked edema, ulceration, and regional lymph node enlargement are present (See "Carcinoma en Cuirasse" in Chapter 18).

Erysipeloid occurs in meat and fish handlers, showing itself as relatively fixed, purplish red, nontender, erythematous plaques, most often on the palmar surfaces. The advancing border is slightly elevated, smooth, and sharply defined. Arcuate borders may be present. Rarely, disseminated forms with systemic symptoms occur.

Other morphological varieties of hemolytic streptococcal infections involving the skin should be mentioned here to define more clearly my concept of erysipelas.

Scarlet fever is a generalized erythema and does not show tumid plaques.

Streptococcal cellulitis can be observed as a diffuse, tender, edematous erythema with gradually sloping edges. An injury or other portal of entry is usually visible, and if central necrosis occurs, pus formation may be present.

Streptococcal infections of the skin with pus formation or superficial streptococcal pyoderma have as basic lesions pus formation and, frequently, lymphangitis and lymphadenitis (e.g. impetigo, ecthyma, secondarily infected eczema). In some cases (e.g. streptococcal infection of blistering tinea pedis), there may be little laudable pus. However, there are no elevated tumid plaques as are seen in erysipelas.

Mitchell's flexural streptococcal pyoderma is an oozing crusted eruption occurring in such areas as retroauricular, axillary, and perianal. Satellite pustules are usually present.

Necrotizing streptococcal gangrene occurs in debilitated patients (e.g. diabetics, alcoholics) as large, deep, penetrating necrotic ulcers, usually on the legs and ankles.

Table 6: Differential Diagnosis of Acute Facial Erythemas	
Erysipelas	*Vascular red tumid plaques, irregular and blotchy, sometimes fever, bullae, and hemorrhage*
Zoster	*Acute tender erythema, unilateral grouped blisters after a few days, mainly unilateral*
Simplex	*Same as zoster, except may be bilateral, lymphadenopathy common*
Contact Eczema	*Acute edema and erythema, often streaking and oozing, no fever, no lymphadenopathy*

Septicemic streptococcal states may produce embolic dermal pustules with deep small, hemorrhagic blisters.

Other nonpyogenic streptococcal related cutaneous changes are erythema nodosum, anaphylactoid purpura (Henoch-Schönlein), polyarteritis nodosa, scleredema adultorum (Buschke's), acute guttate psoriasis, rheumatic erythemas, purpura fulminans, renal edema from nephrosis, and elephantiasis.

DIFFERENTIAL DIAGNOSIS

Table 6 provides a summary of the differential diagnosis of acute facial erythemas.

Abraham Buschke, 1868–1943, German Dermatologist, Berlin
Edouard Heinrich Henoch, 1820–1910, German Physician
James Herbert Mitchell, 1881–1963, U.S. Dermatologist, Chicago, IL
Johann Lukas Schönlein, 1793–1864, German Physician

Miscellaneous

Other causes of localized erythema are the erythema stages of localized erythema calorica and localized erythema actinica as well as the erythema phase of traumatic erosions and excoriations.

Erythema dyschromicum perstans (ashy dermatosis) is seen in the patient who presents with multiple, slate gray, palm-sized areas on the torso. The peripheries of the lesions at onset have palpable erythematous borders. If the border is not visible, the eruption is classified as a postinflammatory melanosis as from a fixed drug eruption.

Chemotherapy-induced acral erythema consists of a progressive evolution from painful, well-demarcated erythema to blistering; eventually desquamation occurs on the palms and soles.

The lid and periocular erythema of neonatal lupus erythematosus is another variety of localized erythema.

References

1. Siemens HW. General diagnosis and therapy of skin diseases. Weiner K, trans. Chicago:University of Chicago Press, 1958.
2. Darwin C. The expression of emotions in man and animals. London: Friedmann, 1979:329.
3. Davies MC, Greaves MW, Coutta A. Nevus oligemicus—a variant of naevus anemicus. Arch Dermatol 1981; 117:111–113.
4. Graham RM, James MP. Exaggerated physiologic speckled mottling of the limbs. Arch Dermatol 1985; 121:415–417.
5. Ziemssen H, ed. Handbook of diseases of the skin. New York:Wm. Wood, 1885:369.
6. Alanko K, Stubb S, Kauppinen K. Cutaneous drug reactions: Clinical types and causative agents. Acta Derm Venereol (Stockh) 1989; 69:223–226.
7. Shear N, Solomon RS. Getting to the bottom of a cutaneous drug reaction. Cdn J Diagnosis 1990; June:101–116
8. Darier J. A textbook of dermatology. Pollitzer S, trans. Philadelphia:Lea & Febiger, 1920:31.
9. Jackson R. Raynaud and Moliére. Arch Dermatol 1983; 119:263–266.
10. Champion RH. Livedo reticularis, a review. Br J Dermatol 1965; 77:167–179.
11. Lewis T. The blood vessels of the human skin and their responses. London: Shaw & Sons, 1927.
12. Wilkin JK. Rosacea a review. Int J Dermatol 1983; 22:393–400.
13. White JW. Gyrate erythema. Derm Clinics 1985; 3:1292–139.

CHAPTER 2

Urticarias

> *A specific type of weal, with many lesions of varying size,*
> *frequently round or oval,*
> *and of a transitory or ephemeral nature.*

Overview

The basic lesion of urticaria is a weal (from or meaning ridge or raised part). A weal is a circumscribed area of fluid accumulation produced by the escape of certain liquid blood products through the small vessel walls (Fig. 2.1). This pathogenesis explains the rapid development and disappearance of the weal, sometimes called hives usually within a matter of hours. This diagnosis can easily be confirmed by outlining several lesions with ink and waiting, after a few hours, the hives may be gone, have a different shape and location, or new lesions may have developed.[1,2] *

A weal (Fig. 2.2) is an elevated, distinctly out-lined efflorescence; light pink in color with a pinkish or whitish areola; of a rounded or oval shape, sometimes polycyclic; of firm consistency and nonpitting. Dimensions of urticaria, usually nummular, vary from the size of a lentil to palm-sized or larger. Rarely is the lesion so small that it can be confused with a papule, but frequently, it enlarges peripherally. At the height of development, the edges of the lesion are well defined; larger

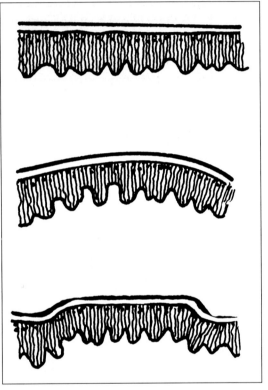

Figure 2.1 *Upper,* Normal skin. *Middle,* Edema. *Lower,* Weal. (Redrawn after Siemens[1].) The fluid causing edema accumulates throughout the dermis and fat, thereby making a sloping, dome-shaped elevation. The fluid causing a weal is more localized, coming from the small dermal blood vessels, and located primarily in the dermis, making a lesion with sharp borders.

weals are not higher in the center than at the edges, but are frequently depressed because of central regression. However, if the subcutis is involved, more rounded dome-shaped swellings (some larger than a hen's egg) with vague edges develop. If the hives involve areas with very loose cutis and subcutis, such as the eyelids, lips, and genitals, then prominent, spherical, somewhat translucent, frequently monstrous swellings develop. These are moderately soft, and the pit left by the pressure of a

Portions of the Overview are taken and modified from Siemens[1] (pp. 40,41) and Darier (pp. 43, 44).

Atopic dermatitis, transient acantholytic dermatitis, papular contact dermatitis, and subacute prurigo ("itchy red bump disease") should also be considered during the diagnosis.[4]

See also Table 7 and under Miscellaneous Lichenified and Papular Dermatoses in Chapter 11.

Table 7: Differential Diagnosis of Widespread Excoriated Urticarial Papular Lesions	
Cat or Dog Flea Bites	*1.0 cm urticarial papules with central puncta, constellation pattern; legs or abdomen*
Cheyletiella	*Small urticarial lesions, not patterned; common on chest*
Bed Bugs	*Solitary, bullous, hemorrhagic, random; torso, thighs, and legs*
Dermatitis Herpetiformis	*Grouped lesions on elbows, knees, small of back, or scalp; occasionally vesicular, symmetrical*
Neurotic Excoriations	*No primary lesion, no grouping; all stages of new, healing, and healed excoriation; accessible sites*
Scabies	*Small discrete crusted papules; sides of fingers, wrists, penis, and torso*
Others	*Mosquito, wasp, ticks, spider, and other insects and arachnids*
Atopic dermatitis	*Lichenification, flexural involvement (including ear lobe crease); hypopigmentation; symmetry; nickel sensitivity*
Transient Acantholytic Dermatoses	*Upper torso, scattered tinged, or vesicular papules, old men, exposure to heat and sun*
Contact Dermatitis	*Caused by such materials as sheets, nickel, fiberglass, neomycin; often papular; follicular and disseminated*

References

1. Siemens HW. General diagnosis and therapy of skin diseases. Weiner K, trans. Chicago:University of Chicago Press, 1958.
2. Darier J. Textbook of Dermatology. Pollitzer S, trans. Philadelphia: Lea & Febiger, 1920.
3. Wong RC, Fairley JA, Ellis CN. Dermographism: A review. J Am Acad Dermatol 1981; 11:643–651.
4. Scherertz EF, Jorizzo JL, White WL, Shar GG, Arlington J. Papular dermatitis in adults: Subacute prurigo. J Am Acad Dermatol 1991; 24:697–702.

CHAPTER 3

Purpuras

> *Extravasation of red blood cells into the skin*
> *(minute = petechia; extensive = ecchymosis; massive = hematoma).*

Overview

The escape of blood from the vessels into the dermis causes purpura,[1,2] an eruption of hemorrhagic purple-colored macules of various sizes and shapes. The spots of purpura do not fade on diascopy.

When blood escapes from the blood vessels, as in a bruise, a deposit of yellow-brown pigment, hemosiderin, derived from hemoglobin develops. Depending on the size, bruises are slowly absorbed and disappear after days or weeks. Purpuric spots may be punctate or very small (petechiae), coin-sized (suggillations), or very extensive (ecchymoses). At first, superficial extravasations are the dark red color of blood. Then gradually, by decomposition and absorption of the hemosiderin, they turn black, purple, green, yellow, and then brown. If situated fairly deep below the surface, purpuras are the same blue color that any area of dark pigment would be if viewed from the surface through the translucency of the overlying skin. The intense dark blue color of a deep cutaneous blood deposit changes to greenish and yellowish hues as the blood pigment becomes altered and resorbed. Purpuric macules may develop into palpable lesions or form blood-filled blisters. Nontraumatic purpura are more or less symmetrical; the lower limbs are most commonly and most extensively involved.

A hematoma is extravasation of blood within tissue in the form of a sizable swelling. Large hematomas on the shin and dorsum of foot from trauma may become semicystic and develop a bloody necrotic-looking area 1 to 2 cm in size on the apex of the bulging hematoma. At times, hematomas closely mimic an abscess with a necrotic surface and edema; pain and swelling are often present. When such large hematomas develop, becoming localized and cystic, the differential diagnosis between an abscess and a necrotizing pyoderma may be difficult. On the scalp, large hematomas may form a boggy subcutaneous cystic swelling. All large hematomas that form semicystic tumors require months to resolve.

Local

Traumatic black petechiae present as a macule or papule, generally circular, sharply defined, and less than 0.5 cm in diameter. Toes, heels, fingers, nail beds, and foreskins are common sites. Suction or shearing purpura may occur on the heels of players of court sports. There may be some surrounding yellowish, greenish, purplish bruising surrounding the central black petechiae. An unusually patterned suction purpura may be seen on the back or buttocks from the pressure and/or suction of the small (1.0 cm) cups on rubber bath mats. This is more common in the elderly. A similar phenomenon can occur following "cupping"* or from electrocardiograph leads. Tight-fitting trousers may cause purpura on the anterior thighs. Purpura also may

---

Portions of the Overview are taken and modified from Siemens[1] (pp. 21).

*Cupping is the application of suction cups, usually to the torso, to draw blood to the surface.

be seen in thrombosed capillary angioma, in which the outline of the original angioma can usually be clearly seen. These black petechiae must be distinguished from other black lesions (e.g. tattoos, in which coloring is more diffuse and less black; black malignant melanomas, which are usually less well defined, are less evenly pigmented, show some evidence of epidermal change, and may show evidence of a pre-existing lesion). Ordinary bruising passes through the shades of purple, brown, green, and yellow, for example "black eye". Large areas may be involved. Bruising on the hips and thighs of women is fairly common. Purpura can be factitial in origin. A vibex or "hickey"* is a linear ecchymosis. Scratch marks may have a purpuric component. In the elderly, blotchy areas of hemorrhage on the sun-damaged backs of the hands, V of neck and upper anterior chest, and forearms are common (Bateman's purpura). A more appropriate name might be actinic or solar purpura. In certain conditions (e.g. blood dyscrasias such as hemophilia, or long-term systemic corticosteroid therapy), large, usually superficial ecchymotic areas develop at sites of minor trauma, especially on the dorsa of the forearms and hands. Autoerythrocyte sensitization is an eruption consisting of 2 to 10 cm areas of purpura, erythema, edema, and painful ecchymoses at sites of trauma (i.e. accidental, venipuncture sites, or self-induced). The autoerythrocyte sensitization lesions are most common on the accessible areas of the upper extremities, torso, head, and neck; early lesions are reddened, warm, edematous, and painful. Then a large ecchymosis develops, and later lesions are a yellowish bruise color. The late lesions may show a boggy light-purple color and may not resolve. Frequently, all stages may be seen at the same time. These lesions may have the distribution of the wounds on the crucified body of Christ (stigmata).

Secondary to Other Eruptions

Many diverse skin conditions may have a purpuric element. In some cases, the purpuric element is minor, in others it may be quite pronounced. Blistering diseases (e.g. poison ivy, variola, zoster, blistering tinea pedis, and pemphigus), erythema nodosum, and some insect bites are examples. In the elderly, many conditions, which elsewhere on the body are not purpuric, are purpuric on the legs (e.g. toxic erythemas and eczema craquelle). The descriptions of these conditions are covered elsewhere.

Disseminated

Gonococcemia or Meningococcemia

The basic lesion observed in patients with gonococcemia or meningococcemia is a purpuric indurated pustule. A few early lesions may be inflammatory dermal papules, and a few lesions may be of a cloudy vesicular nature. The eruption is located on the soles, ankles, legs, elbows, and ears, but spares the torso. In some cases,

Thomas Bateman, 1778–1821, English Dermatologist, London

*A hemorrhagic spot, usually on the side of the neck, from enthusiastic kissing and biting.

the purpuric element predominates, in others, the pustular predominates, and in still others, ulcerative lesions occur. Arthralgia is a common finding in patients with gonococcemia.

The differential diagnosis includes other septicemic conditions, especially of the coccal type. These tend to have a more frankly pustular, or ulcerative element.

In the immunosuppressed patient, disseminated palpable purpura may be a manifestation of infection from many causes.

The rickettsial pox eruption (including Rocky Mountain spotted fever) is more vesicular, and some lesions should be poxlike, although in some only a purpuric element is obvious. These eruptions are not acral in distribution.

Various drug eruptions may produce a purpuric eruption, especially on the lower legs, but these eruptions (except for the pigmented purpuric ones) are basically toxic erythemas.

Cutaneous polyarteritis nodosa and Wegener's granulomatosis may be present with acral purpuric ulcerative lesions.

Various virus infections can have a purpuric component. An unusual one is the papular purpuric gloves and socks syndrome due to parovirus B19.

Leukocyctoclastic Vasculitis (Venular Vasculitis)

Leukocytoclastic vasculitis causes the following dermatological changes: small urticarial lesions that become purpuric, then bullous, and then necrosis, which results in scarring, develops.

The most common basic lesions in leukocytoclastic vasculitis are numerous dark-red to violet-red, round, well-defined petechial macules all under 3 mm in diameter. These are symmetrically located on the dorsa of the feet, the anterior aspect of the lower legs and knees, and on the buttocks. Appearing on the same areas are rather diffuse, irregular-shaped, light-brown macules, some up to 2 cm in diameter. Also on the feet, ankles, and lower legs are irregularly shaped areas of intervening skin with no lesions. There may also be round, 1 to 2 mm, discrete, hemorrhagic crusts on the same areas. Violet round papules (purpura papulosa, palpable purpura) 3 to 5 mm in diameter are present over the anterior aspect of both knees. Early lesions are small erythematous papules. All of these lesions may form arcuate patterns of varying size.

Variations include the presence of larger (up to 1.5 cm) lesions, which have much more of a brownish cast. Varioliform scars are sometimes present. In some cases, purpuric necrotic centers are observed (Fig. 3.1). Occasionally, hemorrhagic vesicles or bullae are present, with large areas of necrosis of the skin. The extremities and buttocks are usually involved, with the larger and more pronounced lesions occurring

F. Wegener, German Pathologist

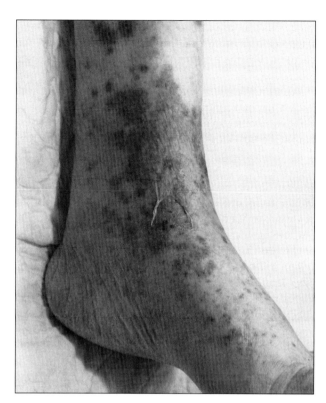

Figure 3.1 Drug-induced vasculitis with purpura and bullae on foot and ankle.

on the lower aspect of the legs. Symmetry is a striking feature. Urticarial lesions and nodules are occasionally present.

Other variations include ulcers of varying sizes and a livedoid pattern. Occasionally the process may be localized to one extremity.

In vasculitis of the Henoch-Schönlein type (rheumatic purpura), there may be, in addition to the skin lesions, arthralgias, abdominal pain, and hematuria. This type usually occurs in teenagers or young adults and may follow a sore throat.

Miscellaneous

Minute purpuric lesions are seen in the nail beds and conjunctiva in subacute bacterial endocarditis and in trichiniasis. Many blood dyscrasias and some of the dysproteinemias, as well as scurvy and Ehlers-Danlos syndromes, may present with fairly extensive purpuric eruptions. In systemic lupus erythematosus, the basically erythematous lesions may have a purpuric element. Purpura is also a feature of the

H.A. Danlos, 1844–1912, French Dermatologist
Edvard Ehlers, 1863–1937, Danish Dermatologist

cutaneous lesions of amyloidosis. The cutaneous manifestations of cholesterol crystal embolization include livedo, gangrene, cyanosis, ulceration, nodules and purpura. It is most frequently associated with anticoagulant therapy or vascular procedures.[3]

Acute pityriasis lichenoides, in addition to blistering, scaling papular, and scarring lesions, may have a purpuric component. At times when the eruption is most extensive in the extremities, this purpuric element may lead one to classify it as a disseminated purpuric eruption. Rarely, pityriasis rosea may have a purpuric element.

Pigmented Purpuric Eruptions

I cannot distinguish between Schamberg's progressive pigmentary disorder, angioma serpiginosum of Hutchinson (this lesion shows no purpura and is better classified as a telangiectatic angioma or perhaps even as a variety of port wine stain), Majocchi's purpura annularis telangiectodes, and the pigmented purpuric lichenoid dermatitis of Gougerot and Blum.[4]

The following characteristics may be found in these conditions: bright-red pinpoint dots (cayenne pepper spots), areas of diffuse uniform redness, slightly raised vascular papules, delicate vascular rings, networks or irregular curved and crooked lines representing ectatic blood vessels (forming annular and serpiginous shapes), atrophic spots, smooth, slightly elevated round or polygonal lichenoid papules 0.25 cm in diameter, and varying shades of brown and reddish brown areas of pigmentation of varying size, sometimes labeled as blotchy, mottled, patchy, retiform, or spotty, and sometimes areas of fresh purpura. In summary, then, the basic lesions are varying shapes and combinations and degrees of telangiectasia, purpura (and its subsequent staining), minute lichenoid papules, and occasionally epidermal atrophy. The eruption is essentially symmetrical and located from the knee down, often starting on the dorsa of the foot or beneath the ankle below the shoe line.

DIFFERENTIAL DIAGNOSIS

The differential diagnosis should include several other conditions.

Itching purpura, in which the basic lesion is eczema or dermatitis, which following scratching, becomes purpuric. Epidermal changes such as lichenification and scaliness are usually present. Telangiectases are not prominent.

Stasis purpura appear in patients with obvious, large varicosities or other evidence of venous stasis, usually sparing the portion of the foot supported by the shoe. These entities are difficult to differentiate from pigmented purpuric eruptions. Where definite stasis changes are present—edema, confluent areas of brown and brownish black pigmentation, and sclerosis—the diagnosis is easier. Frequently, the stasis

Paul Blum, 1878–1933, French Dermatologist, Paris

Henri Gougerot, 1881–1955, French Dermatologist

Domenico Majocchi, 1858–1925, Italian Dermatologist

Jay Frank Schamberg, 1870–1934, U.S. Dermatologist, Philadelphia, PA

purpura is worse on the leg with the most prominent varicosities. Telangiectases are not prominent, although venous stars may be present.

Diethylbromoacetylcarbamide *drug eruptions* are indistinguishable from the pigmented purpuric dermatoses. The drug-induced eruptions, of course, have a rather rapid onset and fade (in time) after the drug is stopped. Involvement of areas other than the legs is common. Telangiectases are not prominent.

Purpuric eruptions from the dye in *clothing* (especially stockings) will present a diagnostic problem. The exact symmetry, sudden onset, young age group, and popliteal fossa involvement helps with the diagnosis. Again, telangiectases are not a common finding.

Dysproteinemia purpura start as erythematous papules and rapidly progress to small petechiae and later more confluent, persistent, and larger areas of frank purpura. There is no telangiectasis.

In some cases, *lichen planus* results in an extensive degree of gray to brown to black pigmentation. This pigmentation is spotted, each spot measuring up to 2 mm in diameter with a somewhat rectangular shape. These spots, of course, represent sites of prior lichen planus papules. In some areas, the pigmentation becomes confluent, although the basic spotted nature can be seen at the periphery. In most cases, some lichen planus papular or annular lesions or mucosal lesions can be found. However, in the late stages, the pigmentation may be the only characteristic present. On the legs, the presence of stasis pigmentation as well as lichen planus pigmentation may make diagnosis difficult. Lichen aureus shows scattered plaques or persistent grouped lichenoid papules with a rust, copper, or burnt orange color.

It is best to remember that some cases of the classic variety of *Kaposi's sarcoma* may be purplish spots with minimal infiltration for many years before the papular tumor stage occurs.

Hemosiderosis of hemochromatosis occurs as a blue-black, slate, or lead color, which is sometimes generalized, but is always more marked on the face, neck, the extensor of the limbs, and the genitalia. Rarely, disseminated granuloma annulare may be a browning disease, especially in the central portion of lesions. This is not a purpuric eruption.

Atrophie blanche (or *noire* or *rouge*) is the name given to localized ischemic changes on the leg, ankle, and foot that appear as atrophy, sclerosis, varying degrees of brown pigmentation, and telangiectatic blood vessels. The ischemic changes may be from complicated stasis, organic occlusion, or vasculitis.

Acro-angiodermatitis of the feet is a variety of stasis, with Kaposi's sarcoma-like changes, involving primarily the toes.

Table 8 summarizes differential diagnosis of pigmented purpuric eruption on the legs.

Moritz Kaposi, 1837–1902, Austrian Dermatologist, Pupil and follower of Hebra in Vienna

Make sure the lesion you call purpura is from the hemosiderin of extravascular blood and not overproduction of melanin. Make sure you do not miss an underlying lesion. For example, some lichen sclerosus et atrophicus can have a large purpuric element, which may mask the underlying changes.

Table 8: Differential Diagnosis of Pigmented Purpuric Eruption on the Legs	
Classical Variety	
Drug	*Rapid onset (weeks); non-leg areas involved*
Itching Purpura	*Lichenification and scaliness, no telangiectases*
Stasis Purpura	*Sclerosis, brown pigmentation, edema are present*
Lichen Planus	*Spotted, other lesions*
Classic Kaposi's Sarcoma	*Irregular purplish patches and plaques, no disease between lesions*
Miscellaneous	*Systemic purpuras, clothing dye*

References:

1. Siemens HW. General diagnosis and therapy of skin diseases. Wiener K. trans. Chicago: University of Chicago Press, 1958.
2. Piette WW. The differential diagnosis of purpura from a morphologic perspective. Advances in Derm 1994; 9:3-24.
3. Falanga V, Fine MJH, Kapoor WN. Cutaneous manifestations of cholesterol crystal embolization. Arch Dermatol 1986; 122:1194–1198.
4. Randall SJ, Kierland RR, Montgomery H. Pigmented purpuric eruptions. Arch Dermatol Syph 1955; 64:177–191.

CHAPTER 4

Telangiectases

> *A permanent enlargement in caliber, coiling and sometimes increase in number of small superficial blood vessels of the skin.*

Overview

Telangiectasia or telangiectasis (pl. telangiectases) are the names given to a permanent enlargement in the size and the amount of coiling in the small superficial blood vessels of the skin.[1] Sometimes there is also an increase in the number of vessels. Usually, the small cutaneous venules are the vessels involved in this change. The redness produced by multiple telangiectases of varying size should be distinguished from the redness of an erythema. Telangiectases may be dot-like (macular), or elevated into a small ball of blood vessels (papular) or they may be linear (ramal). All three types are commonly present. A common variety of papular telangiectasia is the senile angioma or Campbell de Morgan capillary angioma, also called cherry angioma. An arborizing pattern of telangiectasia may be seen in necrobiosis lipoidica diabeticorum and a mat-like pattern in systemic scleroderma, especially on the chest.

In the spider naevus (nevus araneus) the vascular branches radiate from a raised papular center to form a papuloramal telangiectasis vaguely resembling the shape of a spider. All three types of telangiectases may be combined in vascular nevi (nevi flammei, "strawberry marks"). More deeply seated telangiectases become visible as livid to purplish, streak-like, macular branches. They are often arranged in the shape of a fan as on the thighs and lower legs. If larger vessels are involved, they appear to be a dark purple color. Of course, larger veins running in the subcutis appear blue. This is normally the case on the dorsa of the hands and forearm flexures, but it becomes especially distinct if the skin is thinned, as in all atrophies, or if the veins are much dilated (varicose veins), although these are not truly telangiectases. The word telangiectasia means end (tel) vessel (ang) dilatation (ectasia).

Pinpoint telangiectases may be difficult to distinguish from pinpoint purpuras. Pressure on most telangiectatic blood vessels will cause them to disappear. Exceptions are the telangiectases in lichen sclerosus et atrophicus and chronic radiodermatitis, where the dermal sclerosis is marked.

Telangiectatic blood vessels produce quite a variation in color in lesions . There is the fire red of the nevus flammeus, the salmon color of the salmon patch, the purple-red of the port wine stain, the bluish color of the venous stars, and the dusky purplish erythema of lupus erythematosus and dermatomyositis.

Two groups of telangiectatic conditions can be found: primary, in which the telangiectases are the only or major visible skin lesion, and secondary, in which other skin lesions are also present.

Primary

A spider nevus (stellate angioma) is a lesion with a red and prominent central point from which radiate telangiectatic vessels resembling spiders' legs. The total

Campbell de Morgan, 1811–1876, English Physician, London
Portions of the Overview are taken and modified from Siemens[1] (pp. 28, 30).

diameter is up to 2 cm. In some cases, the central point may be absent; in others, the central point may be papular and sometimes finely pulsatile; in others, there is considerable erythema. The spider nevus blanches with pressure. These structures are common on the face, upper torso, and upper extremities, especially in fair-skinned children.

Numerous small spider nevi may be seen in patients suffering from cirrhosis of the liver. The livid red palms are due to numerous telangiectatic blood vessels that because of the thickness of the stratum corneum, do not appear as clearly definable vessels. The redness is due to a diffusion effect of the red from all the dilated vessels into the stratum corneum. This is more clearly shown in the acute or subacute varieties of lupus erythematosus where the periungual telangiectases are easily seen in the dorsa of the finger at the base of the nails and the erythema from the telangiectases on the palmar surfaces of the finger tips and the palms. Pregnancy may be associated with numerous stellate angiomas, which may disappear following delivery.

Hereditary hemorrhagic telangiectasia (Osler-Weber-Rendu disease) shows numerous small-to medium-sized telangiectatic vessels, especially on the skin and mucosa of the face and neck.

Salmon patch ("stork bites") is a collection of fine linear telangiectases, often located on the nape of the neck, eyelids, or on the glabella. The color is light fawn, and in some cases, the telangiectatic element on the glabella is not very obvious. These usually disappear in infancy.

Cutis marmorata telangiectatica congenita is a very rare telangiectasis, present at birth, with a widespread livid network on the abdomen, chest, and limbs. Ulceration and crusting with subsequent atrophy are present in a few areas.

Port-wine stain consists of a fixed, usually dark red or purple, maplike area caused by an accumulation of small dilated capillary vessels in the upper dermis. Ocular, nasal, and oral mucosa may also show this change. Other abnormalities may also be present. On the face, the port-wine stain may be a component of the Sturge-Weber syndrome.

Nevus flammeus is a telangiectatic nevus on the nape of the neck, more common in women, on which occasionally a lichen simplex chronicus develops. It is more red than the salmon patch.

I also include under primary telangiectasia extensive blotchy telangiectatic red areas (often linear in the same pattern as an epidermal nevus — unilateral nevoid telangiectasis) that are present at birth and remain unchanged throughout life. Occasionally, in later life, small angiomatous papules may develop in these red areas.

Sir William Osler, 1849–1919, Canadian Physician

Henry Jules Louis Marie Rendu, 1844–1902, French Physician

William Allen Sturge, 1850–1919, British Physician, London

Frederick Parkes Weber, 1863–1962, British Physician, London

There also is a tendency for portions of port-wine stains to become angiomatous by adulthood.

Venous stars or fans are areas of 1 to 3 cm diameter with small venule dilation, usually occurring on the thighs or legs of women, and in patients with some form of venous stasis of the legs. Because venules are involved, the venous stars are blue. They can be obliterated by pressure. These structures have also been called thread veins.

Following excessive grenz ray exposure, especially to the areas of the body having a thin skin, (e.g. dorsa of hands, and vulvar and perianal areas), an extensive mottled eruption appears, consisting solely of superficial fine telangiectatic blood vessels, with no appreciable atrophy.

Venous lakes are 1 to 3 mm diameter dark blue or purplish areas, usually compressible. On the lips, the area is macular, on other parts of the face or ears the lesion may be papular with a smooth, dome-shaped surface. They also occur on the semimucosa of the vulva and genitals, where they may be confused with angiokeratomas.

"Petechial" telangiectases are multiple, small (1 to 2 mm), bright red to brown macular dots, widely disseminated, compressible, and having at times a striking relationship to minute petechiae. In contrast to petechiae, this type of lesion has no internal significance. They may represent early spider angiomas but they tend to occur on the extremities, in a younger age group, and may be seen in patients with no spider nevi. They may represent a type of essential telangiectasia.

Angioma serpiginosum consists of red-pepper colored punctate macules showing linear, mottled, or netlike patterns of telangiectatic blood vessels. Peripheral extension may result in a serpiginous outline. Morphologically this could be related to the pigmented purpuric eruptions.

Generalized essential telangiectasia consists of extensive linear or large patches of telangiectases on the trunk and limbs. It appears in young adults.

Costal fringe consists of a bandlike pattern of telangiectases across the anterolateral part of the thorax, often near the costal margins. The bandlike pattern can be bilateral, unilateral, or segmental, and it typically occurs as an acquired finding in elderly men.

Tufted angioma presents as purple macules, papules or plaques on a mottled background, usually involving the trunk or neck, and extending over months to years before stabilizing.

Secondary

The second group of telangiectatic conditions consists of the large purplish and smaller red telangiectases over the alae of the nose in rosacea, the innumerable large (up to 3 cm) stellate angioma in the CREST syndrome (i.e. calcinosis cutis Raynaud's phenomenon, esophageal dysfunction, sclerodactyly, and telangiectasia), and the abnormal telangiectasia (often peripheral) in radiation sequelae (Fig. 4.1).

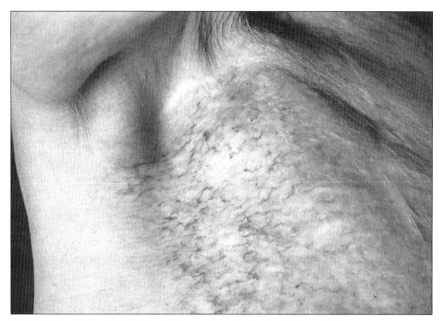

Figure 4.1 Telangiectases in sclerotic radiation sequelae on the chest wall, flank, and axilla.

Figure 4.2 Telangiectases produced by habitual exposure to the sun.

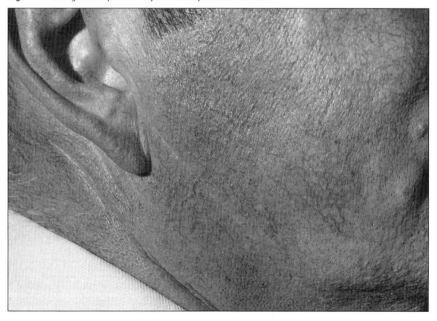

Patients with telangiectasia macularis eruptiva perstans (adult urticaria pigmentosa) present with a widespread brownish mottled macular eruption, more extensive on the torso, with varying degrees of faint telangiectasia. Occasionally dermatographism is present. Urtication is not necessarily present.

Sometimes, it may be difficult to distinguish between telangiectases and small papular angiomatous tumors.

The fine diffuse telangiectatic blood vessels on the cheeks and the fine linear telangiectatic blood vessels in skin damaged by habitual exposure to the sun may be seen in secondary telangiectases (Fig. 4.2).

Other examples are the telangiectatic blood vessels overlying the peripheral areas of certain skin tumors (e.g. basal cell carcinoma) where they are of broad and varying diameter, senile sebaceous adenoma, and telangiectatic blood vessels associated with discoid lupus erythematosus on the face and on the periungual tissues and palms in the acute or subacute systemic type. There is also a type of widespread telangiectatic lupus erythematosus involving the V of the neck and upper back where only telangiectases of various sorts and a minor degree of erythema are present. In some cases, the erythema is more pronounced and the telangiectases are less prominent. Dermatomyositis may present a similar picture.

A permanent flush and telangiectatic blood vessels develop in the late stages of the carcinoid syndrome. Carcinoma en cuirasse (forming a breastplate) may have a telangiectatic component.

In the various forms of poikiloderma and in the semimucosal old lesions of lichen sclerosus et atrophicus, compressible or uncompressible telangiectatic blood vessels may be seen through the atrophic epidermis and situated in the sclerotic dermis. In some cases, actual small linear or telangiectatic purpura may be present.

Arborizing telangiectases and other irregular dilated small venous channels are often seen in patients with venous stasis of the legs. Other changes of venous stasis (e.g. edema, brown pigmentation, sclerosis, and atrophy) are usually present. Arbitrarily, I have defined varicose veins as being over 1 mm in width; telangiectases, under 1 mm in width. One could also define varicose veins as conduits and telangiectases as end vessels.

The pigmented purpuric eruptions may have a telangiectatic component, but as the main lesion is purpura, these conditions are discussed in Chapter 3.

Telangiectases and atrophy may be seen following prolonged topical use of potent fluorinated adrenocorticosteroids, especially on the face and in the large body folds (particularly axillae and groin).

Telangiectatic Syndromes

The following conditions should be considered.

Bloom syndrome is characterized by erythema and diffuse telangiectatic blood vessels on the forehead, cheeks, lips, chin, and dorsa of hands. In addition, dwarfism and photosensitivity are present.

David Bloom, 1892– U.S. Dermatologist

In Rothmund-Thomson syndrome, there are telangiectases on the face, buttocks, arms, and extremities. Mottled brown pigmentation, fine atrophy, scant hair with loss of eyebrows, cataracts, and stubby fingers are among the characteristic features.

Hereditary hemorrhagic telangiectasia shows numerous, rather large, telangiectatic blood vessels on the skin and mucosa, especially on the tongue and lips.

In Cockayne's syndrome, facial erythema with mottled brown pigmentation and scarring are typical findings. Bullae are often present. Retardation, loss of subcutaneous fat on the face, and "Mickey Mouse" ears may also be present.

Ataxia-telangiectasia is characterized by ataxia and dwarfism, as well as telangiectases on the conjunctiva, eyelids, ears, and cheeks.

Focal dermal hypoplasia (Goltz syndrome) is a rare congenital condition in females with dwarfism, linear streaks of telangiectasia, atrophy (absence of dermis), and soft fatty nodules on the trunk and limbs. Digit malformations are also present.

Port-wine stain has been described earlier and may be associated with several syndromes.

DIFFERENTIAL DIAGNOSIS

It must be stressed that the clinician remember that some ordinary conditions are so telangiectatic that, as with the purpuras, the underlying lesion may be missed. Examples are the telangiectasia in radiation sequelae, some forms of lupus erythematosus, rosacea, and lichen sclerosus et atrophicus.

Reference

1. Siemens HW. General diagnosis and therapy of skin diseases. Weiner K, trans. Chicago:University of Chicago Press, 1958.

Edward Alfred Cockayne, 1880–1856, English Physician

Robert Goltz, 1923– U.S. Dermatologist

August von Rothmund, Jr., 1830–1906, German Ophthalmologist and Physician

Matthew Sidney Thomson, 1894–1969, English Dermatologist

CHAPTER 5

Eczemas

A clinical process that is clearly superficial in form and that, early is erythematous, papulovesicular, oozing and crusting and, later, is red purple, scaly, lichenified, and then, brown or hypopigmented. Clinically vesiculation and histologically spongiosis must be present at some stage.

Overview

Eczema is a reaction pattern of the skin characterized by a series of elementary lesions which succeed each other, combine, or coexist in neighboring localities. These elementary lesions are erythema, edema, papulation, vesiculation, exudation, crusting, lichenification, desquamation, and sometimes brown pigmentation (Fig. 5.1 and Table 9). Eczematous pores are the denuded vesicles from which serous fluid exudes.[1]

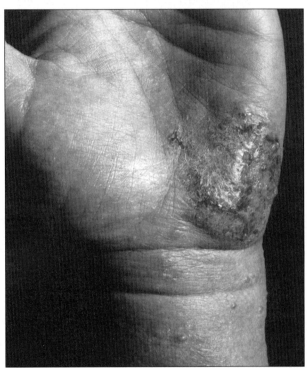

Figure 5.1 Acute contact eczema with blisters, oozing, and edema.

Because many causes of eczema can evoke a similar morphology, it may be difficult to make an etiological diagnosis, although this is not always the case. I should stress that I regard eczema as a morphological and not an etiological diagnosis.[2]

A simplified and often typical course of an eczematous eruption has been given by Darier.

The erythematous stage consists of a vivid reddening with diffuse margins showing a finely edematous papular surface that is pruritic. Sometimes this redness disappears, leaving a fine lamellar or furfuraceous desquamation. This peeling is a useful clue in doubtful cases. In these cases the vesicles or extensive spongiosis are visible only on microscopic examination.

Portions of the Overview are taken and modified from Siemens[1] (pp. 69–71).

vermilion border of the upper and lower lips; the trunk where the long axes of the oval plaques tend to follow the lines of cleavage, particularly noticeable at the regressing scaly and lichenified stages, at which time the resemblance to the later stages of pityriasis rosea is striking.

The discoid exudative lesions disappear, or more often become lichenified, sometimes after going through several exacerbations. The weeping and oozing of this eczematous phase, which occasionally persists, often lasts only a very short time and develops within a day or two into the dry lichenoid stage.

Lichenoid Phase: Scattered lichenoid papules appear on many areas, some irregularly distributed, some appearing in larger and smaller groups. The majority are follicular. While their appearance suggests lichen planus, the papules are smaller and less violaceous and do not have the typical striae, umbilication, flat tops, or polygonal shapes and straight sides of lichen planus papules. The similarity to lichen planus is most noticeable on the glans penis.

In addition to the isolated lichenified papules, large areas of skin show varying degrees of diffuse lichenification. There seems to be not only lichenification but also a nonpitting edema in these lichenified plaques, as shown by the rapid changes in consistency. This edema is most noticeable on the lower legs. Wrists and dorsa of the hands are frequent sites of lichenification.

The lichenoid phase lasts longer than the exudative, premycotic, or urticarial phases, and hence it is more often seen.

Phase Resembling Premycotic Stage of Mycosis Fungoides: In this phase the infiltration of the discoid and oval lesions dominates the picture, while the lichenoid papules and the exudative and crusting eczematous features are less prominent. Intervening clear areas of normal skin, the sharply marginated border and the map-like bizarre borders also tend to make one think of a premycotic eruption.

Urticarial Phase: From time to time showers of small round itchy prurigo-like papules appear. Occasionally some are large and resemble hives. They may appear anywhere or everywhere and last from thirty minutes to several hours. Usually these lesions are part of the previously described eruption, but in some cases they may be the most obvious lesion.

In all stages, goose flesh appears upon exposure to slight changes in temperature, as when undressing, and the nipples may show a persistent and abnormally marked erection.

Miscellaneous Features: Varying shades of brown pigmentation are often seen as the eruption subsides. Deep seated vesicles of varying size, some with brownish hue, are seen in the instep areas of the soles and (smaller vesicular lesions) in the center of the palms. Varying degrees of a moderate, soft, non-tender axillary and inguinal lymph node enlargement may be noted. This waxes and wanes with the eruption. The distal portions of the patient's fingernails are shiny and smooth, more in the center and less laterally, with a considerable degree of wearing off of the distal free edge. Occasionally this wearing off produces a V-shaped groove in the center of the distal border. In general, although no part is immune, most lesions occur on the extensor rather than flexor surfaces. The perimammary areas, the anterior and posterior aspects of the axillary folds, the scrotum, the circumoral region, the bridge of the nose, the abdomen, and the scapular areas are the site of the most numerous and persistent plaques. The penile lesions are seen in most cases.

An impressive feature of the various types of eruptions in this eczema is the dramatic and apparently spontaneous changes in appearance from week to week, and even sometimes from day to day.

DIFFERENTIAL DIAGNOSIS

As has been implied in the original description, all sorts of conditions must be considered in the differential diagnosis of oid-oid disease.

The persistent penile papules and similar lesions on the areola, nipples, and axillary folds are suggestive of scabies, but of course there are no burrows identifiable, the finger webs are clear, and wrists show a lichenified, not an excoriated, papular eruption. On close examination, the penile and axillary lesions are basically eczematous in nature.

Lichen planus was also discussed in the original description. I only add that the sides of the papules in lichen planus eczema slope, with perhaps a partially flat top. In lichenoid eczema, there are no typical lichen planus papules; in lichen planus they can always be found somewhere.

Portions of the eruption of lichenoid dermatophytids, especially on the torso, may appear as follicular papules showing no grouping and having a rather flattened top. Also, there must be a primary tinea focus (often acute). As well, of course, other areas in this disseminated eczema reveal lesions of eczema.

In blistering trichophytids, the sterile instep lesions and those on the palms could represent an id. However, again an acute primary focus would have to be shown. Also, the lesions in other sites are those of eczema.

Portions of the premycotic-like phase of exudative discoid and lichenoid chronic dermatosis may resemble the premycotic phase of mycosis fungoides. However, other areas show lesions more typical of eczema. It must be admitted that time and numerous biopsies may be necessary to definitely exclude mycosis fungoides.

The polymorphism of the eruption, the blistering and urticarial lesions, the tendency to some type of grouping, the involvement of the extensor areas, the symmetry of the eruption, the exacerbations and partial remission, and the residual brown pigmentation certainly suggest dermatitis herpetiformis. However, the presence of numerous satellite lesions, the lack of distinct and intact vesicles or bullae at any time, and the involvement of the palms or soles tend to exclude this diagnosis. It must be said that at times a therapeutic trial of sulfapyridine or diamino-diphenylsulfone may be necessary to confirm diagnosis.

Nonspecific eczematous and follicular ids, resulting from some underlying internal carcinoma or leukemia, are excluded by a general examination and by the passage of time. In general, the extensiveness and acuteness of the eruption means that the underlying condition is usually symptomatic.

Adult atopic dermatitis is basically a lichenified flexor eruption, and has no weeping or blistering except in areas of secondary eczematization due to trauma.

Nummular eczema must also be included in the differential diagnosis.

Fungal Eczemas

It is with some trepidation that these conditions are classified under the eczemas. I do so for two reasons. First, the basic lesion is a vesicle with spongiosis (Lever[11]), that undermines the periphery of the lesion, and other features of eczema such as erythema, crusting, lichenification, desquamation, and brown pigmentation may be present. Second, there seems no other place to put them. Should I group them with the erythematopapulosquamous eruptions? Again, this does not seem reasonable, when true vesicles are the hallmark of the eruption. (Of course, the nonblistering fungal infections, e.g. those due to Trichophyton rubrum, are included in the erythematopapulosquamous group.)

Fungal eczemas that are almost entirely regional, (e.g. fungal eczema of the groins, fungal eczema between the toes, and yeast eczema of the finger webs), have been included under the appropriate discussion of those regional varieties of eczema.

This leaves the disseminated blistering fungal eczemas for discussion here.

Blistering (vesiculating) tinea of the relatively hairless parts (herpes circinatus) appears usually on the face, neck, hands, and forearms. Not all of the lesions are vesicular. Large erythematosquamous spots are present, with a sharply demarcated orbicular circumference and distinctly outlined, clean-cut, vesicular borders, and clearing centers. It is exceptional for the disk to be incomplete or the circle broken. The area is pink or red, with a dusky center covered with powdery, flaky, or crusted scales; it is marginate or plainly circinate through healing from the center. Vesiculation may be present only at the periphery, throughout the lesion, or in concentric circles. The areas are sometimes more or less edematous or infiltrated. The downy hairs may be dull and brittle or encased in scales at the base. The lesions are quite large (up to 10 cm in diameter).

DIFFERENTIAL DIAGNOSIS

This condition (fungal eczema) must be distinguished from the trichophytoid patches of common eczema, which are less regularly outlined and accompanied by scattered eczematous lesions; from pityriasis rosea, which has a characteristic pattern and which does not have blistering; and from the various forms of seborrhea.

Rarely, there is a circinate papulovesicular variety of favus of the hairless regions (favus herpetiformis). It closely resembles circinate trichophytic eczema, but the lesions are less regularly circular, and cup-shaped crusts (scutula) are usually seen in some other areas.

Also, rarely, some of the acute follicular tineas have widespread, lichenoid, follicular, and even more rarely, vesicular ids. These are more common on the torso.

Although unusual, I have seen blistering tinea corporis mimic localized bullous pemphigoid and Sneddon's disease.

Ian Bruce Sneddon, 1915–1987, English Dermatologist

Microbial Eczema (Infectious Eczematoid Dermatitis)

Microbial eczema is a variety of eczema characterized by sharply demarcated areas, usually with polycyclic configuration and continuous peripheral extension.

The areas of eczema are crusted, weeping, scaly, inflammatory eruptions that extend out from the periphery through formation of vesicles or pustules, usually by splitting up or undermining the peripheral epidermis. These lesions are apt to be combined with those of impetigo.

Microbial eczema commonly develops about varicose ulcers, draining ears, or chronic discharging wounds.

Microbial eczema in children may be of a type in which a considerable amount of the secondary eruption is frankly eczematous in nature. The primary lesion (often retroauricular) looks raw, eroded, and fissured, with some scaliness at the periphery. Small peripheral pustules are often present. At times, this condition may be confused with atopic dermatitis and secondary pyoderma.

Microbial eczema is distinguished from eczema with secondary pyoderma.

Specific Patterns of Eczema

Poison Ivy

This is a particular type of eczema with a specific cause, which is diagnostic on examination alone and so should be outlined here.

The basic lesion of poison ivy is an erythematous and edematous linear vesicular or vesiculobullous eruption. The areas are sharply demarcated and, in addition to lines, appear as unusual, irregular areas with varying degrees of erythema, vesiculation, and bullous formation. On the soft tissues (e.g. eyelids and genitalia), edema and erythema are prominent. On the face, weeping from the ruptured vesides occurs. In some cases, vesiculobullous formation is very marked; in others, edema and erythema predominate.

Sometimes, late in the course of the disease, widespread urticarial lesions appear.

Follicular

Table 11 provides differential diagnoses of follicular eczema.

FORMALDEHYDE PRODUCTS IN SHEETS

The basic lesion caused by formaldehyde is follicular and perifollicular, red to skin-colored papular eruption. The papules have steeply sloping sides with a rounded top. They are 2 to 3 mm in diameter, and surprisingly uniform in shape and size. The eruption is most intense and severe on the lateral aspects of the thighs and arms, but also may be present in varying degrees on all areas except the palms, soles, dorsa of fingers and toes, face, scalp, and genitalia. Rarely, erythema papules are present on the instep and palms. On areas where the follicular surfaces are prominent (e.g. lateral arms and thighs), the papules appear to be follicular, but in other areas, e.g. the abdomen, the follicular arrangement is not marked, and in some areas the lesions are definitely not follicular. Varying degrees of traumatic, blotchy, and linear bright

Table 11: Differential Diagnosis of Follicular Eczema	
From Sheets	*Widespread, symmetrical, clearly follicular, eczema on pinnas, very itchy; covered torso areas are spared*
From Nickel	*At sites of contact–but many have secondary lesions, lichenified, excoriated*
From Fiberglass	*Torso mainly, looks follicular (although it's not), very itchy*
From Atopic Dermatitis	*In blacks and asiatics; torso, history of atopy*
From Seborrhea	*Center chest, back, usual seborrheic color, not itchy, may be associated with pustules, occasionally petaloidal on sternal area*
From Neomycin	*Like nickel, this eruption may have a follicular element*
From Kerion	*This is a follicular papular eruption on the torso usually occurring in children; it is an id*

red erythema are also present. On the rims of the ears, eyelids, tip of the nose, and cheeks, the process presents as an erythema, with some areas oozing. On the non-hairy torso, frankly eczematous areas may be seen. After a week or so, the papules flatten down, the blotchy erythema disappears, and the facial areas show a scaly erythema. In 2 to 4 weeks the eruption is gone. Lichenification is not unusual.

The mucosae and lymph nodes are normal.

NICKEL SULFATE

Although there are many kinds and stages of eczema, a few (some already described) have reasonably specific patterns that allow the cause to be almost certainly determined by inspection alone. Eczema from nickel sulfate is one of these. The crusted, oozing, eczematous eruption on the fronts and backs of the ear lobes, the rather poorly demarcated excoriated papular and papulovesicular plaques on the anterior and posterior aspects of the thighs and on one side or other of the back, along with a symmetrical diffuse excoriated papular id on the forearms, elbows, arms, and knees, added together, make a diagnosis of eczema due to nickel sulfate most likely.

Miscellaneous

Another pattern of eczema is that of phytophotodermatitis. Contact with wild parsnips, celery, lime juice, or gas plant, in some cases followed by exposure to sunlight, produces an eczema on the sun-exposed areas at the sites of contact.

A rather characteristic eruption of contact dermatitis eczema is an acute oozing edematous eruption involving the scalp, ears, face, and neck. The amount of edema is often quite marked, with the ears swollen and the eyelids being swollen shut. The degree of oozing is also marked, so much so that the serum may actually drip off. On the scalp, particularly, it becomes crusty and matted. The serum gives off a sweet fruity odor. There may also be an urticarial eczematous id on the upper torso. On the scalp, secondary pyoderma is common. This picture is seen in contact dermatitis from paraphenylenediamine, a frequent component of hair dyes. In less acute cases, hair-covered areas are much less involved than the surrounding nonhairy areas, such as the forehead or ears.

Localized Varieties
Hands and Feet

In general, in dealing with the differential diagnosis of the blistering eczemas,* it is useful to remember that exogenous eczemas are usually on the dorsa of the hands and fingers, and feet and toes, whereas the endogenous eczemas are found on the palmar surfaces or sides of the hands and fingers, and feet and toes.

Eczema of the palms and soles has the same basic characteristics of eczema elsewhere, except that the anatomy of the area and frequent movement may modify the eruption. For example, because of the thick stratum corneum, the appearance is different; because of frequent movement, fissures are extremely common in any eczematous process in these areas. In certain occupational eczemas (e.g. those due to cement), tremendous lichenification may be seen. Hyperhidrosis is a common finding in certain varieties of eczema on the hands and feet (e.g. blistering epidermophytosis and pompholyx). At times, the end stage of palmar or plantar eczema may have flattening of the skin surface, resembling atrophy.

I have seen two cases of pollenosis and photosensitivity eczema that have had a recurrent blistering eruption on the palms and soles. The eruption sometimes flares with a flare of the pollenosis and photosensitivity and sometimes it does not.

In some cases, there may be no morphological difference between many varieties of eczema of the hands and feet. Clinical course and other findings (especially examination of skin scrapings for fungal products) may be required for a final diagnosis.

The purely hyperkeratotic or tylotic eczemas of the palms are really keratodermas and are classified as such. To call these eczemas when there never is a blistering phase does not seem logical.

Pompholyx

Pompholyx[12] is a reaction pattern, not a diagnosis. It may occur as part of or in association with atopic dermatitis, irritant and allergic contact dermatitis, allergy to nickel sulfate, blistering tinea (i.e. primary on feet, id on hands), and rarely pemphigus and bullous pemphigoid.

Symmetrically on hands and/or feet, numerous small or medium-sized vesicles, deeply set in the thick (palmar or plantar) epidermis appear with or without redness and edema. The vesicles are common on lateral surfaces of fingers. The blisters are pinhead-sized, not grouped, and occasionally may become larger or confluent. A clear stringy fluid escapes on puncture. The vesicles may not open spontaneously but disappear by internal absorption leaving a small scaly collarette; usually the blister tops are rubbed off by the patient. Peripheral undermining is not a feature of pompholyx. As the eruption subsides, more scaling appears. Hyperhydrosis is frequently present.

A childhood variant is a recurrent pinhead-sized vesicular eruption occurring primarily on the pulpy tips of the fingers and toes (occasionally extending onto the

*If you are uncertain as to whether or not a small swelling on the thick plantar or palmar skin is a papule or a vesicle, puncture the swelling with a fine needle. If it is a vesicle, a pinhead-sized drop of sticky fluid can be expressed.

anterior portion of the soles). Collarettes may follow absorption or a scaly fissured eruption, in which a diffuse exfoliation is the main finding, may follow. The eruption is much worse in the winter, and usually occurs in the age group of 5 to 10 years. It is rare after puberty. Most cases are not atopic dermatitis.

Peridigital dermatitis of Enta is basically a scaliness with rather large areas of the pulps of the fingers and toes involved. Extension of the scaliness onto the anterior soles (sometimes heels) is common. The affected areas are denuded centrally, and the amounts of peripheral scale vary. In some areas, the eruption is calloused or tylotic with fissures over areas of movement No peripheral undermining is obvious. No blisters are seen. The intertoe web spaces are usually clear. The nails are not involved. Most patients are not atopic. Hyperhidrosis is not often a feature. As there are no blisters, this condition must be included in the differential diagnosis of the palmar and plantar keratodermas, and is not a blistering eczema.

Atopic dermatitis in the classical areas, with the classical clinical findings, and with the classical personal and family history of atopy may be present on the sides of the fingers and on the palms, on the insteps and soles, with a fine blistering eruption, alone quite indistinguishable from the clinical reaction pattern called pompholyx.

Blistering Tinea (Eczema Parasitica)

Blistering tinea[13] is located on the floor of the interdigital folds (especially between the fourth and fifth toe), in the flexion folds of the toes, and on adjacent areas of the plantar skin. The great majority of fungal eczemas appear first either between or under the lateral three toes, or on the part of the sole which, when wet, leaves no print on the floor. When the big toes and dorsa of the feet are predominantly affected, a fungal causation is unlikely. In blistering tinea, macerated horny layer is present and becomes detached in the form of white shreds, leaving a bright red surface or a cheesy material with a peripherally undermined border. Circumferentially, a few deep vesicles,which may dry or coalesce into an eczematiform surface, are sometimes seen. This eczema may extend to the dorsal aspect of the foot as well as to the sole, extending to the arch and heel. Deep bullae, occasionally hemorrhagic and up to 2.0 cm in size, may be seen, especially on the plantar skin. As these bullae dry up, a circular thick red-brown area may be left. Occasionally, blistering tinea may be primarily pustular, but even then a few vesicles can be found. The pustules in blistering tinea do not contain greenish pus and are not present as small lakes of pus.

Pustules with peripheral inflammation, lymphangitis and lymphadenitis representing secondary streptococcal pyoderma does occur A fine sterile vesicular eruption may be present on the sides of the fingers. This id-type eruption is not as extensive or severe as on the toes and soles. Rarely, a figurate erythema occurs on the torso. Blistering tinea of the feet is rare before puberty. Hyperhidrosis is a common associated finding. The toenails are commonly involved and show principal involvement at the free border or under the lateral margins of the nail. The nail plate is thickened with opaque, yellowish, powdery debris in the involved areas. In more

Thomas Enta, 1932–   Canadian Dermatologist, Calgary, AB

severe infections, loss or partial loss of plate, splintering, and lamellated desquamation may be present.

Blistering tinea does not occur on the hands.

The necessity of repeated mycological examinations cannot be stressed enough. There are times when even the expert morphologist cannot clinically distinguish between plantar eczema and blistering tinea on the feet.

When penicillin is given to some patients with blistering tinea pedis, a blistering trichophytid-like eruption appears on the hands and feet.

Blistering tinea of the feet must be distinguished from pustular psoriasis. This is a fixed vesiculopustular eruption, usually occurring on the pressure areas of the palms and soles. There may be an arcuate border with peripheral undermining. A mixture of vesicles and pustules is usually present. The vesicles are small (1 to 2 mm), and when drying up, they tend to have a dark brown color. They are never large as in dyshidrosis or blistering tinea. The pustules are superficial, flaccid, with little erythema. They predominate over the vesicles and are large, sometimes forming lakes of yellow-green pus. They are not tender and there is no objective evidence of lymphangitis or lymphadenitis. When the pustules unite, larger superficial lakes of pus may be seen. When the pustules and vesicles dry up, a red glistening surface may be seen. Psoriasis is usually not found elsewhere. Under the term pustular psoriasis of the hands or feet, I include the entity commonly referred to as pustular bacterid. Acrodermatitis continua of Hallopeau and dermatitis repens are probably varieties of infectious eczematoid dermatitis. Ordinary keratotic and plaque-form psoriasis may occur on the palms and soles, but it is not vesicular or pustular.

DIFFERENTIAL DIAGNOSIS

The differential diagnosis between pompholyx, blistering tinea, and pustular psoriasis on the hands and feet includes the following.

Certain kinds of eczematous dermatitis (contact, irritant) may present with a blistering scaly eruption. However, there is usually no peripheral undermining, satellite lesions are common, and the eruption is usually mainly on the dorsa of the foot and toes, although it may extend to the web spaces. Poison ivy produces an explosive, acute, sharply marginated eruption, usually with lots of edema and vesiculobullous lesions, usually linear or square. Sometimes the fingers are separated by the bullae. The onset is acute, and the total course is about three weeks. Large sheets of exfoliation occurs after the bullous lesions subside. Lesions elsewhere are common. This is one of the rarer causes of acute bullous formations on the palmar and plantar skin.

Atopic dermatitis is basically an excoriated lichenified nonblistering eruption, usually located on the dorsa of the toes and feet, which has no deep-seated blisters on the soles and no peripheral undermining.

François Henri Hallopeau, 1842–1919, French Dermatologist, Paris

Patients with intertrigo and macerations due to hyperhidrosis may present with an erythema with whitening of stratum corneum due to absorption of moisture. No other lesions are present.

Moist white intertriginous psoriasis, especially in the fourth intertoe web skin, has some of the typical psoriasis scaling at the periphery, usually along with lesions of psoriasis elsewhere, especially in other flexural areas. There is no exfoliation, as with the blistering tinea, and there is no undermining of the periphery.

Occasionally, a soft corn on the medial aspect of the fifth toe may be confused with the above-mentioned lesions. It is a solitary circular white keratosis, with a central brownish yellow core of homogenous keratin (the eye of a partridge). It is exquisitely tender on pressure to the lateral side of the fifth toe. As with all hyperkeratotic or keratotic lesions on the plantar surface, paring is necessary to make a correct diagnosis.

Microbial eczema (infectious eczematoid dermatitis), may also occur on the hands and feet and may partially resemble other dyshidrotic eczematous patterns.

Candidiasis may produce a rather sharply demarcated, persistent, vesiculopustular eruption on the hands and paronychial areas, as well as about the orifices and on the elbows and knees in microcutaneous candidiasis. The lesions are moist and have a whitish, scaly, serous crust with a bright underlying erythema. Some of the lesions may be amazingly psoriasiform. Interdigital candidiasis occurs in the web spaces when the areas are habitually moist.

It is best not to forget consideration of scabies in the differential diagnosis. True vesicular lesions, scattered, patchy, and forming a mostly dyshidrosiform pattern, may be seen in addition to the more characteristic sharply marginated and isolated scratched papules and, of course, the typical burrows. Lesions elsewhere (e.g. wrists, elbows, genitalia) are almost always present.

Rarely, even pemphigus and bullous pemphigoid may masquerade as pompholyx. Table 12 provides a summary of the differential diagnosis of blistering eruption of the hands.

Table 12: Differential Diagnosis of Blistering Eruption of the Hands	
Pompholyx	*Areas of fine blistering on the sides of fingers and palms, itchy, various stages present at once*
Nummular Eczema	*Dorsa of hands, 2 to 3 cm in diameter, studded with blisters*
Recalcitrant Vesicopustular Eruptions	*Mainly pustules–large and superficial; blister tops have a brown color when they are old*
Acute Explosive Contact	*Swelling, redness, vesico- or vesiculobullous formation, poorly demarcated*

Keratolysis Exfoliativa

The basic lesion may be a subcorneal "vesicle" or bulla occurring mainly on the palms and occasionally on the soles, usually in the summertime.

The fluid is quickly absorbed and leaves a collapsed thin horny roof, which rapidly falls off, leaving a peripheral scaly collarette varying in diameter from a few millimeters to a few centimeters and various degrees of peripheral undermining. In recent lesions, the yellowish-white separated stratum corneum may still be present. In older lesions, about one-third to one-fifth of the surface may be covered by the scaly collarette, and in still older lesions, only the very periphery of the collarette remains. Confluence of the remains of individual blisters results in the formation of arcuate borders. After desquamation the denuded central area has a bluish-purple tinge. At this stage there is no blistering, either centrally or peripherally. The eruption is symmetrical. There is no fissuring.

Erosio Interdigitalis Blastomycetica

Interdigital candidiasis is a sharply marginated purplish-red erosive lesion with a loosely adherent, yellowish-white, thickened, horny layer. If the horny layer is removed, especially at the periphery, a small amount of peripheral undermining is evident. The lesion is usually located in the second or third finger web space and on the sides of the adjacent fingers where the lesion has an inverted-U shape. The other finger web spaces are less frequently involved. If the hand of the patient with erosio interdigitalis blastomycetica is held up to the light, it will be seen that there is no space visible between the adjacent proximal metacarpal areas, hence the areas stay moist for long periods of time. Erosio interdigitalis blastomycetica is common in orthodox Jewish women who are exposed to double dishwashing and who come from Eastern Europe. The above described metacarpal finding is always present in these patients. Barbers, housewives, bartenders, charwomen (and men) may also develop this condition.

DIFFERENTIAL DIAGNOSIS

The differential diagnosis for erosio interdigitalis blastomycetica includes the following. Eczematous dermatitis starting beneath the ring on the ring finger, shows more scaling, is less well defined, has no frank erosions, and is present more on the sides and top of the fingers rather than in the finger web spaces. Moist psoriasis, which has the characteristic white scaly papules at the periphery and is frequently fissured with lesions elsewhere. Mitchell's flexural streptococcal pyoderma is a red oozing painful eruption, sometimes with secondary peripheral pustules.

On the skin of the toe web spaces, in addition to moist psoriasis, flexural streptococcal pyoderma and both blistering and nonblistering interdigital tinea pedis must be included in the differential diagnosis. For additional differential diagnosis information, see Table 13.

Scalp

Eczema of the scalp is not very common. Whether this is due to increased resistance of the scalp to eczematogenic factors or due to a shielding effect of the hair is not clear. In some cases of primary irritant eczema, as from hair "permanent" solutions,

Table 13: Differential Diagnosis of Nonblistering Eruption of the Hands and Feet	
Glazed Foot (Peridigital Dermatitis of Enta)	*No blister, not itchy, red shiny glazed surface, fissures, gone after puberty*
Keratolysis Exfoliativa	*No blisters, varying sized circles of in-toeing scale*
Trichophytosis	*Diffuse red scaling, nails involved*
Psoriasis	*Plaque variety; vesiculopustular; guttate*
Various Keratodermas	
Eczema	*Usually are blisters at one stage or another, itchy*

the eczema is located on the upper exposed areas of the pinnae, on the mastoid area, and along the hairline skin of the forehead, while the scalp itself is relatively free of lesions.

Eczema of the scalp has a tendency to be predominantly a scaly eruption with excoriations. Although frank oozing and crusting, usually diffuse and without eczema pores, are occasionally seen in severe acute contact allergic eczema (as from chemical hair dyes), in most cases the process is quite indolent with only a minor degree of oozing, but with much scaling, lichenification, and excoriation.

DIFFERENTIAL DIAGNOSIS

Extensive acute eczemas in the scalp may quickly become pyodermatous, with sticky crusting, more inflammation, occasional peripheral pustules and tenderness, and regional lymphadenitis in the postauricular area. Pyodermatous lesions may also develop in the scratch marks of neurotic excoriations or of pediculosis capitis. In these last two cases, scaling is not prominent, and the seropurulent oozing is different from the oozing of acute eczema. Kerion of the scalp is basically a boggy follicular pustular circular eruption with hair loss and is described in Chapter 20. Occasionally, in the subsiding phase, it may resemble a scaly scalp eczema.

The remaining differential diagnosis of scalp eczema is really a differential diagnosis of erythematopapulosquamous eruptions of the scalp, covered in Chapter 6. This list includes seborrhea, psoriasis, atopic dermatitis, lichen simplex chronicus, nonblistering tinea, and neurotic excoriations.

Beard and Hairy Areas

This type of eczema is not common, and presents little difference from scalp eczema. There is a tendency to early scaling, and frank oozing is unusual. Pyoderma can be distinguished because its crusts are more juicy, the lesions are more sharply demarcated, and an occasional pustule can usually be seen.

In the axillae there are usually no blisters, even in very acute cases — usually only varying degrees of oozing. In eczema caused by clothes, the apex is often spared; in eczema from deodorants, the apex is involved. The differential diagnosis of other axillary eruptions is the same as outlined under erythema intertrigo or under papular axillary dermatoses.

Face

Most facial eczemas have the characteristics of eczema anywhere else. A few variations and interesting differential diagnostic situations exist.

Many eczemas on the face take on the follicular, pustular, or seborrheic basic features of facial skin, and so do not look frankly eczematous, but may be papular and occasionally pustular with a fair amount of greasy scale. This is especially true in the nasolabial folds, eyebrows, and chin. Facial allergic contact dermatitis from preservatives is commonly patchy in its distribution on the facial skin. Almost all eczemas on the face develop some prominent peeling as they subside.

Acute contact dermatitis as from a caine containing preparation may cause considerable edema of the face, particularly on the eyelids.

The various clinical forms of photosensitivity (e.g. urticarial, erythema multiforme type, vesicular, and plaque-like) do occur on the face as well as on other sun-exposed areas (see Chapter 1 for classification and description).

The patient with solar eczema (eczematous changes induced by the sun, eczematous polymorphous light eruption) presents with eczema with erythema, papulation, oozing, crusting, scaling, and lichenification. Intact blisters are not usually present. The eczema, characteristically, is worse on the tip of the nose, the malar cheeks, the pinnae, and the sides of the neck. Other sun-exposed areas may also be involved. The location depends in part upon which areas were exposed to the sun and which were protected by clothing, hats, and hair styles. Lichenification is often a feature, especially on the neck. In papular photodermatitis of the North American Indian (Birt), there is an eczematous phase, especially in infancy and childhood. In adults, this eruption is primarily papular.

Hydroa vacciniforme is a bullous eruption, described in Chapter 9.

Pollenosis (phytocontact dermatitis due to pollen) is presented by patients as a markedly and extensively lichenified eczematous eruption on the exposed areas of the face, particularly the eyelids. Other flexural areas such as the neck, antecubital fossae, and popliteal fossae may be involved. In some patients, photosensitivity is a factor, so a combination of the oleoresin fraction of the pollen and the sun's rays causes the eruption. Morphologically, the eczematous portion may be so dominated by the lichenification that one may be tempted to classify pollenosis as a purely lichenified (or papular) eruption. In such cases, the distinction between pollenosis and adult atopic dermatitis may be difficult.

External contact with plants or their extracts followed by sun exposure to cause an eczema is called phytophotodermatitis. The eruption, as expected, occurs on areas contacted by both the plant and sunlight and is usually found on the extremities or neck.

Arthur Birt, 1906–1995, Canadian Dermatologist, Winnipeg

DIFFERENTIAL DIAGNOSIS

Acute eczema of the face is to be distinguished from erysipelas, which shows unilateral, sharply defined, edematous and erythematous tumid plaques, sometimes with blebs (hemorrhagic) and ulceration. Early herpes zoster is unilateral, acute, and edematous, but pain is more a feature, and some linear element may be seen. Eventually, of course, grouped vesicles on an erythematous base may be visible. Early primary herpes simplex has similar findings, but is not unilateral. Poison ivy on the face produces few bullae or vesicles, but much edema, especially of the eyelids, and some oozing, usually in linear or other artificial shapes. Typical linear vesiculobullae may be present on the neck or elsewhere. Acute reaction to hair preparations (e.g. dyes) may produce intense edema, swelling, and oozing of the forehead, eyelids, and other hairline areas, as well as the pinnae of the ears.

Nipples and Areola

Eczematous (blistering) eruptions on these tissues are common in patients with extensive eczema, particularly patients with widespread ids. Morphologically, the thin epidermis means that early rupture of vesicles occurs with much oozing and later crusting. Scaling is not a feature, although lichenification may be. Fissures are common. Small satellite papulovesicles (usually excoriated) are often present. The eruption is commonly bilateral. Eczematous eruptions are common in the pregnant or nursing female.

DIFFERENTIAL DIAGNOSIS

The differential diagnosis includes psoriasis, where there is more scaling than crusting and where the lesion is sharply marginated, salmon-colored, and without satellite lesions. A search elsewhere for other psoriatic lesions should be made. Atopic dermatitis* produces mainly a poorly demarcated excoriated lichenified slightly scaly eruption. This lesion can be called lichen simplex chronicus.

Scabies in this area cause bilateral excoriated papular traumatized eruptions with some oozing. The lesions are poorly demarcated, with scattered satellite lesions. Burrows on the usual sites should be sought, along with the excoriated papular eruption elsewhere among the usual scabies sites. I have never seen scabies only on the nipples and areolae.

A persistent, unilateral, sharply demarcated, erosive, crusted, and scaly patch is suggestive of intraepithelial carcinoma (Paget's disease) arising from the ducts of the lactiferous glands of the breast. Sometimes a minor degree of peripheral papulation may be felt; sometimes a bloody crust is present. Rarely, a distinct hard mass may be felt in the underlying breast tissue and, even more rarely, enlarged firm to hard lymph nodes in the ipsilateral axilla. In some, a deeper erosive or ulcerative lesion may be present. Also, in some, the defect due to loss of epithelium may be seen.

Sir James Paget, 1814–1899, English Surgeon, St. Bartholomew's Hospital, London

*My concept of atopic dermatitis and its relationship to eczema is outlined in Chapter 11.

Legs and Ankles

As with most regional types of eczema, leg and ankle eczema may have the different types as seen with eczema in general (e.g. scaly, lichenified), though the anatomy dictates certain differences and may actually produce "noneczematous" lesions. Also, the differential diagnosis is somewhat different from that of general eczema.

Features common to leg and ankle eczema include edema, asteatosis, and purpura.

Edema is common in acute eczema of the legs and ankles, because of hydrostatic pressure. In some cases, the edema appears on the lower leg and ankle, despite the fact that the eczema is above the knees. Also, the edema worsens after standing. This edema must not be confused with that from cardiac or renal causes. As the eczema subsides, so does the edema.

Asteatosis is by itself not a rare finding on the legs, especially in the elderly during winter. Asteatosis may precede the eczema ("eczema craquelé") or develop as a part of it. Drying lotions may cause asteatosis. A crazy paving pattern with purpura in the superficial fissures sometimes occurs. This cracking desquamation has been likened to the glaze of old Chinese pottery.

Purpura is a common finding in any lower leg and ankle eruption, and eczema is no different. The problem in making a diagnosis is that when the eczema subsides, becoming slightly lichenified and scaly as well as purpuric, it may not be distinguishable from scaly purpuric eczema and the scaly phase of the various pigmented purpuric eruptions. The purpura of the eczema is usually not as marked, severe, or extensive as the purpura in the purpuric eruption. Eczemas, of course, may have a lichenoid aspect, as may the pigmented purpuric eruptions. Telangiectases are not a feature of purpuric eczema.

DIFFERENTIAL DIAGNOSIS

The differential diagnosis of leg and ankle eczema in the early acute erythematous and edematous stage includes erysipelas and phlebitis. Erysipelas lesions are presented as red edematous plaques with sharply marginated ovoid or gently sloping borders. There are no satellite lesions and no primary epidermal changes. Also, tenderness, chills, fever, and regional lymphadenitis are usually present. Phlebitis can have similar findings, although the red area may have a linear aspect, a tender enlarged vein may be palpable, there is no basic epidermal change, and the systemic effects are less obvious than in erysipelas. As time passes, the distinction between an early acute contact eczema (e.g. poison ivy), an early erysipelas, or an early phlebitis becomes clearer, but at the beginning it may be difficult to discern the difference.

Stasis sequelae have four basic findings: dermal sclerosis, epidermal atrophy, varying degrees of brown and reddish brown pigmentation, and edema. Many other findings, such as white atrophic areas, telangiectases, healed ulcer scars, and ulcers may also be present. Also, of course, an eczematous process may develop on top of stasis dermatitis, but it is important to distinguish between the two conditions.

Eczematous processes do not, of course, show atrophy, sclerosisor ulceration (see also Chapter 18).

Lichen simplex chronicus on the legs is basically a lichenified eruption, but it may at times be scaly and excoriated with oozing from abraded areas. In most cases, it can be distinguished easily from eczema.

Orificial

The epithelium and epidermis about various body openings on the head and neck react differently than other skin to ordinary eczematogenic stimuli, and I plan to discuss briefly the differential diagnosis in these areas.

In all of these orificial eczemas, the cavity must be examined for underlying morphological mucosal abnormality or change.

The eyelids show an edematous, finely fissured, slightly scaly reaction to contact (irritant or allergic) dermatitis. The eruption rarely weeps and is almost always bilateral. The upper eyelids are more often and more extensively involved than the lower eyelids. It may be impossible to distinguish this from atopic dermatitis of the eyelids, although lichenification and pigmentation are more pronounced in atopic dermatitis. The epicanthic fold on the lower eyelids is often affected. Other eyelid eruptions such as lichen planus or psoriasis should not be confused with eczema.

Upon observation, the mucosa of the lips and the adjacent skin may show a persistent fissured scaliness. Weeping is unusual. A traumatic irritant eczema is usual in children who habitually suck their lower lip. Some cases of persistent red lip scaliness are associated with severe seborrhea. Actinic cheilitis exists only on the lower red lip. Discoid lupus erythematosus has a central depression, a raised indurated border, and often involves the adjacent skin. Angular cheilitis is considered under the erosions. Lichenified perlèche is usually atopic in origin.

The external auditory meatus, because of its enclosed nature, often has a nonspecific, edematous, fissured, crusted, excoriated, poorly marginated eruption. This symptomatic picture can be from seborrhea, lichen simplex chronicus, psoriasis, or contact eczema, and often only time or other lesions may clarify the diagnosis.

The external nares may be the site of eczema, particularly the primary irritant type, in association with exudative conditions of the nasal mucosae (e.g. coryza).

Genitals and Anal Area

Patients with eczema of the genitalia and perianal area as well as the semimucosa may present with a few unusual features. When acute, erythema with excoriated, eroded papulovesicles and crusting are seen. Also, edema (especially of the vulva or penis) is common. Because of maceration of the eczematous skin, superficial fissures in the groin folds and interbuttock area may be seen. The perianal mucosa is turgid, lichenified, and excoriated. Maceration, in addition to causing fissuring, also gives the eruption a whitish color. This whitish excoriated inflamed skin must not be confused with leukoplakia, which is a sharply marginated, nonedematous, noninflamed keratosis appearing only on the mucosal or semimucosal surface. When the eczema is chronic, the parts are thickened, excoriated, and the folds fissured. Erythema, edema, and oozing are not so pronounced, although there may be a lichenified hypertrophy of the vulva and genitalia. (See also "Intertrigo" in Chapter 1.)

References

1. Darier, J. Textbook of dermatology. Pollitzer S, trans. Philadelphia: Lea & Febiger, 1920.
2. Jackson R. Eczema due to mites and micro-organisms. Can Med Assoc J 1977; 116:156–161.
3. Johnson R, Nusbaum BD, Horowitz SN, Frost P. Transfer of topically applied tetracycline in various vehicles. Arch Dermatol 1983; 119:660–663.
4. Kipping HF. Molluscum dermatitis. Arch Dermatol 1971;103:106–107.
5. Whitfield A. Lumelian lectures on some points in the etiology of skin diseases. Lancet 1921; 2:122–127.
6. Haxthausen H. Generalized ids (autosensitization) in varicose eczemas. Acta Derm Venereol 1955; 36:271–280.
7. Fisher AA. Excited skin syndrome. Cutis 1982; 30:599.
8. Puig L, Alomar A, Randazzo L, Cuatrecasas M. Erythema multiformlike reaction caused by topical application of thuja essential oil. Am J Contact Derm 1994; 5:94–97
9. Sulzberger MB, Garbe W. Nine cases of a distinctive exudative discoid and lichenoid chronic dermatosis. Arch Dermatol Syph 1937; 36:247–272.
10. Sulzberger MB. Distinctive exudative discoid and lichenoid chronic dermatoses (Sulzberger and Garbe)—re-examined 1978. Br J Dermatol 1979; 100:13–20.
11. Lever WF, Lever CS. Histopathology of the skin 5th ed. Philadelphia: Lippincott, 1975; 308.
12. Pompholyx: A still unresolved kind of eczema. Editorial. Dermatologica 1993; 186:241–242.
13. Zais N, Battistini F, Gomez-Urocuyo F, Rojas FR, Ricart R. Treatment of tinea pedis with griseofulvin and topical antifungal creams. Cutis 1978; 22:196–199.

CHAPTER 6

Erythematosquamous Dermatoses

Erythematosquamous eruptions are equally scaly and red.

Overview

I have been rather strict in my interpretation of the erythematosquamous eruptions, so you will find detailed descriptions (with differential diagnosis) of some diseases usually classified as "the papulosquamous eruptions" in other areas of this handbook.[1] I do not consider the adjective papulosquamous a sufficiently accurate term for determination of the differential diagnosis of these eruptions. The morphological difference between, for example, extensive flat warts (a papular eruption), and tinea versicolor (a scaly eruption), is so great that to put them under one morphological grouping is not logical. The diseases covered elsewhere are lichen planus (see Chapter 11), lichen simplex chronicus (see Chapter 11), pityriasis rubra pilaris (see Chapter 20), scaly eczemas (see Chapter 5), and drug-induced eruptions with scale (see Chapters 1, 2 and 3). It is important that these be considered in the differential diagnosis, as at times the erythematosquamous aspect may be prominent.

Two aspects of the concept of an erythematosquame must be enlarged upon.

First, there is the distinction between a red scaly spot or patch (which I have called an erythematosquame) and a papule with scaling. In the glossary I have defined macule, spot, and patch as a "circumscribed deviation from normal skin color without other changes", but I see no reason why a macule, spot, or patch cannot be covered with scale; this does not make it a papule.

Second, it must be realized that some diseases fall into two categories: psoriasis perianally is a scaly erythema (or erythematosquame); on the shins it may be lichenoid or papular with little scale. So, at times one must consider in the differential diagnosis both erythematosquames and papular eruptions.

Normally, imperceptible shedding of the horny layer proceeds. When this process is interfered with (e.g. a plaster of paris cast), a considerable buildup of normal scale occurs. Apart from this, scale usually indicates epidermal dysfunction.

Scales (*escale*, Old French for "husk") are the visible peeling or shedding of groups of coherent horny cells. They occur in any size from fine, flour-like dust to thick laminated disks and extensive parchment-like sheets. The following terms are used to describe the eight common varieties of peeling scales: bran-like, psoriasiform, ichthyosiform, cuticular and lamellar, peeling, collarettes, seborrheic, and exudative (crusted and macerated) scales.

1. *Bran-like scales:* Branny, pityriasiform desquamation (pityron, Greek for "bran"), has very small scales, comparable to dust, flour, or bran. This type of scaling is found mainly in dandruff, pityriasis capitis, superficial nonblistering tinea, tinea versicolor, and in erythrasma. Furfuraceous is also a synonym for bran-like.

2. *Psoriasiform scales:* If the scales are bigger, silvery-white, and mica-like*, they are called platelet-like or psoriasiform desquamation. As the name indicates, this type of scaling is found mainly in psoriasis, but it may also occur in a great

Portions of the Overview are taken and modified from Siemens[1] (pp. 100–110).

*A mineral with small glittering scales

variety of other diseases. Therefore, one speaks of psoriasiform eczemas, psoriasiform syphilis, psoriasiform lupus, and so on. Psoriasiform desquamation appears wherever layers or horny matter have piled up and become dry and brittle so that air can easily enter between the layers. Sometimes the desquamation is brittle on the surface only but is firmly attached below, a combination that causes white, hard, silvery spots not easily scratched off.

If the accumulation of keratinous substance is heavy and the individual layers are bound together by a quantity of exudate, the scales do not crumble off. Thus, thick masses may pile up. This is frequently the case in lesions that periodically enlarge in one area, so that the initial mass of scales is lifted up by a new, larger one, and this again by another one of still larger circumference. By this method of growth, cone-shaped piles of scales with horizontal layers reminiscent of oyster shells develop (psoriasis ostracea, ulcerosquamous syphilis). This oyster-shell-like desquamation is such a striking phenomenon that dermatologists of former generations considered it an entity and called it rupia.

Inter toe-web space psoriasis can produce thick milky white scaling.

Psoriasiform scales on the hairy scalp do not easily break down to a fine powder, as in pityriasiform dandruff (pityriasis capitis), but rather cling to the hair like large platelets (tinea amiantacea*). These scales may sheathe the hairs and look like pieces of asbestos (amiantacea scales or asbestos-like desquamation). It is not a fungous infection. Tinea amiantacea is usually seen in psoriasis.

3. *Ichthyosiform scales:* It is characteristic of some desquamations to form regular, smooth, roundish or more polygonal, lentil-sized and also larger, shields, which are attached in the center and loose at the edges, where they become most visible. These shield-like or fish-scale-like** ichthyosiform desquamations are found especially in ichthyosis, in which, in the affected areas, the shields are arranged in parallel rows or diamond patterns. Shield-like scales may also be encountered in eczemas and erythrodermas. A somewhat similar desquamation is etat craquelé, in which only the thin horny layer cracks, forming a coarse network of superficial hair-thin-rhagades, faintly reminiscent of the glaze of old Chinese pottery. See also eczema craquelé or asteototic eczema. Icthyotic scales often have a dirty dark gray color.

4. *Cuticular and lamellar scales:* In contrast to the scales of ichthyosis, which are attached in the center, cuticular scales adhere on one side, leaving the other side loose, ragged, or even slightly rolled up. The scales, before being shed, cling like a hangnail or cuticle. This common type of scale formation is called cuticular desquamation. Sometimes these cuticles are large (fingernail size or larger) and are called lamella or leaf-like scales. Blistering dermatophytosis between the toes, post ankle edema scaling, and post furuncular scaling are examples of lamellar scaling. This variety of lamellar desquamation is seen in

---

*In the nature of asbestos.

**Actually the scales are not like fish scales. Fish scales are overlapped and attached at one end as are shingles on a roof. Shield-like is a better term than ichthyosiform.

pemphigus foliaceus and in some erythrodermas. If a new scale forms at the base of each scale before it detaches, accumulations suggesting the appearance of a piecrust develop, frequently accompanied and enhanced by exudative processes. A peculiar form of cuticular desquamation is the wood-shaving-like desquamation of tinea versicolor, described later.

5. *Peeling:* If a horny layer comes off in still larger sheets, it is called membranous desquamation or peeling. Peeling may be artificially induced by peeling agents (salicylic acid, resorcinol). In post streptococcal conditions, entire casts of fingers, palms, and soles may be shed. Peeling may also occur in confluent-bullous eczemas (e.g. poison ivy), in erythrodermas, and in toxic epidermal necrolysis.

6. *Collarettes:* A special kind of scale formation is the collar-like desquamation in which, after exfoliation of the centers of lesions, ring-shaped collars remain. Such scaly collars (collarettes) are mostly found in eczemas (following flattening of vesicles), in superficial mycoses, in tinea imbricata, in secondary syphilis, and in the characteristic lesions of pityriasis rosea. They may also appear as "giant collarettes", or as several concentric rings.

7. *Seborrheic scales:* Scales may acquire a peculiar aspect by virtue of a high sebum content. This is a fairly regular occurrence in the pityriasiform desquamations of the scalp, the center of the face, and the central areas of the chest and upper back, because the sebaceous glands of these areas are especially large and numerous. In such instances, one refers to seborrheic desquamation (seborrhea, excessive secretion of sebum). Seborrheic scales are varying shades of a yellowish-brown, look dull, and feel greasy. Squashed between cigarette papers, these secretions leave a greasy spot. These scales may contain up to 30 percent lipid substances. Eczematous eruptions with scaly features in regions with large sebaceous glands, such as the scalp and the central parts of the face and chest, have particularly fatty scales. They are called seborrheic eruptions.

8. *Exudative scales:* The accumulated deposits of scales mixed with serum or pus or exudate-containing scales, look dull, are yellow or brownish-yellow, and feel moist and sticky. Exudative scales are most frequently found in pemphigus foliaceus, but also occur in many desquamating and oozing eczemas. These formations have also been called scale-crusts.

Besides sebum and seropurulent exudate, scales may be saturated with sweat, saliva, or other liquids, which causes a state of maceration. This soaked deposit occurs especially where skin touches skin (i.e. axillae, groins, intergluteal folds, intertoe–web spaces) and on the semimucosa.

It should be emphasized that characteristic scale formation can sometimes be recognized only after scratching the lesion, because the pathologically thickened horny masses are still coherent, even though the horny layer is more fragile, which is revealed on scratching. The fragility, however, is not pronounced enough to manifest itself from the ordinary insults of movement and rubbing by garments. Such latent desquamation is regularly found in the early stages of the lesions of pityriasis rosea. We may then see only a lentil-sized (approximately 0.5 cm) red spot with a slightly brownish center, which desquamates in branny particles after scratching (central scale formation). Also, fresh, not more than lentil-sized lesions of psoriasis often appear as smooth, brownish-red, hard prominences that may be mistaken for papules until gentle scratching suddenly lights them up with a silvery-white scale. This results because scratching permits air to enter between the horny cells and cause the brownish, smooth material to fall apart into mica-like scales. This has also been called a micaceous scale. In parapsoriasis guttata, the horny layer, which covers the lentil-sized lesions, does not disintegrate into silvery platelets on scratching, but rather comes off as a whole lamella (wafer-like desquamation). The latent desquamation is different again in tinea versicolor. In this disease, which forms brown circular maplike spots on the chest and back, the fungi grow between the horny layer and the rete, so that the horny layer generally detached from its base, but is still coherent. If the apparent macule in this disease is scratched with a vigorous stroke, lentil-sized ragged pieces are torn away. The scale, however, is often still adherent at one end (wood-shaving desquamation). It is true that one may elicit the same phenomenon by scratching normal skin, but it is not so easily accomplished, and the scales are not so typically big as in tinea versicolor.

If an erythematosquamous eruption occupies very large areas of the body surface, i.e. if it is generalized or universal (or nearly so) and persistent, it is spoken of as erythrodermic scaling. Such eruptions are encountered in extensive skin diseases (generalized psoriasis) and are also characteristic of the erythrodermas. Secondary erythrodermas are rare complications of dermatoses usually occurring only in circumscribed and widespread forms. Primary erythrodermas form a separate class of diseases. Erythroderma means red skin, but, as already pointed out, the involved skin is not only red, but also scaly and often lichenified. Thus the disorder might better be called an erythrosquamia (see also Chapter 7).

Lesions in which the primary finding is very small, localized accumulations of horny material, are not usually called scales but keratoses (see Chapter 15). When keratoses involve mainly the pilosebaceous unit, they are called folliculoses (see Chapter 20).

Psoriasis

It is important to realize that although most cases of psoriasis are easily diagnosed, a wide spectrum of changes may be visible, depending on the location (e.g. nails, external auditory meatus, interdigital webs of the toes, perianal mucosa and adjacent skin, vermilion border of lips), extent (e.g. psoriatic erythroderma), nature (e.g. pustular psoriasis), and precipitating or aggravating factors (e.g. poststreptococcal guttate psoriasis, and psoriasis with superimposed eczema or moniliasis).

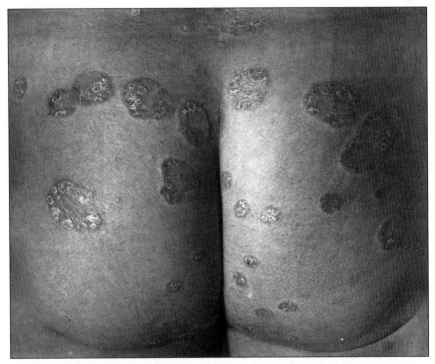

Figure 6.1 Psoriasis on the buttock. Note the shapes of lesions. Usually, more scale is present.

Continued observation may be necessary to diagnose psoriasis in cases in which some secondary change is present. As the secondary change disappears, the characteristic psoriatic lesion appears.

The basic lesion of psoriasis is a bright or deep red, sharply circumscribed, circular, slightly thickened area covered completely with dry mica-like laminated, friable, and abundant scales (Fig. 6.1). Psoriasis, at times, may be basically a papular eruption. The feel of papulation is caused by the presence of scale with a slight thickening of the epidermis. A few psoriatic lesions may exhibit papulation of the epidermal papular variety.

The thickened or papular aspect of psoriasis is minimal compared to the squamous element and compared to the papular aspect of lichen planus or verrucae planae. Hence, classification of psoriasis as an erythematosquame, although, at times, it may be erythematopapulosquamous in nature. In other words, the lesion may be a scaly spot or a scaly papule.

Scratching the lesions with the fingernail causes two characteristic signs: first, the scale breaks down into a fine micaceous dust; and second, after the removal of the scale, fine punctiform capillary hemorrhage occurs (Auspitz's sign). A pale halo of

Heinrich Auspitz, 1835–1886, Austrian Dermatologist

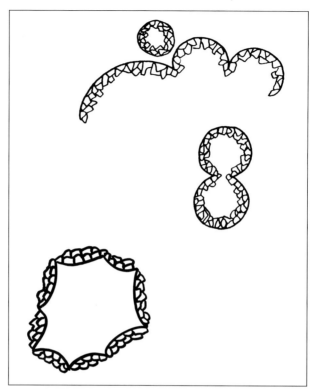

Figure 6.2 Scales of psoriasis with circular and arcuate lesions *(upper);* figure-8 lesions *(middle);* and concave borders *(lower).*

blanched normal skin may be present about each lesion (Woronoff ring), especially after ultraviolet light therapy.

The lesions are basically circular; however, confluence of these circles can lead to gyrate, circinate, or arcuate borders, and with central clearing, marginated plaques can occur. Usually convex (and figure-8 shapes) arcs are produced, but with extensive involvement, concave edges may occur (Fig. 6.2). Psoriasis is a symmetrical eruption with a predilection for bony prominences. In large plaques or patches, especially on the torso, lichenification and coffee-brown pigmentation may result.

The Koebner phenomenon[2-4] (provocation by irritation) occurs in some cases of psoriasis. Three aspects are recognizable.

The first is the appearance of psoriasis in areas related to one localized external traumatic event; that is, in a scratch, in a surgical scar, at a venipuncture site, at allergy test sites, or in a severe sunburn. This is the classical concept of the Koebner phenomenon.

The second is psoriasis from repeated nonspecific traumatization on elbows, knees, and nails. Psoriasis may also be precipitated or perpetuated by scratching on the scalp, external auditory meati, genital and perianal area, and the palms; from occupation, such as palmar psoriasis in a plumber or painter; or from personal habits such as leg psoriasis from leg shaving.

The third aspect is development of psoriasis in the lesions from systemic disease. Psoriasis can occur in the lesions of a drug eruption, measles, or chicken pox. The localization of acute guttate psoriasis lesions is presumably determined by where the circulating streptococcal toxin is deposited in the skin. One might call this third group systemic Koebnerization.

Guttate psoriasis refers to an acute eruptive variety characterized by the sudden appearance of innumerable drop-sized lesions, most easily seen on the torso and extremities. These lesions are from 2 to 4 mm to start with, and palpable. As the condition evolves, the lesions flatten and enlarge to about 2 cm and then disappear. This type is most often seen following streptococcal throat infections, especially in children. In adults who develop this variety of psoriasis, other more common varieties (such as flexural psoriasis, elbow, knee, or scalp psoriasis, or nail psoriasis) are often present before and remain after the guttate lesions have disappeared. In children, this is less often the case.

The plaques or patches of scalp psoriasis are sharply demarcated and have an abundance of white or grayish scales. The hairs are normal, pass through the scale, and do not come out on traction. Hair may be held together by the scale (pityriasis amiantacea). Frequently, a psoriatic corona along the hair line appears on the forehead. The scalp may be universally involved, in which case typical lesions can be seen at the periphery. Usually, though, completely clear and normal areas of scalp are present between the plaques or patches of psoriasis (see seborrhea). Scalp psoriasis is often itchy, and the trauma from scratching may produce oozing. Sebopsoriasis is the term used when psoriatic lesions exist on the scalp, face, presternal, and retroauricular areas in patients who have seborrhea. The scale is thinner and greasier. Localized scalp psoriasis is common in children.

Flexural psoriasis in patients is presented as vivid red plaques, denuded of scales, oozing, and sometimes crusted, usually with sharply marginated arcuate borders. All the large articular folds may be involved as well as the retroauricular crease, the perianal area, the umbilicus, between the toes (so-called white psoriasis), and the inframammary areas. There are no satellite lesions; central clearing is rare; and the circumcised glans penis may have a number of small scaling papular lesions. Periungual and ungual psoriasis is not uncommon in flexural psoriasis.

In the genital and perianal areas, psoriasis may form a red and/or hypopigmented, scaly, sharply marginated circle about the anus, along the median raphe, to the underside and over most of the scrotum, which will have a lichenified, scaly, sharply marginated plaque with broken off hairs.

Erythrodermic psoriasis is absolute and total (although some authors include those nearly universal, e.g. with sparing of palms and soles), with a vivid redness from head to toe. The desquamation loses its stratified and micaceous character (except perhaps in the scalp or other sites of predilection). The hairs of the scalp and body become scanty; the skin is generally thickened; and the nails are thickened and ridged. Ankle and leg edema is common. Nontender, soft, enlarged lymph nodes may be visible in the inguinal and femoral areas and can be felt in the axillae and cervical areas. A characteristic mousy odor from oozing dried serum and the action of the various skin organisms on the serum is evident. When fully developed, all erythrodermas may look the same, although individual psoriatic papules may be found, if carefully searched for (see also Chapter 7).

Palmar and plantar psoriasis have three subvarieties.

1. A common variety where the psoriatic lesions look like psoriasis elsewhere, with a deep red color, marginated arcuate borders, and a micaceous scale, which may be thicker than on other parts of the body. These foci of small annular lesions may line up along the sides of the fingers. Fissuring is often a problem. The Auspitz sign is not positive. Guttate lesions may also occur on the palms and soles. At times it may be very difficult to distinguish between tylotic palmar and plantar eczema from psoriasis. A useful finding is that eczema responds to treatment more easily, more quickly and more completely than psoriasis.

2. A basically vesiculopustular variety (see also Chapter 10), where the palmar and plantar surfaces show sharply demarcated, deep red areas with rather large white scale which, when removed, shows a raw glistening surface. The border is often arcuate; central clearing is not a feature; and on this glistening surface, there are innumerable 1 to 2 mm vesicles and pustules. When these dry they leave a dark-brown horny spot with a small scaly collarette (Fig. 6.3). Often, too, some of the pustules become confluent and form 0.5 cm lakes of yellow-green pus just below the stratum corneum. The pustular variety often has undermined edges. No inflammatory halo forms about the pustules. The eruption may be almost entirely composed of small vesicles or small pustules, or lakes of pus, or combinations thereof, with or without the deep red areas described above. The sequence may be vesicle to dark-brown horny area to pustule. Often no other psoriasis lesions can be found.

3. A keratotic type of palmar and plantar psoriasis also exists. In this variety, the palms and soles may exhibit a patchy distribution of 1 to 2 mm keratoses with a hard yellow scale. On the weight-bearing areas, these keratoses may be up to 1 cm in diameter (cf. keratoderma-arsenical keratoses).

Periungual psoriatic lesions, subungual keratoses, and other nail changes are often present in association with the various forms of palmar and plantar psoriasis. On the dorsa of the hand, solar keratosis and Bowen's disease should be considered in the differential diagnosis; on the palms and soles, the scaly form of mycosis fungoides should be considered.

John Templeton Bowen, 1857–1941, U.S. Dermatologist, Harvard, Boston

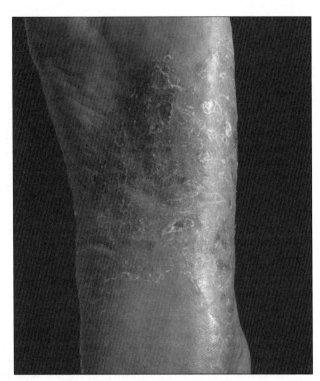

Figure 6.3 Pustular psoriasis. Note the scaly collarettes.

Psoriatic nails are characterized by dotted cup-like depressions (pits), onycholysis, subungual keratotic material, thickening and yellowing mainly at the distal end, and occasional loss of the nail plate. The oil-drop sign refers to the linear yellow-brown streak seen under the distal nail plate. It also frequently occurs at the edge of areas of onycholysis or juxtaposed to areas of onycholysis. Various patterns of transverse or longitudinal ridging may also occur. Often, the periungual skin may show typical psoriasis. In severe and disabling ungual psoriasis, psoriatic arthritis involving the terminal interphalangeal joints and spine may be present (see also Chapter 13).

Morphological Patterns and Variations

Other patterns of psoriasis that have been given names based on the predominance of certain morphological characteristics abound. The features of these are outlined below.

The larger plaques of psoriasis do not arise as such, but are the result of peripheral growth from an originally small lesion; as the growth of the lesion may stop at any time and remain stationary for a shorter or longer period, or almost indefinitely, it can be readily understood how the so-called clinical varieties or patterns of disease may arise.

Psoriasis punctata is the term used for psoriasis when most of the lesions are pinhead-sized. If the lesions stop growing when they reach drop size, the term used is psoriasis guttata. If the lesions become coin-sized, nummular psoriasis is a term that can be employed. When coin-sized lesions start showing central involution, and therefore show clear centers with a peripheral inflammatory scaly band, the term psoriasis circinata or psoriasis annulata may be used. If several of these centrally clearing ring-shaped lesions expand and touch each other, with the coalescing portions disappearing, only serpentine, arcuate, inflammatory scaly bands or psoriasis gyrata are seen. If several large, closely situated plaques join together, they may form larger areas of varying dimensions, sometimes sufficiently large to cover a part or an entire region (psoriasis diffusa). When these diffused areas cover over a joint, become fissured, very thickened and resistant to therapy, the term psoriasis inveterata may be applied. When the entire cutaneous surface is covered (or almost covered), the term psoriasis universalis is appropriate (see erythrodermic psoriasis). Rarely, on some plaques there is a tendency to central heaping up of the scales, which may also become hard and horny (psoriasis rupioides or ostreacea—oyster-shell-like). When there is marked papillary overgrowth (as on the lower legs) the designation is psoriasis verrucosa (see Fig. 16.2). In a small percentage of psoriatic patients, a severe sunburn erythema, especially on the back, will slowly disappear as usual, but will then develop into a large patch of psoriasis. This sun-induced psoriasis spares areas not exposed to the sun. Follicular psoriasis may be seen on the torso and thighs, especially in women.

In distinguishing between psoriasis and psoriasiform eczemas, it is useful to remember that in psoriasis the lesions are usually all psoriasis-like, while in psoriasiform eczemas only a few lesions may be so.

In childhood, there may be a follicular psoriasis, particularly on the anterior tibial and olecranon areas. If more characteristic psoriatic scalp lesions are present, the diagnosis is easy. If not, the distinction from pityriasis rubra pilaris may be made only with difficulty. Guttate psoriasis is more common in children, as is localized scalp psoriasis. Pustular psoriasis or dermatitis repens may be persistent on a single digit in children. The various forms of erythrokeratodermia should also be considered in the differential diagnosis.

Nuchal psoriasis always offers a diagnostic problem, especially when there are no other areas involved. The plaques are dry, scaly, and have arcuate borders without hair loss. Excoriations with dotted crusts are often present, with areas of oozing. The scale is not that typical in the scalp. As with lichen simplex chronicus, this condition is much more common in females and may have an underlying nevus flammeus.

Generalized pustular psoriasis may begin as classic psoriasis or may appear de novo. The pustules are superficial, from 2 to 4 mm in diameter, and either studded over areas or in nummular clusters. Often, large arcuate borders are present.

Frequently, larger (up to 1 cm) superficial lakes of pus are present. In some cases, both ordinary and pustular lesions may coexist. There is a surrounding erythematous halo. Fever, erythema multiforme mucosal lesions, moist oozing pustular periungual and glans penis lesions with a urethral discharge are often factors. The entire diagnostic picture resembles Reiter's disease or keratoderma blennorrhagicum.

Psoriasis of the external auditory meatus is really a form of moist psoriasis, often aggravated by scratching and irritating or sensitizing topical applications. The lesions are basically those of psoriasis, with the scale more greasy and less nacreous, due to the nature of the skin in that area. Usually, only the most outside portion is involved, but be sure to check in the triangular fossa of the pinna, as scaly lesions are often found there. The lesions are distinctly outlined as compared with seborrhea, where the eruption is less well demarcated.

Inflamed psoriasis (rarely arising de novo) attributable to a superimposed irritant or contact dermatitis, following withdrawal of systemic adrenal corticosteroids or methotrexate, or developing in dermatitis medicamentosa, may present a bizarre picture. Features can include vividly red indurated lesions that come out in crops and rapidly increase in size; acute perilesional and lesional dermatitis with eczematous features; and purpura, pustules, and bullae in the psoriatic lesions.

An uncommon variety of drug reaction from a systemically administered drug (e.g. beta-blockers, gold, lithium) may be a psoriasiform eruption. In these instances, the lesion may be more erythematous (and even purpuric), have a nonmicaceous scale, have a more sudden onset, lack the classic distribution, and there will be no psoriasis of the scalp or nails. Also, there may be no pre-existing psoriasis. It does happen that a drug eruption may turn into or act as a Koebner phenomenon in localizing true psoriasis. In this case, of course, it may not be possible to make a diagnosis of a systemic drug eruption.

Seborrhiasis (sebopsoriasis) is psoriasis occurring on the scalp, retroauricular fold, triangular fossae, external auditory meati, glabella, eyebrows, nasolabial folds, and presternal area. The scales tend to be greasier and the lesions less red. Some oozing may develop; however, many psoriatic features are present, such as sharply marginated borders, arcuate borders, clear areas in the scalp, and mica scale with bleeding points in some lesions.

The differential diagnosis of psoriasis is long and complicated, and even the most astute clinician will be mistaken from time to time. Most of the conditions with which psoriasis can be confused are listed in this chapter on the erythematosquames.

An epitome of the differential diagnosis is provided in Table 14. The differential diagnoses in Chapter 5 for the scaly disseminated eczemas should also be considered.

Hans Conrad Julius Reiter, 1881–1969, German Physician

Pityriasis Rosea

The herald scaly patch is a 2 to 4 cm, circular, rarely ovoid, uniformly scaly area, preceding the more extensive eruption that follows. The herald patch may be located anywhere (e.g. face or leg). Central clearing with faint whitening may be seen, but not always. When seen alone, the lesion may be impossible to exclude a scaly eczema. Trichophytoses can be excluded by potassium hydroxide (KOH) examination. Other variations in the herald patch can include a gigantic herald patch, multiple herald patches, and a herald patch appearing 2 to 3 months or 1 to 2 days before the general eruption.[5]

Ovoid pinkish lesions of pityriasis rosea average 1 cm in length, with a peripheral erythematous halo in the center of which is an ovoid, slightly brownish center. When scratched, the center reveals a branny desquamation. Earlier lesions are smaller and may show only a pinhead-sized central scaly area (Fig. 6.4). Later lesions become larger and may be scaly throughout. At the periphery of the central scaly area, a collarette of scales may be seen in older lesions, presumably, once the central scaly portion has fallen off. All lesions except the herald patch tend to occur with the long axes along the skin lines, giving a Christmas tree effect.

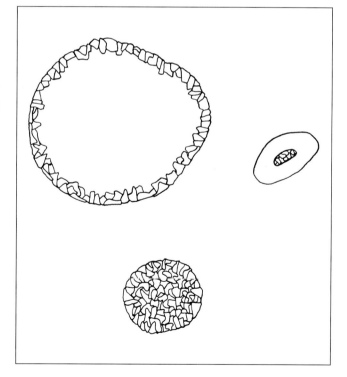

Figure 6.4 Shape and scale of blistering tinea *(upper left)*; pityriasis rosea *(upper right)*; and psoriasis *(lower)*. The scale is relative.

The eruption involves mainly the torso, thighs, and arms, in that order, with new lesions appearing on the neck and extremities as the torso lesions fade. Rarely does hypopigmentation occur. Suntanned areas may be less extensively involved, but sometimes the reverse is true, and the extremities are the main areas of involvement. This has been called inverse pityriasis rosea.

In the occasional very acute and extensive eruption, an evenly distributed blistering eruption may be present on the palmar and plantar areas. These blisters are 2 to 4 mm in diameter. Also, the eruption may develop into a generalized confluent erythematoscaly eruption involving the face, scalp, and lower legs—areas normally spared.

In the occasional widespread case, some of the lesions, especially on the medial aspect of the arms and thighs, and especially in fair-skinned patients, become inflamed and may present with an eczematized and/or asteatotic component. Oozing lesions may be seen in the herald patch and in the central area of other ovoid scaly lesions. However, if examined carefully, the typical oval scaly lesions can be found, particularly on the sides of the neck and in the subaxillary area. Rarely, there may be a purpuric element to this eruption. Even more rarely, the total eruption may be purpuric without scale, but having the round primary lesion, the ovoid secondary lesions, and following the usual course.

Hemorrhagic areas have been reported in the oral mucosa, especially in children. In adults, discrete or confluent plaques 1 to 2 cm in diameter, some with superficial erosion, have been reported.

In the natural course of events, the herald patch arrives a few weeks before the generalized eruption. Rarely is there more than one herald patch. The generalized eruption emerges rather quickly over a period of 2 weeks; it stays for 2 weeks, then over the next 2 weeks it gradually fades. As the generalized eruption fades, the lesions that came out first disappear first and so on. Frequently, the herald patch has almost disappeared if the eruption is seen in its late stage. Sometimes only a few large lesions are present. Sometimes the lesions are mainly centrifugal. Other variations reported are papular lesions in blacks; a preceding urticarial eruption; vesicles on the palms and soles; bullous lesions; browning following the disease; localization to one side of the body; localization to the axillae, groins, and neck; and localization to the hands and feet, eyelids, and penis. Rarely, the disease may recur (sometimes more than once). The problem is that no cause is known, and so on a purely clinical (or morphological) basis, how wide you cast your net depends on what you mean by the term pityriasis rosea.

DIFFERENTIAL DIAGNOSIS

The differential diagnosis is most important. Pityriasis rosea can and must be distinguished from other conditions.

In psoriasis, the lesions are always circular, darker red, more sharply demarcated, have a micaceous scale throughout the lesion, and show capillary bleeding on removal of the scale.

Blistering tinea of the hairless parts (as from Microsporum canis) lesions are larger (up to 4 to 6 cm in diameter), circular, fewer in number, less symmetrical, show peripheral induration and scaliness, and usually pinhead blistering, with a tendency to central clearing (just the opposite of pityriasis rosea). A pseudopsoriatic scaly trichophytid has been reported on the elbows and knees.

Nonblistering tinea of the hairless parts (as from Trichophyton rubrum) lesions are similar to those of blistering tinea, except that there is no peripheral blistering. Also, the lesions frequently have a residual brown pigmentation and are more common on the medial thighs and buttocks. Also, involvement of palms and soles, toe-web skin, and the nails is typical. This process is persistent.

Syphilitic papulosquamous lesions are round, not basically scaly, and have a slight purplish hue; they are indurated and often present on the palms and soles. Mucous patches or glandular enlargement may also be present.

Presternal and interscapular seborrhea lesions are polycyclic, sharply marginated, with elevated papular borders, and covered with a yellowish scale and crusts of a fatty consistency. Locations are usually the forehead, presternum and center of upper back.

Some of the varieties of pityriasis lichenoides (e.g. guttate) have a more round lesion than pityriasis rosea, the lesions of which may be purpuric with central necrosis. Occasionally acute parapsoriasis may have a Christmas tree distribution. Parapsoriasis en plaque should be considered in the differential diagnosis of pityriasis rosea. (See also pityriasis lichenoides and parapsoriasis in this Chapter.)

Pityriasis-rosea-like drug eruptions may occur following injection of gold salts or occasionally from other drugs. The lesions are less numerous, larger, and more scaly than those of classic pityriasis rosea. They are not uniformly scaly in the center, many are poorly defined, and others in the folds may be superficially erosive. The Christmas tree effect is not often seen. Also, photosensitivity aggravation and erosive oral mucosal lesions are often concomitant. The natural slow increase in size of the herald patch, rapid initial spread, and slow spontaneous clearing in from 6 to 8 weeks is not followed. Bjornberg and Hellgren in their classic review describe pityriasis-rosea-like eruptions following the use of gold, salvarsan, bismuth, and methopromazine.[6] Occasional transformation into lichen planus, subsequent pronounced hyper-pigmentation, and histologically, the appearance of lichen planus are also reported.

Rarely, a patient with asteatotic nummular eczema can present with features reminiscent of pityriasis rosea. Some cases of pityriasis rosea have a tendency to become eczematized.

Tinea versicolor rarely mimics pityriasis rosea as the scale color and natural course are so different.

Pityriasis Alba

An area of pityriasis alba takes the appearance of several to numerous, rounded, oval furfuraceous areas that are poorly demarcated with a normally colored or slightly pinkish or hypopigmented color. When the complexion is tanned or sunburnt, the involved area is more obvious. This condition occurs in fair-skinned children and young adults, particularly on the cheeks and lateral arms. In asiatic patients, the hypopigmentation may be quite noticeable. Pityriasis alba is sometimes a manifestation of atopic dermatitis. In this case, usually some itching as well as lichenification is present. (See "Melanin Decrease" in Chapter 17.)

Pityriasis Rotunda

Pityriasis rotunda (pityriasis circinata, acquired ichthyosis in circular plaques) consists of circular sharply demarcated patches of dry shield-like scaling up to the size of a palm. The patches are located on the buttocks, thighs, and abdomen. This afflication has been reported in Japanese, Egyptians, Bantus, and British West Indians. Occasionally, a debilitating chronic illness is also present.

Syphilis

The roseola of syphilis is never squamous or scaly, whereas pityriasis rosea and psoriasis are always scaly.

The papular syphilides of secondary syphilis are only slightly scaly, but may become so to a degree that entitles them to the designation psoriasiform. They vary in size from 2 to 3 mm to 1 to 2 cm, and they are round and, in late secondary lues, annular. They are pink or dull red purplish and not so vivid as the lesions of psoriasis. Scaling is not nearly so pronounced as in psoriasis; scratching reveals no mica scale. The big difference is the degree of firm resistant infiltration of these syphilides as opposed to the pliable and nonindurated lesions of psoriasis. Really, the syphilis lesions are squamous papules, whereas the psoriasis lesions are more squamous than papular. Secondary lues is irregularly scattered everywhere, including the palms and soles. Syphilis lesions are confluent on the face, back, or nape of neck, but not on the elbows, knees, and scalp. Not all lesions are squamous papules, some may be purpuric and some ulcerative. Of course, enlarged lymph nodes, mucous patches, and a positive serological test for syphilis should be present.

The papulonodular syphilides may be abundantly scaly and psoriasis-like. However, they are firm to the touch, usually circinate, always segregated, regional, not very numerous, and always produce a scar on healing. These are not erythematosquamous or papulosquamous lesions; these are nodular or nodal lesions.

Discoid Lupus Erythematosus

Discoid lupus erythematosus is an erythematous, follicular, telangiectatic, scaly, atrophic eruption. Persistent redness of a light pink or carmine shade is characteristic.

Fine reticular or stellate telangiectatic capillaries are usually present. The scaling is adherent and may vary in extent. On removal, the underside of the scale shows carpet tacking where the hyperkeratosis has extended into dilated pilosebaceous units.* The infiltration is prominent and consists of a turgescence of the borders, the central area being depressed. The scarring atrophy is both diffuse and follicular. Scarring may be extensive on the ears and nose. The lesions are sharp, rounded, oval, or polycyclic. Brown pigmentation may occasionally be present as may excoriations. Cheeks, forehead, scalp, nose and ears are the sites of predilection. Lesions below the neck without head or neck involvement are uncommon.

Discoid lupus erythematosus may at times have a verrucous and papillary component, particularly in patients with extensive lesions on the head and neck. This may take the form of 1 to 2 cm verrucous superficial rounded nodules located in areas of purplish erythema and scarring sometimes resembling keratoacanthomas. Or, rarely, a papillary verrucous diffuse change may occur on the ears, eyebrows, nose, and cheeks.

Oral lesions are present, especially on the buccal mucosae, in about one-quarter of patients with numerous skin lesions.

There are many other varieties of skin involvement in lupus erythematosus. These are listed here for completeness although they also can be found in other appropriate sections.

Neonatal lupus erythematosus is usually on the face and particularly on the eyelids and periorbital areas. Starting as irregularly sized and shaped patches of erythema, it rapidly becomes atrophic and slightly scaly. Faint scarring with a livido pattern may remain. The main feature may be telangiectasia.

Hypertrophic lupus erythematosus can be seen on the extremities, particularly in blacks. As implied, the lesions are verrucous and papillary, resembling at times prurigo nodularis, keratoacanthoma, and even verrucous squamous cell carcinoma.

Superficial cutaneous lupus erythematosus appears as half-palm sized circular, peripherally scaly red purplish areas usually on the upper torso. Atrophy is not a big feature. The main differential is nonblistering tinea corporis and pemphigus foliaceus.

Bullous lupus erythematosus is quite rare and usually concomitant with other findings of some form of cutaneous and systemic lupus erythematosus.

Telangiectatic lupus erythematosus is described Chapter 4. Other varieties include a patchy, sharply marginated, follicular scarring on the scalp, lupus erythematosus profundus, and localized scarring of buccal mucosae.

DIFFERENTIAL DIAGNOSIS

Discoid lupus erythematosus should be distinguished from the following entities.

Solar keratoses are smaller, sharply marginated keratotic lesions located on the sun-exposed areas of the face and hands. The scale is whitish, firmly adherent, and does not show carpet tacking. The variety with epidermal atrophy may have only a

---

*The appearance of spiny processes that project from the undersurface of detached scale and correspond to follicular openings has also been reported as the 'tin-tack' sign in pemphigus foliaceus drug-induced lichen planus, seborrheic dermatitis, and on the scalp recovering from cancerocidal doses of ionizing radiation.[7]

small amount of scale and may show some telangiectatic blood vessels. The atrophy is never follicular and does not involve the dermis. The lesions are not carmine in color. Problems exist when discoid lupus erythematosus occurs in skin damaged by habitual exposure to sunlight.

Rosacea is not a scaly atrophic disease, is not carmine in color, and presents as a diffuse erythema. Follicular pustules are usually present; pustules are not present in discoid lupus erythematosus.

In some cases, excoriated discoid lupus erythematosus may be confused with excoriated acne but nontraumatized lesions usually show the features of lupus erythematosus. Neurotic excoriations often have a linear or unnatural border and show residual brown pigmentation.

Certain varieties of polymorphous light eruption (plaque-like solar eczema, persistent solar erythema), granuloma faciale, insect bites, sarcoidosis, Jessner's lymphocytic infiltration, and lymphocytoma cutis must be considered in the differential diagnosis. Basically, none of these are scaly telangiectatic atrophic disorders. The main confusion arises because they may have the purplish red or carmine color of lupus erythematosus.

Discoid lupus erythematosus may be confused with the facial lesions of subacute cutaneous lupus erythematosus. The latter, of course, is an erythema with some scale. The findings and differential diagnosis of discoid lupus erythematosus of the scalp are discussed under "Alopecias" in Chapter 21.

Pityriasis Lichenoides and Parapsoriasis

The terminology* of the various forms of pityriasis lichenoides and parapsoriasis has for many years been quite a dog's breakfast.[8-12] It now seems that we can make some sense out of some of the terms and biological concepts. I am going to make two large groupings and fit as much as possible of the gross description under these two headings: Pityriasis Lichenoides and Parapsoriasis (small and large plaque). Where a subvariety of one of the larger groups appears to have significant morphological validity, it will be pointed out.

It is fascinating that the synonyms that have been used for both groups morphologically describe many of the major characteristics.

Pityriasis Lichenoides

The former terms for this grouping were pityriasis lichenoides et varioliformis acuta, Mucha-Habermann disease, parapsoriasis varioliformis, pityriasis lichenoides chronica Juliusberg, guttate parapsoriasis, and dermatitis psoriasiformis nodularis.

The terms that I use are: pityriasis lichenoides et varioloformis acuta (PLEVA) and pityriasis lichenoides chronica. The second group includes guttate parapsoriasis.

Rudolph Habermann, 1884–1941, German Dermatologist
M. Jessner, U.S. Dermatologist
Fritz Juliusberg, 1872–1936, German Dermatologist
Viktor Mucha, 1877– 1919, Austrian Dermatologist
*For a historical review of how we got where we are, references 8 to 12 are of some interest.

I should stress that for years it has seemed to me that these conditions are a spectrum with pure PLEVA at one end and guttate parapsoriasis at the other.

Patients with PLEVA present with five different sorts of lesions.

1. Numerous scaly macules scattered on the torso and extremities.
2. Flattish, skin-colored papules appear with regular, but not angular border, some of which have no scale, and no particular grouping or linear arrangement.
3. Some of the lesions, nondescript in type, have a mica scale, which may be attached at the center and free at the edge. The scales may be on a papule or on a small erythematous macule. Classically, the wafer-like scale comes off easily and reveals a brownish-red papule beneath.
4. Some of the papules show a purpuric element, i.e. they are brownish-red in color, and this color does not fade completely on pressure.
5. A few of the lesions are small vesicles or the crusted remains of small vesicles. These old lesions are often the reddish-brown purpuric papules described above. A few vesicular lesions in some very acute cases may show necrosis and varioliform scarring as part of their evolution.

The distribution of lesions is mainly on the torso and limbs, with no definite pattern and no confluence to form arcuate borders. PLEVA is more common in children and young adults. At times, only six or so lesions may be present.

All of these lesions may be present at the same time; some lesions involuting while other lesions are appearing.[13] In the beginning, the eruption has a more blistering and purpuric element; later on, it is more lichenoid and scaly. At this stage it probably represents parapsoriasis guttata. When there are no purpuric, vesicular, necrotic lesions and no varioliform scarring, it is easy to see why some authors have classified this condition separately from the other forms of acute parapsoriasis. Guttate parapsoriasis is very rare. Some lesions resemble those of lymphomatoid papulosis. Secondary syphilis also should be considered in the differential diagnosis.

Parapsoriasis: Large Plaque

Other names used for varieties of large plaque parapsoriasis have included atrophic parapsoriasis, retiform parapsoriasis, parapsoriasis lichenoid, parakeratosis variegata, lichen variegata, poikiloderma atrophicans vasculare*, erythrodermia pityriasique en plaque disseminée (Brocq), mycosis fungoides, and cutaneous T-cell lymphoma.

On the arms, legs, and trunk, numerous (about fifteen) oval-shaped, macular, fawn-colored, scaling lesions vary from 5 to 10 cm in diameter, often with arcuate borders suggesting an artifact. Frequently symmetrical, especially on the arms, thighs, buttocks, and sides of the torso, and particularly on the girdle area of the lower torso, the lesions are usually sharply marginated and persistent. Some patches are irregularly yellow-brown to coffee brown, with a fine reticulated erythema and telangiectasis throughout. Some patches show epidermal atrophy with loosely

Jean Louis Brocq, 1856–1928, French Dermatologist, Paris

*The term poikiloderma atrophicans vasculare has been used to describe similar finding in chronic radiation sequlae, lupis erythematosus, dermatomyositis and two rare congenital conditions – Bloom's syndrome and dyskeratosis congenita.

adherent scales. The scale is really quite unremarkable, and, unlike many other erythematosquamous eruptions, may not be of diagnostic value. In some, the scale is only slight and of the lamellar type, whereas in others, it is thicker. Scratching does not lead to pinpoint bleeding. Some lesions are scaly only in the center. In other cases, a moderately adherent white scale has large flakes that become smaller in size as the periphery is approached. In dark-skinned patients, the lesions may be hypopigmented or hyperpigmented.

The lesions become quite scaly, sharply marginated, and persistent on the palms and soles. The scale is often attached at the periphery. The lesions are 1 to 2 cm in diameter, usually numerous, and may be fissured. They should be distinguished from other forms of erythematosquamous diseases, especially psoriasis, and from some forms of keratoderma.

Sharply demarcated scaly plaques are common on the eyelids.

In some cases, the atrophy and telangiectasia are marked, and when associated with alternating white and brown patches, the eruption assumes the characteristics of a poikiloderma. Atrophic lesions may be quite extensive, and in fact, may predominate. Involvement of the upper chest and breasts is particularly common (atrophic parapsoriasis or premycotic poikiloderma vasculare atrophicans).

Rarely, black or dark-skinned patients can present with chronic lichenoid parapsoriasis as a widespread hypopigmentation on the proximal parts of the limbs and axillary folds.

The plaques become infiltrated and even tumorous in some cases. Mycosis fungoides is the name usually used for these tumors. These plaques are of moderate consistency and a fleshy red colour. Oozing, ulceration, and crusting occur. Sometimes these lesions arise on pre-existing scaly patches or plaques; other times they arise on normal-appearing skin. These infiltrative plaques and tumors are basically circular and arcuate in shape. There are also some central uninvolved areas.

It should be noted that in a small percentage of cases, the onset of mycosis fungoides in large plaque parapsoriasis may be heralded by the appearance of small ulcerative vasculitis-type lesions. These lesions usually occur when the en-plaque aspect is quite obvious and should not be confused with the varioliform lesions of acute parapsoriasis.

Parapsoriasis lichenoides or parakeratosis variegata is a lichen planus-like type of parapsoriasis. The eruption consists of an infiltrated eruption of papules and streaks, which assumes a coarse retiform pattern on flanks, abdomen, thighs, and forearms. The eruption has a purplish tint with slight scaling.

Granulomatous slack skin is now considered a variant of mycosis fungoides.

Parapsoriasis: Small Plaque

Other names for varieties of small plaque parapsoriasis have included parapsoriasis maculata, xanthoerythroderma perstans, chronic superficial dermatitis and digitate dermatosis.

Apart from the size (rarely over 5 cm in diameter), the small plaque variety has a similar basic lesion and distribution to the large plaque variety of parapsoriasis. The palms, soles, and eyelids are rarely involved. Also, in the small plaque variety, atrophy, telangiectasia, and lichenoid change are usually not present. Progression to larger infiltrative plaques and frank tumorous mycosis fungoides is very unusual in the small plaque variety.

Digitate dermatosis is the name given to a variety that has elongated ovals or finger-shaped lesions on the torso, particularly easily seen on the flanks.

When the yellow-brown color predominates, usually with little scale and no atrophy, one can use the name xanthoerythroderma perstans.

Although the clinical features, natural course, and prognosis of the two types of parapsoriasis are normally what has been described, I must add a caveat that this is not always so. I have had two patients in whom the original lesions were the size of pityriasis rosea lesions and in both cases, lesions progressed to classical mycosis fungoides over a 25-year period. Xanthoerythroderma perstans may be made up of rather larger plaques.

Tinea Corporis (Nonblistering, Literally Nonvesiculating)

There is a variety of tinea in which the peripheral border has essentially no vesiculation (as from *Trichophyton rubrum*).

The eruption consists of a small number of fairly large (4 to 10 cm diameter) erythematosquamous plaques. They are all circular or arcuate, and occasionally have a figure-8 appearance where two lesions join together. A bomb-explosion pattern may be present. The border is sharply demarcated and palpable. The lesion is a dusky red color, with more redness and even faint telangiectasis at the periphery. A dusky brown colors the central clearing portions and in areas where the lesion has resolved. The scale is fine and light except at the border, where it is more extensive. The buttocks and groin are common locations, but it may also be seen on the face, lower extremities, and torso. This eruption illustrates the tendency of infections to have central clearing with spreading borders. In the groin, nonblistering tinea frequently has a superadded follicular pustular eruption. On the lower extremity, the lesions may be eczematized.

A scaly erythema may be seen, particularly between the fourth and fifth toes. Also, a diffuse, sharply marginated, sometimes unilateral erythematosquamous eruption may be present on the palms or soles (the so-called "moccasin" type[14]). This is sometimes manifest as "two feet-one hand" (or rarely "one foot-two hand") tinea. In addition, changes caused by tinea of the nails may be seen. Very rarely, a small number of 1 mm deep vesicles may be present on the instep area.

In general, the old maxim "if you see a scale, scrape it for fungi," has much to recommend it.

DIFFERENTIAL DIAGNOSIS

These torso and extremity lesions must be distinguished from the following lesions.

Psoriasis lesions are smaller and more numerous, have a mica scale throughout, rarely show browning sequelae, and do not have a border distinct from the rest of the lesion.

The basic lesion of nummular eczema is a vesicle, the top of which has been rubbed off. The border is less well marked, the lesions are smaller, usually all are nearly the same size, rarely arcuate, and more numerous, and residual brown pigmentation is rare, compared with parapsoriasis.

Secondary syphilis lesions are smaller and more widely disseminated, less scaly, uniform throughout, and often infiltrated. These lesions display no fusing and no clearing centers. Other types of lesions such as ulcerations, mucous patches, alopecia, and regional lymphadenopathy are commonly present.

Pityriasis rosea lesions are ovoid, more numerous, with a central scaly collarette, peripheral erythema, and no color change on clearing.

Parapsoriasis en plaque lesions are a lighter red color, are less scaly, and have no definite peripheral border.

Disseminated discoid lupus erythematosus lesions are more erythematous with telangiectasis, atrophy, and more adherent scale. Lichen planus, lichen simplex chronicus, and pityriasis rubra pilaris are basically papular eruptions. The subsiding brown erythematous patches of a fixed drug eruption are not scaly and do not have a palpable border.

Other vesicular tineas may present a diagnostic problem when the degree of blistering is minimal and not easily seen. Most of these types, e.g. due to *Microsporum canis* and *Epidermophyton floccosum*, tend to have the same general type of lesion as regards shape and size, but of course their borders do show blistering and their speed of onset and rapid growth put them in a different group compared to the nonblistering type. Rarely, favus may occur as scaly patches without "cups" on the torso.

Patients with candidiasis present with lesions of a bright red, well-defined oozing area with ragged undermined and scalloped borders. Peripheral vesiculopustules arise at the edges of the area, and small satellite lesions decrease in number and size as one moves away from the central area. At times, the degree and type of scale may resemble psoriasis, especially in nonintertriginous areas in patients with extensive candidiasis.

Tinea incognito is the name given to nonblistering tinea treated by potent topical corticosteroids. The degree of erythema and scaliness may be markedly reduced. On the face, the distinction between tinea faciale and discoid lupus erythematosus, dermatomyositis, polymorphous light eruption, and psoriasis may be very difficult. The basic arcuate or polycyclic shape is the most important clue.

Digital interspace tinea of the feet may vary from an erythema with low-grade peeling, scaling and fissuring, as found in nonblistering types (*Trichophyton rubrum*), to a soggy, whitish, macerated center with a peripheral blistering border that shows undermining in the blistering types (*E. floccosum, T. mentagrophytes*). It should also be remembered that overgrowth of normally resident skin bacteria may occur.

Seborrhea

Diffuse Seborrhea

This condition has as its basic lesion a heavy greasy or light dry diffuse nondescript scale, with varying degrees of thickening and erythema, but no definite papulation. The border is reasonably well demarcated. The eruption involves the following areas: scalp, retroauricular crease, external opening of the external auditory meatus, eyebrows, glabella, eyelid margins, nasolabial crease, and the presternal area. There may be minor fissuring, but oozing is not present to any appreciable degree.

Extensive seborrhea is more common in the elderly, in the mentally retarded, in some postencephalitic states, and in those treated with drugs inducing a Parkinsonism-like state. Some seborrhea may be present in acne vulgaris and rosacea. Occasionally, one will see a patient who has the tendency to frequently develop pyoderma on top of seborrhea.

Acute flexural oozing eruptions in such areas as axillae, groin, nasolabial folds, and retroauricular creases are in many cases varying types of irritant or contact eczema, low grade pyoderma (Mitchell's flexural streptococcal pyoderma), irritated psoriasis, irritated atopic dermatitis, or irritated forms of erythema intertrigo. To call these conditions seborrheic dermatitis solely because they occur in patients with seborrhea does not make sense. Flexural eczema in a patient with seborrhea is not automatically seborrheic dermatitis. Many of my colleagues and I are impressed by the number of patients with so-called typical seborrhea who show, at some time or other, typical stigmata of psoriasis or atopic dermatitis, especially if these stigmata are looked for in other areas of the body. Most of the flexural eruptions are discussed in detail in the differential diagnosis of "Intertrigo" in Chapter 1. For the differential diagnosis of diffuse scalp seborrhea, see "Persistent Scaly Scalp Dermatoses" in this Chapter.)

Despite what I have explained in the previous paragraph, there are certain oozing flexural eruptions with scale and erythema that could be called seborrheic dermatitis. I find, though, that this condition is greatly misdiagnosed and so, to stress my point, I have labeled the condition seborrhea and not seborrheic dermatitis.

Presternal and Interscapular Seborrhea

An arcuate brownish red scaly lesion with slow peripheral extension and central clearing, and frequently with central browning indicates interscapular seborrhea. The term petaloid is frequently used to describe these lesions. The scale is greasy, and there is often peripheral border papulation. The lesions are nummular in size and shape and may number from 3 to 20 lesions. In some patients, the presternal and

James Parkinson, 1755–1824, English Physician, London

interscapular seborrhea resembles more closely the seborrhea of the scalp or eyebrows, i.e. it is less dark red, less well demarcated, and shows no residual brown pigmentation. Psoriasis must always be considered in the differential diagnosis. Occasionally there are associated follicular lesions on the torso. I call these follicular seborrhea. Some have called them *Pityrosporum* folliculitis.

Cheilitis Exfoliativa

Localized on the vermilion border of the lips, there is rather sharply marginated thin or thick scale formation with occasionally some admixture of crust from underlying fissures. Sometimes it is associated with seborrhea elsewhere. The lack of edema, oozing, and involvement of the adjacent skin excludes an eczematous reaction. Only with great difficulty can this be distinguished from cheilitis due to habitual lip licking.

Tinea Versicolor

The patient presenting with tinea versicolor shows scattered circular or oval areas of light brown scaly macules. These areas are mainly macular, but some are slightly raised. The lesions are irregularly circular in shape, sized approximately 2 by 4 mm. The borders are well defined, but in some areas the lesions run into one another. There is no central clearing. The 2 by 4 mm circular lesions tend to be most easily seen at the periphery. On being scratched, they have an overlying fine wood shaving type of white scale. These lesions are found on the upper chest, neck, and back, extending into the axillae. Lesions may also be present in the groin. On the tanned areas, e.g. deltoid, the lesions are whitish.

Erythrasma

The site of predilection for this eruption is in the genitocrural fold, high in the medial aspect of the thigh. Rarely, it extends to the pubic area or scrotum. Rarely, the axillae and intertoe web spaces are involved. Erythrasma is palm-sized and has a distinct polycyclic and serrated circumference. Only rarely are satellite lesions seen. The color is dark yellowish brown. The surface is level, powdery, finely squamous, and often criss-crossed in very fine folds. Wood's light shows a coral red fluorescence. Erythrasma produces very little inflammatory reaction.

Intertrigo is more inflammatory and has no sharply defined contours. Eczemas are rarely so sharply demarcated. Lichen simplex chronicus is more lichenified. Inguinal tinea corporis is of a brighter red color, is more polycyclical and marginated. Tinea versicolor is less reddish brown, has satellite lesions, and is usually present in areas other than the groin. Inverse psoriasis should be considered.

Robert Williams Wood, 1868–1953, American Physicist

Table 14: Differential Diagnosis of Common Erythematosquames	
Psoriasis	*Sharply demarcated, silvery scale, deep red color, nail involvement*
Pityriasis Rosea	*Round herald scaly patch, oval patches with central scale*
Pityriasis Alba	*Whitish hypopigmented scaly lesions, poorly demarcated*
Syphilis	*Indurated scaly lesions with palms and soles involved, enlarged lymph nodes*
Discoid Lupus Erythematosus	*Carmine color, adherent carpet-tack scale, atrophy with hypo- or hyperpigmentation*
Pityriasis Lichenoides	*Macules, papules, scales with purpuric and vesicular lesions*
En Plaque Parapsoriasis	*Large demarcated scaly plaques or plaques sometimes with atrophy, telangiectasia, and browning*
Seborrhea	*Brown color, greasy scale, arcuate ill-defined border*
Tinea Versicolor	*Small circular brown or scaly macules with a fine wood-shaving type scale with discrete border*
Erythrasma	*Dark yellowish-brown large patches with serrated borders in flexual areas*
Drug Eruption	*Variable*

A useful clinical finding to distinguish between erythemas with secondary scaling and erythematosquamous eruptions is that erythematosquames almost always are scaly from the onset.

Persistent Scaly Scalp Dermatoses

Persistent scaly eruptions of the scalp fit in at this place in my handbook, although they will be covered in part in the descriptions of separate entities (see, for example, psoriasis, discoid lupus erythematosus).

Seborrhea of the scalp presents as a greasy or dry diffuse scaliness, sometimes with extension on the adjoining nonhairy skin, especially at the forehead, temples, and behind the ears. On the nonhairy skin, the eruption tends to have a greasy scale and to be inflamed and rather sharply demarcated. Although scalp seborrhea may vary in extent, it is a diffuse process with much or little free scale. Alopecia of the male pattern type may also be present; when it is, the seborrhea is worse in the hairy areas.

Psoriasis of the scalp is more often patchy, with scaly, sharply demarcated arcuate borders and normal-appearing intervening scalp skin. When the eruption extends onto the adjacent nonhairy skin, the borders show the typical psoriatic papules and scale. Frequently, excoriations with crusting are present. Rarely, the whole scalp may be involved.

The subsiding stage of acute contact dermatitis (primary irritant or allergic) may have a scaly phase, although usually some evidence of oozing or crusting can be found. Also, the scale is more adherent and the border is poorly defined.

Nonblistering tinea of the scalp shows sharply marginated borders, loss of hair and broken-off abnormal hair shafts, prominent follicles, and varying degrees of scaliness.

Pityriasis rubra pilaris may have a diffuse branny scaliness over the whole scalp; in fact, it may begin on the scalp and face and be misdiagnosed as seborrhea.

Atopic dermatitis of the scalp presents as a nondescript, poorly demarcated, slightly scaly, exoriated eruption.

Ichthyosis of the scalp shows a finer branny diffuse scaliness.

Discoid lupus erythematosus of the scalp is an atrophic follicular scarring eruption with a peripheral palpable border. This is a scarring alopecia. Other scarring alopecias occasionally showing scale are lichen planopilaris and favus.

The scalp may be involved in rare cases of extensive pityriasis rosea, as a seborrheic id from acute trichophytosis and in scaly drug eruptions, as well as follicular lichen planus (lichen planopilaris Graham Little's disease).

Lack of adequate shampooing of the scalp may result in a pronounced greasy, dirty, yellow scale throughout the scalp.

Nuchal Scaly Eczemas

This condition is, like many scalp eczemas (see Chapter 5), characterized by scaling, lichenification, and excoriation. Vesicles are rarely seen. The borders are poorly to moderately well defined and are rarely over 6 cm in diameter. The scale is minor in amount and usually has an admixture of serum (either from ruptured vesicles or excoriations). What pure scale there is tends to be branny and adherent. Surprisingly, there is rarely any loss of hair. Nuchal eczema is more common in women, frequently with an underlying nevus flammeus; a classical example of locus minoris resisentiae.

DIFFERENTIAL DIAGNOSIS

Lichen simplex chronicus presents with mainly lichenification and excoriations. Hair loss is more common. Frequently, lesions of prurigo nodularis are also present. Atopic dermatitis presents a similar picture.

Psoriasis shows more silvery scale, especially at the lower nonhairy portion. The lesion is sharply demarcated, often arcuate, and often has a purplish red hue.

Patients with neurotic excoriations present with excoriations and secondary lichenification. Prurigo nodularis lesions may be present.

Nonblistering tinea (with alopecia, deformed broken-off hairs, and circular shape), and seborrhea with trauma rarely present problems in diagnosis, nor does the psoriasiform id of napkin dermatitis.

In some cases, the morphology may not be diagnostic and the diagnosis is made by finding other typical areas of, for example, psoriasis, lichen simplex, or neurotic excoriations.

Sir Ernest gordon Graham Little, 1867–1950, English Dermatologist

References

1. Siemens HW. General diagnosis and therapy of skin diseases. Wiener K, trans. Chicago:University of Chicago Press, 1958.
2. Waisman M. Historical note: koebner on the isomorphic phenomenon AMA Arch Dermatol 1981;117:415.
3. Miller RW. The koebner phenomenon. Int J Dermatol 1982;21:192–197.
4. Boyd AS, Neldner KH. The isomorphic response of koebner. Int J Dermatol 1990;29:401–410.
5. Butterworth T. Pityriasis rosea: Clinical varieties and etiology. Penn Med J 1935; (March) 1–10.
6. Bjornberg, Hellgren. Pityriasis rosea. Acta Dermato-Venereologica 1962; 42 (Suppl):50.
7. Cowley NC, Lawrence CM. Tin-tack sign in seborrheic dermatitis. Br J Dermatol 1991; 124:393–394.
8. Wise F. Parapsoriasis: Suggestions for simplifying its nomenclature and classifying its clinical varieties for teaching purposes. NY State J Med 1928; 28:901–908.
9. Montgomery H. Dermatopathology. Vol.1. New York:Hoeber, 1969:337.
10. Lambert WC, Everett MA. The nosology of parapsoriasis. J Am Acad Dermatol 1981; 5:373–395.
11. Textbook of Dermatology. Rook/Wilkinson/Ebling 5th Ed. Oxford:Blackwell, 1992:569, 1957.
12. Smoller BR. What is parapsoriasis? Med Surg Dermatol 1994; 1:69–71.
13. Gelmetti C, Rigoni C, Alessi E, Ermacorn E, Berti E, Caputo R. Pityriasis lichenoides in children: A long-term follow-up of 89 cases. J Am Acad Dermatol 1990; 23:473–478.
14. Daniel CR, Gupta AK, Daniel MP, Daniel CM. Two feet-one hand syndrome: a retrospective multicenter survey. Int J Dermatol 1997; 36: 658–660.

CHAPTER 7
Erythrodermas

*A persistent inflammatory reddening of all the skin,
with lichenification and scaling.*

Overview

I have defined erythroderma as an inflammatory universal or generalized red skin of a persistent nature, often secondarily lichenified and scaly. Extensive congenital vascular nevi (which are not scaly) are excluded. Generalized exfoliative dermatitis is a synonym.[1]

Two areas of this definition require elaboration. First, what is an almost universal eruption? Frequently, the palms, soles, and scalp are spared, so we need not be concerned if these areas are not involved. What about the patient who has very extensive psoriasis with only a few clear areas of skin on the torso and extremities? I believe that if there are large confluent areas covering most (80%) of the skin surface, the term erythroderma is justified. Second, what is meant by the term persistent? Many toxic erythemas (e.g. from drugs, bacterial toxins,) could be (and have been) considered as erythrodermas. However, many last only a few days. I have decided that a toxic erythema must last at least 7 days to be considered an erythroderma. Another factor bearing on the time element is the advent of systemic adrenocorticosteroid therapy. If a rapidly spreading, widespread, lichen planus or toxic erythema is treated in its early stages, then the therapeutic suppression of the eruption obviously prevents the development of erythroderma. This seems to me to be particularly relevant with regard to drug eruptions. Many previously reported drug-induced erythrodermas, if they occurred today, would be treated and probably never develop into erythrodermas.

Overall Clinical Findings

The patient may be shivering and covered with many blankets. The skin is universally erythematous, warm to the touch, dry and thickened. This thickening is particularly noticeable over the knees and elbows; large lichenified areas with obliteration of the finer skin lines are often present (Fig. 7.1). Scaling may vary from almost none to fine bran-like scales to large lamellar exfoliation (Fig. 7.2). Edema of the dependent parts (feet, ankles, lower legs, rarely sacrum and scrotum) is common and may at times be very severe. Oozing may occur in the intertriginous areas. Scratch marks (from the nails) or eroded areas (rub marks) are present. Several forms of pyoderma may be present, e.g. follicular pustules and crusted honey-scabbed lesions. A deep, tender, papulonodular eruption with erythema may occur in the extremities and represents a deep dermal pyoderma. Incision and expression reveals a small amount of pus. These are, in effect, small dermal abscesses. The semimucosae (lips, perianal area) may be involved, but the true mucosae (oral mucosa, conjunctiva) are usually clear in the secondary type.

The patient has a sweet-rancid odor. The skin may be browner than normal especially in cases of long-standing. A diffuse generalized nonscarring loss of hair is commonly seen, especially in the axillae and pubic area.

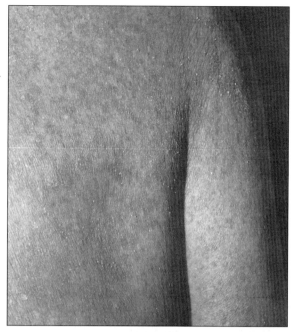

Figure 7.1 Psoriatic erythroderma. Note the diffuse lichenification.

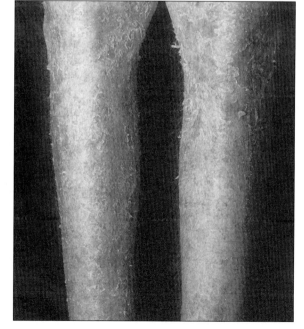

Figure 7.2 Drug-induced erythroderma–exfoliating phase.

The nails may show changes of the erythroderma, of the underlying disease, or of the effects of scratching and rubbing. The erythrodermic changes may vary from complete loss of nails, to thickening and yellowing, to ridging with subungual keratoses. Psoriasis may be indicated by the presence of pitting and subungual keratosis formation. The scratching and rubbing produce a buffed nail which is shinier in the central portion. If severe, actual central loss and indentation of the nail occur.

Firm, nontender, fleshy, freely moveable lymph nodes of varying size are usually present, particularly in the groin and axillae (dermatopathic lymphadenopathy).

Primary

Primary erythrodermas (no pre-existing skin disease) have no preceding skin disease and are usually idiopathic (except for those due to drugs); secondary erythrodermas do have a pre-existing skin condition. Occasionally, an underlying cause surfaces as the erythroderma progresses.

Acute primary erythroderma is a generalized erythema with lamellar, leaf-like, or foliaceous desquamation. The eruption starts as a bright red eruption in the large folds of the trunk and the limbs. In a few days, the eruption becomes universal. Before the redness disappears, desquamation begins and gradually extends. This desquamation is locally furfuraceous, but more apt to occur in large collodion-like sheets or on the hands and feet in the form of an incomplete glove or shoe. The skin underneath appears smooth, sometimes scaly, or sometimes oozing in the folds. The mucosae may be affected; redness of the conjunctivae, mouth, and throat with desquamation of the tongue may be noted. Mucosal involvement is unusual except in the drug-induced variety. The nails may be marked with a transverse furrow.

DIFFERENTIAL DIAGNOSIS

This condition is to be distinguished from the erythema of scarlatina, in which the erythema is less extensive, certainly not universal, more transitory, and less desquamative. Also, the fever and general toxicity are greater in scarlet fever; and the angina and the tongue changes are more pronounced.

Acute primary erythroderma is also to be distinguished from the staphylococcal scalded skin syndrome, in which purulent conjunctivitis and exfoliation or peeling of the skin are frequently more marked. In addition, beneath the peeled off skin, the remains of the epidermis are red, slightly moist, and finely granular. Trauma of any sort results in the detachment of the outer layer of the epidermis, hence exfoliation is more common in the skin at and about the large flexures, e.g. axillae and groin. Exfoliation starts while the erythema is still present. It is very tender. The term scalded skin syndrome is a good descriptive term. (See also section at end of this chapter.)

Toxic epidermal necrolysis (nonstaphylococcal scalded skin syndrome) has many similarities to the scalded skin syndrome except that central facial erythema with pus formation is not a marked feature of toxic epidermal necrolysis.

Toxic shock syndrome seen in menstruating women is probably related. It consists of an acute toxic erythema sparing the face and trunk and being particularly marked on the palms and soles, which later desquamate. The mucosae may also be involved with erythema.

In contrast to the secondary erythrodermas, lichenification and scratch marks are usually not present in primary erythrodermas. The distinction between some generalized toxic erythemas and some acute primary erythrodermas is very difficult and may be arbitrarily based only on the duration of the eruption.

Primary chronic (lasting at least 3 months) erythrodermas, resulting from lymphomas and leukemias have always been rare. They are even more so now, because the potent anticancer drugs now available prevent the development of extensive, generalized, or universal skin involvement. Leukemids, leukemic tumors, and infiltration may become extensive, but only rarely are they erythrodermas.

Secondary (Pre-Existing Skin Diseases)

Generalized eczema (allergic eczemtous dermatitis) of long standing may be indistinguishable from other forms of erythroderma. Sometimes, however, certain clues may be seen to reveal the primary diagnosis. If, for example, a stasis dermatitis develops a generalized id, a more acute red weeping portion can be seen at the site of the primary eruption. Patients with generalized eczema sometimes are prone to repeated attacks of pyoderma, and so evidence of this may be present. Also, evidence of scratching and rubbing are prominent. Acanthomata following eczema (see Chapter 15) may be seen after an episode erythrodermatous eczema begins to subside.

Generalized atopic dermatitis may show more lichenification, more excoriation, and more redness in elbow and knee creases and other sites of predilection. In cutaneous pollenosis in adults, a picture similar to atopic dermatitis may be seen. The face tends to be the area showing the greatest degree of lichenification.

Psoriasis is a common erythroderma. Sometimes typical psoriatic lesions may be seen if looked for carefully. The nail changes of psoriasis may be visible. Linear or dotted pitting and subungual keratoses are probably the most reliable findings. The characteristic mica-like scale is often missing. Generalized psoriasis may become eczematized.

Pityriasis rubra pilaris rarely becomes erythrodermatous. Clues that this is the underlying disease follow: small islands of normal-appearing skin, distinctly outlined and sometimes angular are almost always present; peripilar cones may be seen at the periphery of these islands or at the sites of predilection (the dorsa of the fingers); the scalp is covered with a diffuse erythematosquamous eruption without alopecia; the scale is fine, but thick; the palms and soles may show a thickening and have a yellowish-red color; and scratch marks are not usually present. On the face, the erythroderma caused by pityriasis rubra pilaris has a dusky red color and may produce ectropion.

Lichen planus rarely becomes universal. Usually some areas show typical lichen planus papules. The nail changes of lichen planus may be observed. The purplish reticulated network on the mucosae and semimucosae may give a clue as to the diagnosis.

Pemphigus foliaceus may be generalized. Bullous or discrete erosive lesions may be seen. The exfoliation is noteworthy for the moist and even oozing condition of the tissue beneath the scales. The scales are of the lamellar type. (See also Chapter 9.)

Rarely, Norwegian scabies may be almost generalized and scaly. The elderly and infirm, as in those with AIDS, are mostly involved.

Some cases of parapsoriasis en plaque may be very extensive, but these extensive lichenoid plaques are almost never universal. By the time they are, mycotic tumors are almost always present.

Sézary syndrome is an exfoliative erythroderma with intense pruritus, edema, browning, superficial lymphadenopathy, hepatomegaly, leonine facies, alopecia, dystrophic nails, and hyperkeratoses of the palms and soles. It is the leukemic form of mycosis fungoides.

Rarely, extensive ichthyosis and xerosis may develop in the course of a lymphoma. The degree of erythema in this acquired adult ichthyosis is minimal.

Congenital Erythroderma and Erythrodermas of Newborn and Children

Ritter von Rittershain's disease is a generalized exfoliative form of impetigo of the newborn. Large flaccid bullae with an erythematous halo extend rapidly to cover the entire body. There may be a frankly purulent primary source (infected circumcision or umbilical wound). The bullae do not remain, and the skin appears scalded; large sheets of the horn separate spontaneously or with slight trauma. In my opinion, this is the same condition as staphylococcal scalded skin syndrome (SSSS), although there are variations. In SSSS the predominant feature is widespread tender erythema, which rapidly develops into extensive exfoliation of the upper layers of the epidermis, giving the appearance of scalded skin. Frank pyoderma often is not present, except for a mucopurulent conjunctivitis and/or a purulent crusted eruption in the nasolabial folds. The epidermolysis is more extensive in the large joint flexures. The bullous nature of SSSS does not seem to be as prominent as in old descriptions of Ritter von Rittershain's disease. (See also primary Erythroderma.)

Leiner's disease usually occurring in neonates, is a very rare, generalized, erythematosquamous eruption of the trunk and limbs. Flexural involvement is common, with oozing. Scalp and eyebrows are heavily crusted. Face scaling is fine and branny; on the torso and extensor limbs, the scales are large, gray, and opaque.

Karl Leiner, 1871–1930, Austrian Pediatrician, Vienna
Gottfried Ritter Von Rittershain, 1820–1883, Austrian Pediatrician
Albert Sézary, 1880–1956, French Dermatologist

Atopic erythroderma may occur in infants as well. Psoriatic erythroderma and drug-induced erythroderma are rarely seen. Candidal erythroderma has also been reported. It is rarely that pityriasis rubra pilaris and Norwegian scabies cause erythroderma in children.

Congenital ichthyosiform dermatoses (see Chapter 15, "Disseminated ichthyoses") may occur as well.

Reference

1. Adam JE. Exfoliative dermatitis. Can Med Assoc J 1968; 99:661–666.

CHAPTER 8

Vesicles

*A microscopic cavity filled with clear liquid,
pinhead to pea-sized (up to 1.0 cm), spherical in shape,
forming little ring-shaped collars of scales (collarettes) when emptied,
almost always multicocular, and, possibly umbilicated.*

Overview

Vesicles [from the Latin meaning small bladder] are small circumscribed elevations of the epidermis which have a macroscopic cavity filled with a clear liquid [Fig. 8.1]. Since fluid in a cavity exerts equal pressure in all directions, vesicles assume a spherical shape. Larger

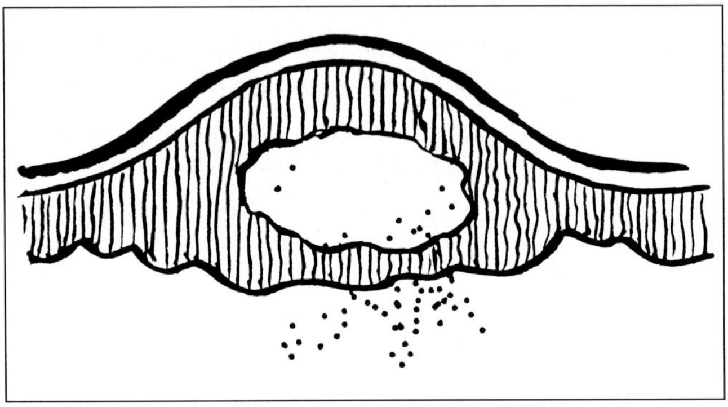

Figure 8.1 Schematic drawing of a vesicle. Redrawn after Siemens.[1]

vesicles may develop by coalescence of several small vesicles. In some cases, they may show polycyclic (composed of several segments of a circle) borders or they may occur in grape-like clusters (herpes). Sometimes the roof of a vesicle is centrally depressed. If the depression is caused by central necrosis (vaccinia), the lesion is spoken of as a pock (plural, pocks or pox), and the depression is called the navel of the pock (umbilicated lesion). Vesicles are usually tense, are elevated, and have a taut and glossy surface. They are firm to the touch. If they are small and imbedded in thick and tough skin, such as on the palms, they may be neither raised nor palpable. However, they can still be recognized by their round shape and the glass-bead-like or the "sago-grain" reflections of their translucent contents, or by the little ring-shaped collar of scales which remains after the vesicle has emptied (collarettes). Older palmar and plantar vesicles may have a brownish tinge. Confirmation that the lesion is a vesicle is obtained by pricking the lesion with a needle and observing whether or not fluid escapes. Vesicles almost always have a hyperemic base.

Vesicles have tops, contents, and floors. Their contents consist mainly of serum and fibrin, a few white cells, and occasionally blood. If the contents dry out, a little round, yellowish brown to dark red or brown crust forms at the center. If the top of the blister bursts or is scratched off, the floor is exposed and appears as a small round erosion. As the exudate dries, the erosion becomes covered with a small, serous or bloody crust, which is not so perfectly round or smooth as the crust of the dried-out vesicle top. It is characteristic of some diseases that the vesicle top bursts very early (mucosal vesicles) or is invariably scratched off (nummular eczema). The vesicles of other dermatoses are more stable, dry without injury, and exfoliate after the healing of the floor or are shed as a crust formed over the entire lesion. In the pock, necrosis involves the connective tissue and causes deep destruction, so that sharply bordered and depressed ("varioliform") scars result (this

Portions of the Overview are taken and modified from Siemens[1] (pp. 44,46).

occasionally occurs in varicella, acne necrotica, hydroa vacciniforme). Mucosal vesicles usually lose their tops soon after they appear and are ordinarily seen as small round erosions whose floors are covered with a little yellowish exudate. They can maintain the grouping or polycyclic borders seen on the skin. Mucosal vesicles or erosions of vesicular origin are called aphthae.

Vesicles are located very superficially and almost exclusively involve various layers of the epidermis under the horny layer. Vesicles have various modes of pathogenesis and are classified into the following types as (1) intercellular, (2) intracellular, (3) necrobiotic, and (4) simple separation.

Intercellular edema (fluid between the cells) pushes the rete cells apart, forming a honeycomb or sponge-like structure whose meshes finally rupture. This process is called spongiosis and is the hallmark of eczema.

Intracellular edema arises within the cells, causing them to burst, and forming a multilocular vesicle. The septa inside the blister are formed by resisting cell walls. Thus unicellular "vesicles" develop which coalesce and form the clinical vesicle or altération cavitaire (French for "change characterized by the cavities"). This process is also called reticular degeneration.

In other cases the edema arises between the cells, but the cells undergo a process of necrobiotic deterioration with loss of the intercellular bridges with resulting acantholysis. There is also giant cell formation. This is termed ballooning degeneration (varicella, herpes simplex, zona).[1]

In some cases, there is more than one method of formation. Vesicles may be pinhead-sized or larger, but if the liquid-filled cavity is larger than a pea, it is usually no longer called a vesicle but a bulla (blister, bleb).

From a morphological point of view, let us work backwards in trying to distinguish the difference, if any, between vesicles and bullae. Table 15 lists some of the conditions commonly called vesicular and those commonly called bullous. It is interesting that many texts do in fact separate these two groups of diseases, despite the fact that in the same texts a bulla is defined only as a large vesicle.

Table 15: Vesicular and Bullous Conditions
Vesicular
Varicella
Herpes Simplex
Zoster
Orf
Bullous
Various forms of pemphigus
Various forms of pemphigoid (including herpes gestationis)
Dermatitis herpetiformis
Various forms of epidermolysis bullosa
Porphyria

What and where are the basic pathological changes that result in the formation of the above listed diseases? In general, the vesicular diseases are those where the vesicle (or, if large enough, macrovesicle) is formed by an ongoing inflammatory epidermal process. The spongiotic intercellular edema and the ballooning interepi-dermal degeneration of the viral diseases are excellent examples of vesicles.

I must admit that I have no absolute answer to those who say that some bullous disorders are an ongoing inflammatory process. I believe however, that the fluid accumulation in vesicles is a more active process than it is with the formation of bullae.

In general, bullae are formed by an accumulation of fluid in a pre-existing space, due to intrinsic or extrinsic damage to the cohesiveness of the epidermal cells or the epidermal–dermal junction or to direct damage to the epidermis and dermis. Thus, we have the subcorneal bulla of bullous impetigo and subcorneal pustular dermatoses, the intracorneal microbulla (not vesicle) of miliaria crystallina, the varying levels of acantholytic bullae of pemphigus, the subepidermal bullae due to degeneration of the basal cell layers (e.g. lichen planus, lupus erythematosus), the subepidermal bullae due to degeneration of the basement membrane (e.g. dermatitis herpetiformis), and the bullae from burns caused by damage to the basal layer and upper dermis.[2]

Therefore, vesicles differ from bullae not only because of a usually smaller volume, but also by mode of formation. In contradistinction to bullae, vesicles are frequently multilocular, at least at their inception. So, although a bulla collapses after a single puncture, a vesicle will not. It should be repeated and emphasized that some large vesicles are not bullae (e.g. poison ivy and incontinentia pigmenti) because in these conditions, the mode of formation is not a passive accumulation of fluid in the upper epidermis, but is a result of an ongoing inflammatory process. Bullae almost always leave a circle of light-brown pigmentation. Table 16 compares vesicles and bullae.

Table 16: Comparison of Vesicles and Bullae		
Characteristic	Vesicles	Bullae
Size	*Usually under 1.0 cm*	*Usually over 1.0 cm*
Location	*Usually intra-epidermal*	*Most often subepidermal*
Structure	*Multilocular, do not collapse when punctured* *May be poxed*	*Unilocular, collapse when punctured* *Never form pocks*
Development	*Usually inflammatory, active*	*Rarely inflammatory, passive*
Sequelae	*Scarring if necrosis of tissue* *Rarely brown pigmentation*	*Scarring of mechanobullous diseases* *Commonly brown pigmentation*

In general, it is not hard to diagnose the presence or absence of vesicles, but a few cystic conditions which may appear to be vesicular, should be mentioned. Hidrocystoma, cyst of gland of Moll, lymphangioma circumscriptum, the obstructive post radiation lymphangiectasias, and the lymphangiectasias of the Klippel-Trenaunay syndrome present as clear, tensely filled structures which contain a fluid. These cysts are not intra-epidermal.

Maurice Klippel, 1858–1942, French Neurologist
Jacob Antonius Moll, 1832–1914, Dutch Ophthalmologist
P. Trenaunay, 1875– French Physician

Also, in miliaria crystallina there are small, pinhead-sized, clear, fluid-filled structures. They are unilocular and have no surrounding erythema at the base. Morphologically, they could be considered as minute bullae high in the epidermis.

Disseminated Vesicular Dermatoses
Hand-Foot-and-Mouth Disease

In the oropharynx, erythematous macules evolve into small, 1 to 2 mm, vesicles on erythematous bases. The distribution includes the pharynx, soft palate, hard palate, buccal mucosa, gingiva, and tongue. These vesicles are scattered and not grouped. The blisters in the oropharynx often remain intact. Similar lesions occur on the hands and feet (including the palms and soles) and buttocks. Fever, headache, and malaise may also be present.

DIFFERENTIAL DIAGNOSIS

The differential diagnosis includes herpangina, which consists of vesicles or ulcers of the posterior part of the mouth, and aphthous stomatitis, in which the lesions may be larger and more painful, but no blisters are present. Primary herpes simplex infections are associated with a high fever and lymphadenopathy. None of the above have hand or foot lesions. Erythema multiforme may have a similar distribution, but target or iris lesions should be present.

Varicella and Varicelliform Syphilis

Varicella (chickenpox) must be compared and contrasted with papulovesicu-lonecrotic secondary syphilis.

Chickenpox is usually more severe in the adult and may be associated with high fever. The lesions may be extensive, large, and hemorrhagic. Chickenpox may also occur on the palms and soles. Death of tissue resulting in scarring (pock marks) is common in both. Occasionally with varicella, I have seen one or two lesions appear 2 or 3 days before the main eruption. These lesions are erythematous urticarial papules with a small central vesicle. The early lesions are often larger (up to 1 cm) than subsequent crops.

In the eruptive period, there is first a hyperemic spot, then a papular erythema with a small central vesicle and then a frank vesicle. The degree of erythema may be quite marked, and in the beginning, it may seem to be the primary lesion since the central vesicle cannot be seen clearly.

Later, some of the larger vesicles may have a central crust with new peripheral vesiculation. The degree of erythema about the vesicle varies from none to quite a marked erythema. In the final stage when crusting occurs, some of the blisters may become turbid and slightly yellowish. This is not pyoderma. Accentuation of varicella has been reported in areas sunburned during the incubation period.

Distinctions between varicella and the pox-like manifestations of syphilis are outlined in Table 17.

Characteristic	Varicella	Syphilis
Spots	*Bright red spots*	*Dull red spots*
Vesicles	*Vesicles cloudy on second day; rarely pustules*	*Transparent vesicles turn into true pustules*
Areola	*Areola at base of vesicles is slight and pink in color*	*Areola at the base of vesicles is dull red or copper-colored*
Crusts	*Crusts small, light colored and easily detached*	*Crusts are dark, thick, and very adherent*
Color	*Light brown residual pigmentation slight and disappears quickly*	*Dark brown persistent stain*
Timing	*Rapid appearance of successive crops of blisters*	*Vesicles appear more slowly and over a longer longer interval*
Distribution	*Vesicles isolated; more on torso than extremities*	*Vesicles occur in groups or clusters*
Sequelae	*Excoriations and pyoderma are main sequelae*	*May develop into papulonecrotic or or noduloulcerative lesion*

Table 17: Differential Diagnosis Between Varicella and Varicelliform Secondary Syphilis

Modified from Liveing R. Handbook of skin diseases with especial reference to diagnosis and treatment. 5th Ed. London:Longmans Green and Company, 1887.

Other varicelliform eruptions include eczema herpeticum and generalized zoster or zoster with a varicelliform eruption.

Eczema Herpeticum

Compared to varicella, the eruption is more extensive, confluent, and acute on the sites of such pre-existing conditions as atopic dermatitis and Darier's disease. The other lesions on noninvolved skin are more typical, solitary, pox-like lesions, but are less numerous, acute, and severe.

Varicelliform Eruption of Zoster

The varicelliform eruption occurring in 20 percent of patients with zoster is relatively sparse, and certainly not classically pock-like.

Disseminated Zoster

In this condition, the eruption is usually extensive in debilitated patients and involves many nerve roots (multidermatomal). It may be purpuric, necrotic, and certainly pock-like. Usually, these patients are obviously very ill. Note that the basic lesion in disseminated zoster is a grouped cluster of vesicles on an erythematous base and not a number of solitary chickenpox-like lesions. Disseminated zoster is very rare.

In all zoster cases a primary, unilateral, two or three sensory nerve distribution area is involved. Even in the debilitated patient, the so-called primary zoster is usually quite obvious.

Miscellaneous Vesicular Eruptions

Some other diseases, may, at times, present with vesicles. Eczema has other lesions such as erythema, edema, and then scaling, burning, and lichenification. Dermatitis herpetiformis and the polymorphic eruptions of pregnancy are discussed under the bullous dermatoses. The blistering tineas are discussed under eczema and under the folliculoses. A maculopapular and papulovesicular eruption may be seen in rickettsial pox. The vesicles are similar to those of chickenpox or smallpox, but are deeper. This eruption is basically an erythema. Rarely, some strains of echo and entero viruses may produce a toxic erythema, one feature of which may be small vesicles. Acute pityriasis lichenoides (Mucha-Habermann disease) may have a vesicular component, but of course papules, macules, scales, and purpuric lesions are also seen. This condition is described in Chapter 6. The early blistering phase of erythema multiforme may at times be a purely blistering condition. Linear lesions, clumps, and patches are the arrangement of these blisters, some of which may be pox-like. The extensive erosive mucosal lesions usually confirm the diagnosis. In a day or two, iris lesions develop.

Vesicles of varying size occur in groups and whorled lines, mainly on the extremities, in the blistering phase of incontinentia pigmenti. There is often an inflammatory base.

Localized Vesicular Dermatoses

Herpes Simplex

This disease in its recurrent or secondary form presents as asymmetrical grape-like clusters of 2 to 3 mm vesicles on an erythematous base. At the beginning, there may be only small clusters of erythematous papules. At the end, there are clusters of small, yellowish, serous crusts. The number of vesicles in each cluster varies from 3 to 10, and the number of clusters from 2 or 3 up to 12. When the vesicles touch each other, they fuse and produce a scalloped or small arcuate border. This is particularly noticeable at the erosive or crusting stage. The lymph glands may be slightly enlarged and tender. Lips, nose, and face are common locations; next are the genitals, either on the skin or the semimucosa. A linear "zosteriform" type can be present on the lower torso and buttocks. This variety is characteristically more painful and more commonly associated with inguinal or femoral lymphadenopathy. The lesions heal in from 7 to 10 days. Recurrent herpes simplex probably does not occur on the oral mucosa (except in the immunocompromised patient) or if it does, it is usually on the hard palate. Recurrent herpes simplex may occur on the fingers. The remains of a sunburn or the flushed florid face of fever may be present, as may be irritated nares due to coryza. Sometimes rather large areas are involved, e.g. the whole side of the face. In such cases, mucosal eye lesions with keratitis and keratitic scarring are common. Herpes simplex does not scar on the skin or in the mouth. Disseminated herpes simplex (eczema herpeticum) has been mentioned in the disseminated pox eruptions. Progressive, purpuric or nonhealing and scarring herpes simplex may be seen in patients who are immunologically deficient.

DIFFERENTIAL DIAGNOSIS

The differential diagnosis of herpes simplex includes impetigo. The basic lesion in impetigo is a yellowish vesicle or bulla, frequently crusted, with a bright red surrounding erythema. Also, whereas herpes simplex may involve only the red border of the lip, impetigo almost always involves the adjacent skin surface, i.e. impetigo is never present on the mucosa or semimucosa alone. The recurrent nature of secondary herpes simplex, which almost always occurs at the same site, and the self-healing aspect are useful diagnostic points. The only other condition that does this is a fixed drug erythema; however, these drug erythemas are basically erythemas with a bulla (approximately 3 cm diameter) and usually (except on the mucosa) leave a lasting brown stain.

Another bullous erythema that may involve the facial skin and mucosa is erythema multiforme bullosum, in which the basic lesion is erythema with bullous formation and iris lesions. Often, the remains of a sun-induced herpes simplex may be seen on the lip. On the semimucosal surface of the penis, vesicles of herpes simplex are rarely seen, only the polycyclic erosions. In contradistinction with a syphilitic chancre, there is no induration, and the depth of the inflammation is much less.

The primary infection with herpes simplex has the same basic morphology as the recurrent form. However, there are certain differences. The extent of the primary eruption is greater, there is more edema and inflammation, enlarged lymph nodes are present, and the eruption lasts from 2 to 3 weeks. In children, primary herpes simplex occurs on the oral and pharyngeal mucosa as well as on the perioral skin and semimucosa. In adults, on the vulva and fingers, the acuity of primary herpes simplex is quite alarming. The differential diagnosis in cases of severe mucosal involvement is that of erosive lesions of the mucosa.

Herpes Zoster (Zona, Shingles)

At the onset of herpes zoster, scattered, slightly erythematous patches with a roughened surface appear, with normal intervening skin. Within a day vesicles form, primarily in the center of the red areas. They rapidly increase in size. They become tense, pearly, and uniform, from the size of a pinhead to that of a pea. They lie close together and are sometimes confluent. The fluid in the vesicles becomes opalescent and turbid, even purulent, by the third day, while at the same time the erythematous plaque fades and flattens. Desiccation then occurs and is complete by about the twelfth day. The crusts fall off in about 3 weeks. The onset is not simultaneous but successive, so that several stages can be seen at one time, and the last part to appear often does not develop frank vesiculation and crusting. At times, the vesicles are hemorrhagic. Usually, the vesicles do not rupture unless they are on areas easily traumatized or on the mucosa. When ruptured, the remnants may present as rather deep ulcerations, polycyclic in shape, with a seropurulent base and an inflammatory halo. The residual erythema may last a few months. Scarring is the rule, especially from the lesions that appear first, as they tend to be larger and deeper. Sometimes gangrenous areas appear and become extensive, especially in patients who are immunologically deficient. Paresthesias and muscle paralysis are occasional symptoms. Recurrences are rare.

The regional lymph nodes are regularly enlarged and tender. The distinction between the secondary varicelliform eruption and disseminated herpes zoster has already been made.

The site of predilection is the torso, like a half-belt (zona = belt) (Fig. 8.2). Cervical zona and ophthalmic zona are also common. Zona of the extremities is more unusual. The mucosa will be involved if it is in the distribution of the sensory nerve involved. Exceptionally, double or bilateral, alternating, multiple or even generalized dermatomal zona are seen.

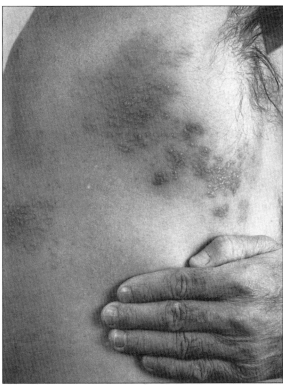

Figure 8.2 Herpes zoster on the flank and chest.

Herpes zoster is unilateral and is located along the distribution of the peripheral sensory nerves, usually spreading over the territory of two or even three neighboring spinal roots. Sometimes there is crossing over for a few millimeters over the midline, and sometimes there are one or two aberrant vesicles. On the face in particular, with the edema and erythema, it may seem at onset that the eruption is not strictly limited to one side. In a few days, however, the vesicles clearly show the lack of cross-over. If the tip of the nose is involved, the cornea will also be involved. The eye lesions are conjunctivitis, keratitis with ulceration, and uveitis.

The diagnosis is usually easy: clustered vesicles, arranged in groups over one or more nerve territories, unilateral, and accompanied by pain. Early in the eruption, especially on the face, the edema and erythema may mimic erysipelas or acute contact dermatitis. Herpes simplex is usually bilateral and recurrent at the same site, and there is little pain. When there is only a single patch of zona, especially in the younger patient, it may not be possible to make a final morphological diagnosis. For some reason, the central forehead is a favorite location for a single patch of zona.

Orf (Sheep Pox, Ecthyma Contagiosum)

The basic lesion is a 1.7 to 2 cm diameter, turgid, elevated, firm papulovesicle with sloping edges and an umbilicated top. On puncturing, the small amount of fluid may be expressed. The lesions are most common on the fingers, hands, and wrists. Regional lymph node enlargement may occur. Scarring is usual.

Aphthae (Mucosal Vesicles)

Mucosal vesicles are very rare. Almost always, these lesions present as erosions or (in the mouth) aphthae. Therefore I have described the mucosal vesicles in Chapter 14.

References

1. Siemens HW. General diagnosis and therapy of skin diseases. Weiner K, trans. Chicago:University of Chicago Press, 1958.
2. Lever WF, Schaumberg-Lever G. Histopathology of the skin. 7th Ed. Philadelphia:Lippincott, 1990:104.

CHAPTER 9
Bullous Dermatoses

> *A liquid-filled cavity, usually unilocular, larger than a pea,
> i.e. larger than 1.0 cm.*

Overview

Bullae differ from vesicles not only in size, but also in (an often deeper) location, structure, and mode of development.[1] See Chapter 8 on vesicles for more details.

Bullae or blisters are localized elevations, usually of a diameter greater than 1 cm, of the epidermis that contain fluid. Large blisters may occasionally be situated directly under the horny layer. More commonly, they separate the deeper epidermal layers or are located between the epidermis and dermis, lifting the epidermis in full thickness from its base.

Bullae may be subcorneal, intraepidermal (acantholytic), and subepidermal (Table 18; Fig. 9.1). Simple separation of the layers, which is rarely found in vesicles, is the most common pathogenesis of bullae. For this reason they are, in contrast to vesicles, usually unilocular. The size of bullae varies greatly, although usually they are at least as big as a pea. An exception is the lesion of sudamina (miliaria crystallina) which can be classified as microbullae. There are, however, vesicles of large size that are inflammatory in nature, which originate from spongiosis (bullous eczemas), or which come about by intracellular edema (altération cavitaire), by ballooning degeneration (herpes zoster) and by interstitial edema with cellular disintegration (burn, frostbite). Some blisters have a remarkably rapid growth, which can be checked by de-roofing and release of the pressure. This is done more effectively with fine scissors than by needle puncture, which seals itself too easily. As vesicles are multilocular, they do not collapse after deroofing.

Table 18: Classification of Bullae			
Type of Bullae	Mode of Formation	Site of Formation	Disease
Subcorneal bulla	*Detachment of horny layer*	*Subcorneal*	*Miliaria crystallina Impetigo*
Acantholytic bulla	*Dissolution of intercellular cement substance*	*Intraepidermal* *(1) Suprabasal* *(2) Subcorneal*	*Pemphigus vulgaris* *Familial benign pemphigus* *Pemphigus foliaceus*
Bulla due to degeneration of basal cells	*Damaged basal cells lose contact with dermis*	*Subepidermal*	*Epidermolysis bullosa, epidermal types* *Lichen planus* *Lichen sclerosus et atrophicus* *Lupus erythematosus*
Bulla due to degenerative changes in the basement membrane zone	*Damage in the structures causing coherence of basal cells with dermis*	*Subepidermal*	*Epidermolysis bullosa, junctional, dystrophic, and acquired types* *Urticaria pigmentosa* *Bullous pemphigoid* *Cicatrical pemphigoid* *Herpes gestationis* *Dermatitis herpetiformis* *Linear IgA dermatosis* *Erythema multiforme, dermal type* *Porphyria cutanea tarda* *Thermal bullae* *Treatment induced*

Portions of the Overview are taken and modified from Siemens[1] (pp. 46–49).

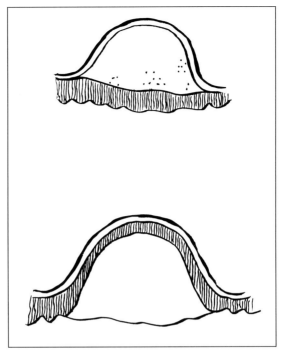

Figure 9.1 *Upper:* Subcorneal bullae.
Lower: Subepidermal bullae.
Redrawn after Siemens.[1]

Bullae can be provoked mechanically by prolonged rubbing (friction blisters on the hands from rowing or on the feet from unaccustomed marching or ill-fitting shoes). In patients with epidermolysis bullosa, minor rubbing or a slight bump is sufficient to provoke such bullae. In these cases, the great ease of mechanically producing bullae confirms the diagnosis. To accomplish this, the examiner rubs a fingernail across the patient's skin in the opposite direction from that of scratching. This is called scratch-rubbing. A suitable place for such scratch-rubbing is the skin over bony prominences, e.g. on the knuckles. In epidermolysis bullosa, after a few strokes of scratch-rubbing, the detachment of the epidermis can be felt by the presence of a shifting little epidermal fold. The potential cavity indicated by this fold fills up in a few minutes to form a blister, which may continue to grow for several days.

In pemphigus, the findings are sometimes similar, but Nikolsky's sign[2] is more typical. This phenomenon, elicited by a vigorous "wiping" pressure of the thumb, involves detachment and shifting of the upper layers of the normal appearing epidermis, leaving a slightly eroded surface. Also by pulling on the ruptured wall of the blister it is possible to take off the upper layers for a long distance even onto seemingly healthy skin. According to Goodman, the fact that blisters may also show lateral spread by pressure, is not part of Nikolsky's sign.[2] This has been called the Asboe-Hansen sign.

G. Asboe-Hansen

Pyotr Vasilyevich Nikolsky, 1858–1940, Russian Dermatologist

Bullae may also be caused chemically (cantharides), mechanically (epidermolysis), thermally (burns, frostbite), actinically (sunburn, X-ray, hydroa), or they may form spontaneously without any obvious external cause (pemphigus). Mechanobullous conditions are primarily the various varieties of epidermolysis and porphyria.

Bullae, like vesicles, have a round or sometimes oval shape. If they are caused by the confluence of several bullae, their borders are more or less polycyclic. Very irregular, jagged, and streaky outlines suggest extrinsic causation (friction, cantharides). Fresh bullae are taut, but soon become soft and wrinkled. If they grow very soft, the fluid may collect at the lowest point, as in a bag of thin plastic film. At the bottom of such a bag, a cloudy accumulation of leukocytes may collect (hypopyon). Bullae may continue to dry more and more, so that the loosely attached top, when it finally tears, exposes an already slightly keratinized blister floor. If the bulla top tears at an earlier stage, the floor is a glossy red, oozing erosion. Serosanguineous crusting is commonly present. The sweet sickly odor of extensive pemphigus vulgaris is due to bacterial colonization of the oozing serum. As in the case of vesicles, the peripheral remnants of the blister top usually persist for some time as a ring of scales (collarette). It is from this coarse collar of scales that one can sometimes recognize that an erosion originated from a bulla. When the erosion heals, it leaves a residual erythema which may still show fine desquamation, sometimes leukoderma, or more likely melanoderma. These residues are strikingly round and vanish slowly after weeks or months.

In general, bullae do not leave scars. Exceptions are scarring mucous membrane pemphigoid, epidermolysis bullosa dystrophica, porphyria, hydroa vacciniforme, and severe burns of whatever cause. Senear-Usher syndrome or pemphigus erythematosus may leave a fine epidermal atrophy; dermatitis herpetiformis lesions probably do not themselves scar (the scars are from fairly violent excoriations); the same is probably true for the scars sometimes seen after bullous insect bites.

The contents of bullae, like those of vesicles, at first are clear or yellowish, or, by admixture of blood, reddish to black red. However, secondary infection with pyogenic cocci may cause such contents to become turbid from leukocytes. In this way, the vesicle or the bulla may become a pustule (pus vesicle or pus blister). To emphasize the origin of a pustule from a bulla or to indicate its size, it can be termed a bullous pustule or a purulent bulla.

Mention should be made of the fact that in infants and young children, there is a tendency for many eruptions of unrelated cause to be bullous, e.g. bullous syphilides, bullous lesions of scabies and impetigo, bullous dermatitis herpetiformis, and so on. This appears to be a characteristic of the lack of "adhesiveness" of the epidermal layers in children.

Francis Eugene Senear, 1889–1958, U.S. Dermatologist, Chicago

Barney Usher, 1899–1978, Canadian Dermatologist, Montreal

Pemphigus Vulgaris

The basic lesion of pemphigus vulgaris is a superficial flaccid bulla that upon light pressure increases in size by spreading peripherally in the direction of applied pressure. When the patient stands up, the upper portion of the bulla becomes wrinkled and collapsed as the yellowish or turbid fluid contents of the bulla fall down to fill the lower portion more.

In pemphigus vulgaris, some of the bullae appear on normal skin; some become confluent, forming figure-8s or arcuate borders with peripheral blistering and central crusting; and some bullae appear on an erythematous base. The bullae may contain a hemorrhagic fluid. Crusting of a serosanguineous type is common, as the flaccid bullae rupture easily. The denuded areas may be larger than the bullae that preceded them. The bullae are 1 to 2 cm in size. There is no particular arrangement, but some of the bullae are clustered. Only rarely is there secondary pyoderma. No area is immune, but torso and extremities are most commonly involved. The middle-chest area is particularly prone to lesions. Flaccid bullae that produce erosions are present in mucosal surfaces, especially in the mouth, on the lips, conjunctiva, and more rarely, nose, genital, and anal mucosa, and in the large creases. The oral mucosa is a common site of onset.

When the lesions heal, they leave a brown or reddish macule. Sometimes the healed areas are hypopigmented; they do not scar. If the bulla roof comes off, a smooth, bright red glistening surface can be seen before crusting occurs. Excoriations are unusual. A rather sweet, sickly odor may come from the room of patients who have florid pemphigus.[3]

By forcible pressure in an area adjacent to bullae, the outer and horny layers of the epidermis can be pushed off (Nikolsky's sign). Intact blisters can be made to spread by pressure. Pemphigus vulgaris is more common in the middle-aged to elderly, especially in the Jewish race.

Pemphigus Vegetans

Pemphigus vegetans shows spongy, papillomatous, moist, and keratotic epidermal thickenings. They are often formed in denuded areas after rupture of bullae. The condition favors the face, axillae, genital region, and oral mucosae. Some of the hypertrophic borders may show a micropustular eruption. Sometimes there are large arcuate verrucous and papillomatous borders.

DIFFERENTIAL DIAGNOSIS

Occasionally, other vegetating diseases such as blastomycosis must be considered in the differential diagnosis (see Chapter 16).

Pemphigus Erythematosus (Senear-Usher Syndrome)

In Senear-Usher syndrome, the basic lesion is an erosion or bulla, located mainly on the face, trunk, and scalp. On the face, the areas most heavily involved are the nose and adjacent cheeks and forehead. On the trunk, the sternal and interscapular areas are almost invariably the most severely affected. Occasionally, the axillae, inguinal, and inframammary areas are involved. Only rarely are lesions present on the extremities. Rarely, bullae occur in the oral mucosa.

On the trunk, the superficial bullae have a wrinkled flaccid appearance with a thin roof. These lesions rupture quickly, resulting in the development of two other lesions. By coalescence or extension of the ruptured bullae, large patches of denuded, reddish, sharply defined erosions develop, sometimes with crusting. These lesions come and go, leaving reddish or brownish areas in which fresh bullae may again appear. If the lesions do not enlarge, they are an oval-shaped with a thick greasy crusty scale. These lesions tend to have the long axis vertically, and at times, the back of the patient is covered with lesions in a Christmas tree distribution. These crusty scales are at times quite dry, at other times quite greasy. There is an inflammatory base. The crusty scales have a dirty yellowish color. Removal of these crusty keratotic lesions reveals an eroded red base. These lesions eventually disappear, leaving brown spots. Minor epidermal atrophy may occur on the torso lesions.

On the face, the eruption consists of sharply marginated scaly patches. They have a dusky red color. The patches vary from 2 to 3 cm in diameter, and sometimes they become confluent with arcuate borders. The central area of the face is most commonly involved. The lesions show varying degrees of inflammation, oozing, scaling, and crusting. Sometimes the follicles are enlarged, but there is no scarring. Sometimes there is an almost purely scaly eruption; at other times there is a moist yellowish crust. Telangiectasia is not normally present. On all areas the eruption is essentially symmetrical.

DIFFERENTIAL DIAGNOSIS

Discoid lupus erythematosus shows atrophy, telangiectasia, carpet tack scaling, a carmine color, and an active indurated border. Crusting is not present.

Seborrhea has a yellowish brown greasy scale, is poorly demarcated on the face, and forms small arcuate areas, often with central brown pigmentation. There are no bullae and no crusting.

On the face, solar keratoses are small, sometimes sharply demarcated irregularly shaped keratotic areas. Removal of the scale produces bleeding.

Impetigo should also be considered in the differential diagnosis.

Pemphigus Foliaceus

Pemphigus foliaceus is a widespread or generalized eruption, which produces flaccid bullae on an erythematous or scaly base. Sometimes bullae are lacking. The skin surface is a mixture of keratoses and dried serous crusting. The face, scalp, and thorax are commonly involved. The conjunctiva may be edematous and inflamed. The oral mucosa is rarely involved. In Brazil, the disease is called fogo selvagem and occurs in children and young female adults and often in families. Fogo selvagem appears to be transmitted by an infectious agent.

DIFFERENTIAL DIAGNOSIS

At times the differential diagnosis must include the various forms of erythroderma.

Familial Benign Chronic Pemphigus (Hailey-Hailey Disease)

Familial benign chronic pemphigus is a bullous disorder occurring primarily on the sides and back of the neck, axillae, groin, and rarely in other flexural areas. The bullae arise on normal skin with fine irregular linear fissuring. They rapidly rupture and become crusted, with a red eroded surface.

The central area often heals, leaving a peripheral, active, blistering, and crusted border. There is no infiltration. The lesions may have a velvety feel. The lesions spread peripherally producing circinate borders. The average lesion may measure up to 4 or 5 cm in diameter. The lesions come and go without scarring. They are worse in the summer. Large bullae are not present. At times it may be clinically and histologically difficult to separate localized areas of Darier's disease from familial benign chronic pemphigus.

Bullous Pemphigoid

If dermatitis herpetiformis is a complex disease morphologically, then bullous pemphigoid[4] is relatively simple. Bullous pemphigoid has one basic lesion: large tense bullae occurring randomly in the elderly, especially on the limbs, trunk, and flexural creases. There is no pattern to the number or size. Excoriations may or may not be present. There is no marked symmetry. The bullae arise on normal or nearly normal skin. There may be preceding or co-existent erythematous or urticarial areas. Clustered early lesions of bullous pemphigoid can at times, closely resemble the clustered bites of cat/dog fleas. Some patients start with small itchy pruritic bullae. There is no pigmentation. Mucosal involvement occurs in about 30 % of cases. When the bullae break, the size of the erosion is the same as the bulla. Nikolsky's sign is usually negative. Localized bullous lesions may occur on the lower part of the legs. As will be seen from this description, morphologically bullous pemphigoid is noted for its unimpressiveness.

Hugh Edward Hailey, 1909– U.S. Dermatologist
William Howard Hailey, 1898–1967, U.S. Dermatologist

Other diagnostic techniques such as biopsy and direct and indirect immunofluorescence, as well as the natural course and response to treatment and presence or absence of underlying disease, are obviously important in establishing the diagnosis. Subtypes of bullous pemphigoid are localized bullous pemphigoid, hyperkeratotic bullous pemphigoid (nodular bullous pemphigoid), dermatitis herpetiformis-like bullous pemphigoid (vesicular, polymorphic), IgA bullous pemphigoid, and epidermolysis bullosa acquisita.

Benign Mucous Membrane Pemphigoid (Cicatricial Pemphigoid, Ocular Pemphigus)

Bullous lesions and denuded areas are present in these variants that appear on the orificial mucosae, especially the conjunctivae and oral mucosae. More rarely, the mucosa of the larynx, esophagus, nose, penis, vulva and anus are involved. Scarring commonly develops on the conjunctivae and, rarely, elsewhere. Fibrous adhesions and shrinkage may cause disability or dysfunction such as entropion and symblepharon. Corneal lesions may heal by vascularization and ingrowth of connective tissue from the conjunctivae. The tear duct may be blocked. Adhesions between lips, between the soft palate and the pharyngeal wall, and between the prepuce and the glans penis may occur, as well as between structures in the esophagus and the vaginal orifice. Rarely, bullae and scarring are present on the skin, particularly on the head and neck (Brunsting-Perry type). The general health of the patient is not impaired.

Chronic Bullous Dermatoses of Childhood (Linear IgA Bullous Dermatoses)

Linear IgA disease, an extensive bullous eruption occurring in the prepubertal child, has as the basic lesion large (up to 1.5 cm), rather tense unilocular bullae, many of which are hemorrhagic. The base may or may not be inflamed. The bullae are in clusters of up to 10, and sometimes more. The bullae often appear in a ring shape producing rosettes or clusters of bullae at the margin of the lesion. Some may be broken, and the eroded red base is obvious. The distribution is symmetrical, commonly involving the large creases of the neck, groin, and buttocks, but they may also occur in other areas. Occasionally there is a superadded pyoderma. The child is obviously healthy. There is no odor. Mucosal lesions are unusual. A few small erythematous vesicles may be present, but basically this is a monomorphous disease. A few scratch marks are present. Annular hypopigmented macules may occasionally be seen.

Linear IgA disease, in adults, may have more of the clinical pattern of dermatitis herpetiformis.

Louis A. Brunsting, 1900– U.S. Dermatologist, Mayo Clinic
Harold O. Perry, 1921– U.S. Dermatologist, Mayo Clinic

The differential diagnosis includes bullous drug eruptions, bullous impetigo, incontinentia pigmenti, and dermatitis herpetiformis. Juvenile dermatitis herpetiformis closely resembles adult dermatitis herpetiformis with such features as symmetry and excoriated papulovesicles.

Dermatitis Herpetiformis

From a morphological point of view, dermatitis herpetiformis is not a clearcut disease entity, therefore the term polymorphous pemphigus as a label has much to recommend it.

The eruption presents as a symmetrical, excoriated, grouped, browning, erythematous papulovesicular, bullous eruption on the elbows, knees, scalp, small of back, and interscapular area. Although rare on the hands, dermatitis herpetiformis has been said to involve areas where the bones are immediately covered by skin and where subcutaneous fat is rare. Considerable brown pigmentation of a post-inflammatory type may be present. The mucosae are usually clear. There is no odor.

The following description discusses additional details and some of the variants of classical dermatitis herpetiformis.

The symmetry of the eruption is usually quite striking, even in patients who do not have many lesions. However, there seems to be a variant called localized dermatitis herpetiformis where a palm-sized, grouped cluster of excoriated papulovesicular areas with brown pigmentation may occur, often on the torso. At other times there may be several of these localized areas.

Excoriations are readily apparent. In some cases they are so numerous and extensive that it is difficult to see the primary papule or vesicle.

The grouping of the lesions varies from case to case. Most show some clustering herpetiform areas, but they vary from patient to patient and also from area to area in each patient. The grouping is in areas about 2 to 3 cm across. Both papules and vesicles and other lesions may show this grouping.

The papular or erythematous phase presents as small (up to 4 mm), turgid, epidermal—dermal red papules. At times they become confluent and may form erythematous plaques-sometimes with arcuate borders and sometimes with a blister surmounting the papule. Frequently, the erythematous papules are all excoriated.

The bullae are usually present at some stage, but in many cases, only small glistening vesicle-like lesions may be present on a plain base, or more likely on an erythematous or papular erythematous base. In other cases, mainly vesicles are present, without much of an erythematous base. In still others, there are mainly bullae. The bullae are not hemorrhagic. However, even then, unilocular bullae, up to 2 cm in diameter, will have some of the previously described features, i.e. grouping, excoriations, symmetry, as well as other lesions such as small bullae or erythematous papules. These bullae of dermatitis herpetiformis are rather deep-seated, feel rather firm and tense, and are not easily collapsible as are, for example, the bullae of pemphigus or bullous impetigo. Rarely, erosive lesions are present on the oral mucosae.

The amount of brown pigmentation present is variable. It is diffusely distributed at the site of prior or present lesions, poorly demarcated, having the light or tan to dark brown color of postinflammatory pigmentation. At times, small areas of whitish depigmentation (the sites of healed excoriations) may be intermingled with brown pigmentation, vesicles, and other lesions.

As described, the morphological mix that has been and will be called dermatitis herpetiformis is quite broad, and mixtures of all the previous findings may be found, or the lesion may be basically monomorphous.

Dermatitis herpetiformis is very rare before puberty. It is basically a disease of those between 20 and 60 years of age. Exacerbations and remissions are the rule, and although there is usually the same morphological pattern to each exacerbation, at times this is not so. Dermatitis herpetiformis may occur during pregnancy, but is not related to or affected by the pregnancy.

DIFFERENTIAL DIAGNOSIS

The differential diagnosis varies, depending on the predominant feature of the eruption. If excoriations are present, then neurotic excoriations and insect bites must be considered. If primarily erythematous papules are present, the various types of erythema, e.g. papular erythema multiforme and drug erythemas, must be considered. If the eruption is primarily vesiculobullous, then think of bullous pemphigoid, pemphigus vulgaris, erythema multiforme bullosum, and bullous drug eruptions.

Polymorphous Eruption of Pregnancy

Polymorphous eruption of pregnancy has also been called herpes gestationis, pruritus without lesions, idiopathic recurrent jaundice of pregnancy, prurigo gravidarum, Spangler's papular dermatitis of pregnancy, prurigo gestationis (of Besnier), prurigo annularis, pruritic urticarialpapules and plaques of pregnancy, and pruritic folliculitis of pregnancy.

Being a lumper rather than a splitter, I agree with Borraderi and Saurat that the "with the exception of pemphigoid (herpes) gestations, we know of no criteria which can be used to differentiate these conditions".[5]

Polymorphous eruption of pregnancy is a disseminated erythema with secondary papulation, urticarial areas, vesicles, and bullae. Like dermatitis herpetiformis, this is a polymorphous eruption that can present with almost a unilesional eruption or one of the above basic lesions.

The lesions are blotchy, common on the abdomen and extremities, and present as somewhat grouped areas of erythema, erythematous papules, urticarial patches, and

Ernest Besnier, 1831–1909, French Dermatologist, Paris

Arthur Spangler, 1916–1975, U.S. Dermatologist, Boston

vesicles and bullae. It commonly starts on, and is worse on, the lower abdomen especially in the striae from previous pregnancies. The eruption often spares the back, face, palms, and soles.

All stages may be seen, and at times there is some intermingling. Residual brown pigmentation may also be present. Excoriations are common. The eruption usually starts in the late months of pregnancy and progressively worsens without treatment. Occasionally, it may start after delivery. It usually begins with the first or second pregnancy and recurs with each succeeding pregnancy, sometimes starting earlier and being more severe in subsequent pregnancies. Recurrences of a minor degree may occur with each of the first two or three menses. Also, birth control pills may cause a minor recurrence of the eruption.

I believe that a variant of polymorphous eruption of pregnancy is prurigo gestationis, in which the basic lesion is a small, occasionally grouped, erythematous papule that rapidly becomes excoriated and prurigo-like, due to scratching. The shins are a common site. It seems most likely that the pruritus of pregnancy without lesions represents a milder variant. Hence, I believe the term polymorphous eruption of pregnancy is more exact than herpes gestationis.

Recent immunofluorescent studies indicate that the blistering form of this condition may be related to bullous pemphigoid.[6] The term pemphigoid gestationis has been suggested.

DIFFERENTIAL DIAGNOSIS

Bullous drug-induced toxic erythema should be considered in the differential diagnosis.

Epidermolysis bullosa is difficult to classify morphologically because there is clinical overlap in the different types.

Epidermolysis Bullosa Simplex

In general, the simplex types include the Weber-Cockayne syndrome, the junctional epidermolysis bullosa, and the epidermolysis bullosa letalis type.

This condition consists of the tendency to formation of tense, subcorneal, serous or serosanguinous noninflamed bullae that can measure up to 3 cm in diameter. These lesions are located at sites of trauma or friction, especially in the palmar and plantar skin, but also on the elbows, knees and on the torso at points of contact with tight clothing. Some have a linear aspect where the original trauma was linear. Blebs may occur in the mucosae, especially oral and especially along the line of occlusion.

All lesions are unilocular bullae that heal quickly and leave no scar. Occasionally, there is a faint purplish brown stain. All bullae occur on normal-appearing skin.

Hyperhidrosis of the palms and soles with maceration of the plantar skin is quite common in patients with this condition. The eruption is usually limited to childhood and often disappears after puberty.

Epidermolysis Bullosa Dystrophica

The principal feature of the dystrophic type, which distinguishes it from the simplex type, is atrophy and scarring. There are dominant and recessive forms of this variant.

Scarring occurs at the sites of prior bulla formation and can be very extensive, leading to loss of tissue such as nails, subcutaneous tissue, and even bone. This loss of tissue can result in a tremendously shortened and deformed hand or foot. Pseudowebs of the fingers and toes or of the hand may develop; club fists and contractures may also be present, especially in the recessive form.

The bullae also result in large superficial ulcers.

The association of congenital deformities of the teeth, hair (sparse), and nails (rudimentary, thickened) is not unusual and patients should be examined for these characteristics.

Also, the extent, size, and frequency of bullae formation and ulceration tend to be greater in the dystrophic type. The same process may produce horrible scarring and mutilation on the face and in the mouth. Milia are commonly present in the scars. Sometimes the scars are thick, almost keloidal, in nature. Rarely do squamous cell carcinomas develop in the scars.

The acquista epidermolysis bullosa (EBA), reported following penicillamine therapy and associated with Crohn's and other diseases, usually scars. The nails are described as being dystrophic.

Porphyria

The skin changes associated with the various forms of porphyria in adults are primarily varying degrees of bullous formation. These bullae occur almost exclusively in the sun-exposed areas of the upper extremities (particularly the dorsa of the hands and forearms), head, and neck. The bullae are large (up to 2 cm), usually flaccid, and easily broken. They are scattered irregularly over the affected areas. In many cases, only crusts at the sites of prior bullae formation may be seen. It seems likely that these bullae arise from trauma, often of a very minor degree. As a result of these bullae and other trauma, rather extensive, severe, dermal fibrosis or scarring may occur. This scarring is irregularly arranged, is usually most fully developed on the face, neck, and dorsa of the hands, and may be associated with a violaceous hue. Alopecia of the sides and front of the scalp may be quite marked. The presence of a considerable degree of mottled light browning with the scarring may suggest sclerodermatous poikiloderma. In some cases the scarring is severe enough to produce mutilations, especially on the fingers. A rather fine terminal hair overgrowth (hypertrichosis) on the sides of the face and dorsa of the hands may also be present.

Pseudoporphyria from drugs or chronic renal failure is clinically difficult to differentiate from porphyria.

Burrill Bernard Crohn, 1884–1983, Gastroenterologist, New York

Porphyria in young children may show similar bullae formation, but usually scarring, browning and hypertrichosis are not present. Smaller vacciniform bullae may be present on the rims of the ears and tip of the nose. In the rare erythropoietic type, the teeth may be pink.

Hydroa Vacciniforme

The eruption in hydroa vacciniforme is symmetrical and usually limited to the uncovered parts of the body; the bridge of the nose, malar cheeks, rims of the ears, and the backs of the hands are the parts most affected. The disease occurs in successive outbreaks. The lesions start as red macules or papules that rapidly form vesicles or bullae, sometimes separate and sometimes coalescent. The bullae dry, the large ones becoming depressed in the center. This central depression is black surrounded by a ring of fluid, while about the whole is a reddened areola. The dark center is converted rapidly into a thick black crust which, when it falls off, leaves a depressed reddened scar that eventually becomes white and almost indistinguishable from that of variola. The disease begins in the first few years of life and disappears at or near puberty.

Juvenile spring eruption (hydroa estivale) is a rare variation with smaller blisters that do not scar. It has the feature of occurring only on the first intensive exposure to sun in the springtime. Sometimes it is confused with Hutchinson's summer prurigo. Both may represent the cutaneous manifestations of porphyria or polymorphous light eruption.

Miscellaneous

A few nodular tumors may have bullae. Bullae are rarely seen on malignant melanoma nodules or Hutchinson freckles. Also, bullae may be seen on the nodular tumor stage of mycosis fungoides. The solitary brown dermal nodule of childhood mastocytosis may produce a bulla on rubbing; frequently there is also a generalized flushing.

Various forms of the toxic erythemas (disseminated erythema, urticaria, and purpura) may have a bullous element. Some examples are bullous urticaria, bullous drug erythemas (Fig. 9.2) (including the vasculitis type), and bullous erythema multiforme. Other disseminated erythemas such as thermal, chemical, electrical, radiation burns, frostbite, or sunburn commonly have bullae as part of the picture. Bullae may also be present in pellagra and other photosensitivity eruptions. Rarely, large flaccid bullae may be seen on old burn scars. Traumatic localized erythemas can also include bullae.

Insect bites may produce discrete solitary bullae, usually on the lower legs. Such bullae are unilocular and usually arise on normal skin, although a faint erythema may be present at the periphery. These bullae maintain the same dit-dit-dit or constellation arrangement and sometimes show a small dimple in the center, the

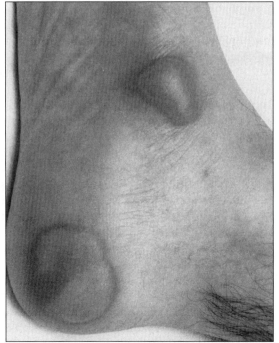

Figure 9.2 Drug erythema with bullae.

remains of the central punctum. Some of the bullae may not be intact. Not all lesions are bullous: some are urticarial papules, excoriated or not. Impetigo in infants is often bullous. When the impetiginous bullae are left quiet and not disturbed, the lower one-quarter of the bullae has a markedly turbid appearance. Erysipelas may have surface bullae, sometimes hemorrhagic. The fixed drug erythema may be bullous. Traumatic erythema may at times be bullous.

Many contact eczemas may have a bullous component. Actually, though, the bullae in contact eczema are really giant vesicles, in that the formation is the result of a basic intraepidermal inflammatory process and not a benign passive accumulation of serum. Poison ivy eczema is a good example. Pompholyx at times may be bullous.

Lichen planus and systemic lupus erythematosus may have bullae as may lichen sclerosus et atrophicus. In the latter, the bullae are frequently hemorrhagic.

Large bullae may present in lazarine or maculoanesthetic leprosy.

The plantar hyperkeratotic lesions of pachyonychia congenita are often bullous. At times, the lesion must be pared to reveal the presence of the bullae.

Bullae may occur in congenital syphilis, usually on the palms and soles. They are large (up to 2 cm in diameter), flaccid lesions that rapidly become erosive or ulcerative. Some produce deep ulcers with a serosanguinous purulent base.

Staphylococcal scalded skin syndrome (SSSS) (Ritter von Rittershain's disease), dermatitis exfoliativa neonatorum, and toxic epidermal necrolysis may present with many large very superficial flaccid bullae that rapidly spread to cover most of the body. However, I have classified the basic morphology as a persistent generalized erythema with bulla formation, and described them under erythroderma. Usually true intact bullae are rarely seen in SSSS.

Rarely, the skin changes in the upper extremities of patients with syringomyelia may show bullae as well as fissures in a bluish, thinned, anesthetic skin.

Cerebral damage (e.g. from tumors, strokes, or coal gas poisoning) may be associated with bullae. These are probably similar to the pressure bullae described later.

Polymorphous eruptions, including erythemas of various sorts as well as bullae, may be seen secondary to some underlying carcinoma.

Flexural ichthyosis with some erythemas as seen in congenital ichthyosiform erythroderma rarely may show a few flaccid bullae on the extremities. These disappear without sequelae.

In pressure bullae due to coma-producing doses of barbiturates and other tranquilizers, the primary lesion is a bulla. The bullae are approximately 4 by 6 cm in size and tend to be oval in shape. They are surrounded by an erythematous border of approximately 1 to 2 mm, with a well-defined margin. Some of the bullae are tense and filled with a clear straw-colored fluid. Others are quite flaccid with only a very small amount of fluid. In these lesions, the underlying dermis shows a punctate erythema. The lesions are unilocular and single. They are distributed randomly on the buttocks and lower extremities (Fig. 9.3). They probably come from ischemia due to constant pressure on one area in a comatose patient.[7]

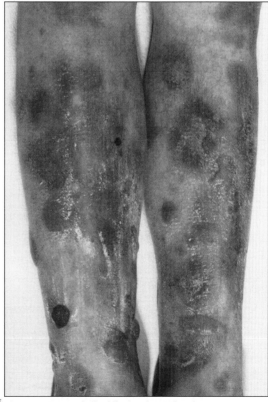

Figure 9.3 Pressure bullae following drug-induced coma.

Other diseases with a bullous component are lupus erythematosus, blistering tinea, bullous amyloid, morphea, urticaria pigmentosa, and ischemic bullae of diabetic feet. For this miscellaneous group, see under the disease mentioned for a complete description.

Remember that bullae can be produced by therapy (e.g. cantharidin, potent salicyclic acid preparations, and cryotherapy).

References

1. Siemens HW. General diagnosis and therapy of skin diseases. Wiener K, trans. Chicago:University of Chicago Press, 1958.
2. Goodman H. Nikolsky sign. AMA Arch Dermatol 1953; 68:334–335.
3. Holubar K. Odor in pemphigus. Dermatology 1993; 187:151–152.
4. Lui HH, Su WPD, Rogers RS. Clinical variants of pemphigoid. Int J Dermatol 1986; 25:17–27.
5. Borradori L, Saurat JH. Specific dermatoses of pregnancy. Arch Dermatol 1994; 130:778–779.
6. Holmes RC, Black MM. The specific dermatoses of pregnancy. J Am Acad Dermatol 1983; 8:405–412.
7. Dunn C, Held JL, Grossman ME, Spitz J, Kohn SK, Silvers DN. Coma blisters. Cutis 1990; 45:423–425.

CHAPTER 10
Pustules and Pustular Dermatoses

An epidermal elevation containing a purulent liquid.

Overview

A pustule is a pea-sized epidermal elevation containing a purulent liquid.[1] The cavity containing the pus may be situated in the epidermis, in the dermis, or in a hair follicle. So we have (1) epidermal pustules, which may be superficial when formed under the horny layer (impetigo) or deep when they involve the basal layer and therefore leave a scar behind them (ecthyma); (2) dermal pustules, which are rare (miliary coccal abscesses of the newborn); and (3) follicular pustules, which are extremely common (see Chapter 20).

It would be correct and logical to reserve the name pustule for primary pustules, namely those in which the lesion is suppurative from the start. But this distinction is not always practical, so the words vesiculopustule, papulopustule, and so forth are commonly used.

Collections of pus in the hypoderm are not pustules, but abscesses. The same may apply to dermal pustules if they are solitary and not disseminated.

Pustules are of rounded, rarely oval, configuration, more or less prominent, hemispherical or flattened, tense or flaccid, of a yellowish-white or grayish color, and surrounded by an erythematous areola. Depending on the color of the pus, the pustule may look white, yellowish white, yellow, yellowish green, or green. Dimensions are variable; they may be punctiform, lenticular, or nummular. Often, they are small at first and enlarge peripherally.

It is usually easy to ascertain the depth by direct examination. If necessary and advisable to do so, puncture with a needle may be performed in order to empty and determine the contents, ascertain the thickness and constitution of the roof, and check the characteristics of the floor of the pustules. The contents may be a more or less turbid and yellowish fluid, or consist of a creamy, thickened substance known in former times as "laudable pus".

Pustules do not persist for a long time; they are terminated by accidental or spontaneous rupture, or by desiccation. In both cases, they are followed by a yellow, brown, brownish-red, or black crust, more or less thickened and irregular, covering an erosion, excoriation or ulceration. Crusts are discussed in detail in Chapter 14.

Pustular dermatoses are dermatoses in which primary or secondary pustules occur. The latter have also been called secondarily or accidently pustular dermatoses.

The pyodermas are characterized by pustules from the start, originating on healthy skin and resulting from a cutaneous infection by pus-forming cocci. Only the impetigos and ecthymas are discussed here. Descriptions of follicular pyodermas are in Chapter 20.

Several infectious diseases are likewise pustular from the start, the pathogenic agent being capable of causing suppuration by itself (e.g. syphilis, tuberculosis, mycoses). Cutaneous diphtheria may exceptionally assume the appearance of impetigo vulgaris. Some exanthemata (varicella) are pustular at a certain stage of their course.

Portions of the Overview are taken and modified from Darier[1] (pp. 160–162).

Some chemical and drug-induced dermatoses are or may be pustular from the start. Mercurial agents, fumes of tar, and resinous plasters sometimes cause erythemas with small scattered miliary pustules. Oil of cade, crude coal tar, and analogous products sometimes give rise to papulopustules. Tar folliculitis, whether occupational or iatrogenic, tends to be more prominent in areas where the hair and hair follicles are larger (e.g. forearms and thighs). Certain toxidermas of internal origin are likewise pustular (iodides, bromides).

Persistent recalcitrant pustular dermatoses of the palms and soles are also included here.

It should be stressed that there are numerous and varied nonbacterial pus-forming skin diseases. The biological response of pus formation may be caused by such agents as viruses, parasites, heat, and systemic and topical drugs.[2] These are listed in the Table 19.

Impetigo

Impetigo (Fig. 10.1)[3] is manifest by small, very transient, turbid vesicles or pustules that rapidly break and become crusted. A few small intact vesicles and pustules may be present at the periphery.

The crusts are the hallmark of the disease. They are gummy, yellowish, and sometimes black due to blood. They are very superficial and have a stuck-on appearance. They extend slightly beyond the active border, and the edges may be curved upward. They are easily removed, leaving a sharply marginated, red, moist, superficial erosion, often with slight bleeding. The amount of pus present varies, but is usually not excessive. They vary, from dime to half-dollar (1.7 to 2.6 cm) sized. Sometimes confluence of small crusted areas produces a figure-8, gyrate, or some arcuate clusters (Fig. 10.2). Rarely, central clearing occurs, and as a result, unusual, large arcuate lesions form. A bright erythematous halo usually appears about the crusted lesions. The lesions heal, leaving light brown spots, but no scarring.

The sites of election are exposed portions of the body, especially the face, neck, and hands. In children, both the skin and mucosal surfaces of the nares are commonly involved, as are the fingers. Periungual lesions, pyogenic whitlow, and other morphological types of pyoderma may be present e.g. follicular pustules on the face and ecthyma on the legs.

Regional enlargement of the lymph nodes is not usually present, except in very extensive and long-standing cases such as impetigo of the scalp associated with pediculosis capitis.

Bullous Impetigo

Very thin-walled, semitranslucent, 1 to 5 cm, flaccid bullae may arise on normal-appearing skin. If held vertically, the dependent parts of the bulla show a more turbid appearance (hypopyon). These bullae rupture easily, shrivelling the epidermis. The lesions extend peripherally, and after rupture, central clearing, leaving a peripheral

Table 19: **Some Causes of Nonbacterial Pus-Forming Skin Diseases**

Fungus	
Deep	*North American blastomycosis*
	Lymphangitic sporotrichosis
	Cervicofacial actinomycosis
Immediate	*Intertriginous candidiasis*
Superficial	*Suppurative ringworm (kerion)*
Virus	*Herpes zoster*
	Varicella
	Variola
	Herpes simplex
	Vaccinia
	Hand-foot-and-mouth disease
Protozoa and Arthropods	*Amebiasis*
	Myiasis
Physical	*Miliaria pustulosa*
Systemic Drugs	*Iododerma*
	Bromoderma
Topical Applications	*Tar folliculitis*
	Sterile pustular patch tests
Injected Material	*Foreign body granuloma*
Miscellaneous	*Pustular acne vulgaris and its variants:*
	Rosacea
	Hidradentitis suppurativa
	Peri-oral dermatitis
	Pustular psoriasis
	Localized (palms and soles)
	Generalized
	Sneddon's subcorneal pustulosis
	Pustular dermatitis herpetiformis
	Furunculoid and acneform lesions in ulcerative colitis, Behçet's disease and early lesions of pyoderma gangrenosum
	Ulcers

ring of a collapsed bulla may occur. Sometimes gyrate or arcuate forms are seen. When the epidermis is removed, a moist area is visible. Later, a small amount of crusty scale forms. After healing, slight browning may be present. In addition to the areas of nonbullous impetigo, the axillae are commonly involved.

This eruption of bullous impetigo may be seen as a mixture with crusted impetigo, but not usually. The bullous eruption is rarely seen after puberty and is usually seen in the newborn.

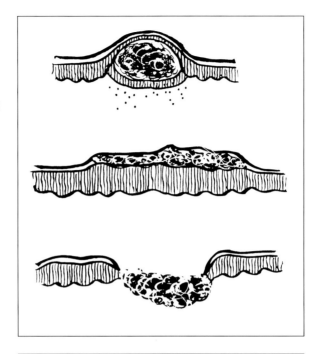

Figure 10.1
Impetigo and ecthyma.
Upper: Bockhart's or superficial
follicular impetigo.
Middle: Bullous impetigo.
Lower: Ecthyma.
Redrawn after Siemens.[3]

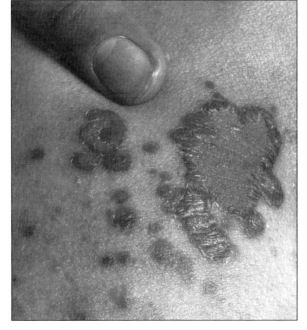

Figure 10.2 Impetigo on
buttocks. Note circular and
arcuate shapes. Peripheral
undermining of the border
can also be seen.

Bockhart's Impetigo

This is characterized by a 1 to 5 mm, superficial, epidermal pustule, sometimes with a hair piercing the center of the lesion. There is a bright-red inflammatory halo. Most lesions are full of thick yellow pus. The follicular nature is common, but not constant. The pustules do not rupture easily. When they do, superficial crusts are found. The hairy areas such as forearms, legs, and thighs are more commonly involved in this variety of impetigo.

Crusted impetigo, bullous impetigo, and Bockhart's impetigo may exist in the same patient, and really they could all be called superficial pyodermas of the skin.

From a morphological point of view, there are a few clues to indicate the causative organisms. Pyodermas due to staphylococci tend to produce more bullae; those due to streptococci tend to be more crusted.

DIFFERENTIAL DIAGNOSIS

The differential diagnosis of impetigo is not a problem, except with the bullous variety. The concern is to maintain vigilance and recognize the initial event or underlying cause. Underlying parasitic diseases, especially scabies and pediculosis capitis, must be considered. Perleche, epidermophytosis, insect bites, varicella, cuts and scrapes, herpes simplex, various eczemas, atopic dermatitis, and hangnails are some of the underlying causes. These impetiginized eruptions are sometimes not clearly recognized until the impetigo has improved or cleared. Sometimes it takes two or three attacks of impetigo before the underlying cause becomes obvious.

The follicular impetigos on the beard area are considered in more detail in Chapter 20. Other follicular pyodermas such as boils and furuncles are also described in Chapter 20, as are other nonpyodermatous follicular conditions such as acne and tar folliculitis.

The differential diagnosis of bullous impetigo is more complicated. Bullous insect bites have central puncta, usually occur in a grouped arrangement, and are most common on the lower legs. Bullous drug eruptions tend to be more disseminated, tenser and deeper, and associated with more erythema and often with erosive mucosal lesions. Bullous fixed drug eruptions are basically an erythema with secondary bulla formation. Brown or slate gray pigmentation is often present. There are usually only one or two lesions. Chronic bullous dermatosis of childhood should be mentioned as a differential diagnosis. In some cases where the bullae are very extensive and occur in the newborn, bullous impetigo is called Ritter von Rittershain's disease. The bullae may rapidly break, forming huge areas of exfoliation, called the staphylococcal scalded skin syndrome. The scalding effect is the result of of an exotoxin released by the staphylococcus.

Max Bockhart, 1887–1941, German Physician

Ecthyma

Ecthyma is a pustuloulcerative pyoderma. It starts as a pustule, usually flattened, with turbid contents. It rapidly reaches large coin size, then shrivels up into a more or less thickened, yellowish or brown, adherent crust, which is flattened or protuberant and sometimes even ostraceous, surrounded at first by a bullous collar and always by a congestive halo. When the crust is removed forcibly or by means of wet dressings, it is seen to cover a rounded or oval ulceration, more or less deeply encroaching upon the dermis. The borders of the ulcer are regular and clean-cut, the floor is red and pultaceous, sloping toward the center in the stage of advance, granulating in the stage of repair. The secretion consists of viscid or clotted brownish and blood-tinged pus. The base is not indurated, but sometimes diffusely edematous. Larger lesions may be malodorous.

Healing occurs by granulation and superficial scarring is common. Brown pigmentation is common throughout the lesion or at the periphery. Glandular enlargement, lymphangitis, and abscesses are rare complications. The lesions are usually multiple, rarely very numerous. They are, as a rule, of different ages, having originated from successive autoinoculation.

The site of predilection is on the legs and thighs, rarely the buttocks and back. It is common in the middle-aged or younger, and in debilitated patients. It commonly starts following trauma and then gradually spreads. Rarely, in some patients, ecthyma may be the starting point of larger pyogenic leg ulcers. "Wine Sores" are deep ulcers, usually with a heaped-up crust, usually not more than three or four, and occurring in the derelict male population of large cities. Trauma, low grade pyoderma, stasis with edema and occasionally ischemia are some of the multiple etiological factors.

Note that examination of this condition requires removal of the thick crust to see the characteristics of the ulcer beneath. This applies to all ulcerative conditions.

DIFFERENTIAL DIAGNOSIS

The differential diagnosis includes a considerable number of conditions, which at one stage or another may have a crusted pyogenic element.

First, there are other forms of common pyoderma, viz. follicular impetigo and infected wounds. Follicular impetigo should show some superficial pustules with centers pierced by a hair. Crusting is unusual. Infected wounds usually occur only at the sites of trauma.

Second, there is a group of proliferating ulcerating conditions with polycyclic borders, minute peripheral pustulation and a thick undermined advancing border behind which extensive scarring occurs. These are called pyoderma gangrenosum.

Third, gangrene, whether due to systemic septicemic conditions or local infections, in an unduly susceptible host may at times have an ecthymatous element.

Fourth, certain uncommon tropical or semitropical conditions such as diphtheria and leishmaniasis should be considered.

Fifth, consider other infectious diseases such as the malignant ecthymatous syphilides, the pustular aspects of fungating or ulcerative tuberculosis, and occasionally sporotrichosis. Ecthymatous acne is described under the acnes (see Chapter 20).

Flexural Streptococcal Pyoderma of Mitchell

The lesion of flexural streptococcal pyoderma is red, erosive, and moist, with a sticky yellowish exudate which accumulates at the periphery.[4] It was first reported between the toes, but is also frequently seen in the retroauricular folds of children with atopic dermatitis, and in the peri-anal area. It frequently is quite tender. It can be very difficult to distinguish from an acute weeping contact eczema. Occasionally, regional lymph nodes may be enlarged, or there may be more easily recognized pustular or yellow crusted lesions elsewhere. It has recently been discovered in the peri-anal area of children. (Other pyogenic and nonpyogenic cutaneous manifestations of streptococcal skin diseases are outlined and discussed under erysipelas in Chapter on erythemas.)

Persistent Pustular Dermatoses of Palms and Soles

Localized

Basic lesions of pustular psoriasis are pinhead to 1 to 2 mm flaccid pustules which exist in very large numbers in association with a tremendous erythema. The pustules arise on the erythematous skin, and even when they are not on areas of erythema, there is a halo of erythema about the isolated peripheral pustules arising on essentially normal skin. In some areas the pustules become confluent, but they never become larger than 0.5 cm in diameter. In some cases, at the borders, small 1 to 2 mm deep-seated vesicles may be seen. The borders are arcuate, and in some areas there is peripheral undermining, although this is not marked. Some of the lesions are circular. The confluent red areas containing some pustules also contain a micropapulation, which presumably is the start of more pustules. When the lesions resolve, they leave dried up pustules with a tan brown cover. The degree of erythema is variable, and in some areas appears dusky red in the center, almost like erythema multiforme. Often there is a fair degree of scaling, which seems to originate by a confluence of the scaly collarettes that develop as pustules or vesicles dry up. On the palms, it starts in the midportion and then spreads to the thenar and hypothenar eminences. On the soles, the eruption often starts in the instep and extends peripherally to the heels or the balls of the feet. Occasionally lateral and medial sides of the palms are involved; occasionally small groups of pustules are noted on the tips of the fingers and toes. There is almost never any involvement on the sides of the fingers and toes or in the web spaces, but the periungual and ungual areas may be involved. The eruption spreads both by peripheral extension and by the development of new outlying areas. Relative symmetry is quite a striking feature. Other evidence of psoriasis on the skin or nails is usually not present, but should be looked for on examination.

DIFFERENTIAL DIAGNOSIS

The differential diagnosis of pustular eruptions of the palms and soles includes the idiopathic type, including the pustular bacterid of Andrews and pustulosis palmaris et plantaris. Whether these two conditions actually exist is open to question, and I would not object strenuously if one were to delete this idiopathic group. Certainly from a morphological point of view, there is no reason to maintain them as a separate entity from pustular psoriasis.

Infectious eczematoid dermatitis (see Chapter 5) is a type of eczema. It usually is a solitary lesion up to 5 cm in diameter with an active peripheral vesiculopustular undermined border.

Acrodermatitis continua of Hallopeau and dermatitis repens are classified as varieties of infectious eczematoid dermatitis. Coincident with the introduction of potent antibiotics, these two conditions have almost disappeared.

While pompholyx may have a few pustules, the vast majority of the lesions are rather deep-seated and sago-grain-like blisters. When pustules are present, there are often other signs of pyoderma—erythema, swelling, and tenderness—findings usually rare in pustular psoriasis. The distribution of pompholyx is different, occurring on the sides of fingers and toes as well as the volar skin.

Blistering tinea with pustules is mentioned in the miscellaneous group.

Disseminated

1. Psoriasis, generalized pustular psoriasis
2. Reiter's disease
3. Keratoderma blennorrhagica*
4. Acrodermatitis enteropathica (hereditary or parenteral nutritional zinc deficiency)

The basic lesion is a subcorneal superficial pustule that rapidly forms superficial, small (1 cm) lakes of pus. The pus is yellow and moderately thick. Often a few small (1 to 2 mm) deep-seated vesicles are present on the pulps of the fingers and toes. When these pustules or vesicles coalesce, the lesions are sharply demarcated and have undermined edges.

The lesions form palm-sized or larger arcuate areas, which grow in an outward manner over quite large areas within 1 week. The advancing border is studded with hundreds of 1 mm or smaller subcorneal pustules on a bright red erythematous base. In places this erythema is diffuse with only a few small pustules. In areas, the erythema

George Andrews, 1891–1978, U.S. Dermatologist, New York

*This term is now (1997) used to describe the psoriasiform eruption of Reiter's. Formerly it referred to the late disseminated pustular keratotic sequelae of gonorrhea.

and pustulation may be linear. The skin is often also edematous. Aggregates of these minute pustules that have formed subcorneal lakes of pus of various size are then seen, followed by a shaggy irregular superficial exfoliation, which represents the loss of stratum corneum over the pustular lakes. In the central portion of the exfoliated areas, which is often a deep purplish color, the scale is gone and more small scattered pustules may be present.

The eruption is symmetrical and involves hands, feet, thighs, arms, lower torso, and the inguinal and axillary areas. The face and scalp are spared. Rather marked ankle edema is usually present. More than 80 percent of the body is frequently involved. When the process subsides, a purplish scaly erythema can be seen. The hands and feet are the last to clear up and the nails may never return to normal.

On the top and sides of the anterior portion of the tongue, on the lip, and on the anterior undersurface in the sulcus beside the inner aspect of the lower lip, circular and arcuate whitish bordered patches of up to 2 cm in diameter can sometimes be found. The border is just palpable, and with the hand lens, seems to be made up of minute subepithelial pustules. This is called annulus migrans. The central area is free of pustules, but looks redder and slightly more glossy than the surrounding mucosa. The border of these lesions is neither as wide, nor as white, as the border of the lesions of geographic tongue. Both eruptions can change markedly in size and shape in 1 week. I have never seen lesions of geographic tongue on any area but the tongue, but annulus migrans is common on the mucosal lip.[5]

About and under the nails, seropurulent scale accumulates beneath which free pus with a foul smell may develop. Also at the edges, pus may be seen underneath the undermined border. The nails are lifted up by the process, especially in the distal half, and in some cases the nail plate itself is mixed in with this process. At times this resembles subungual keratosis formation, but the material lifting up the nail plate is composed of pus and serum as well as stratum corneum. The nail plate may not be elevated much, but may show a yellowish onycholysis, which on examination is seen to be due to a pus lake. In some, there is more keratotic material; in others, there is more oozing and crusting.

On other areas of the palmar and plantar skin, e.g. heels, instep, and palms, the lesions are more keratotic, often with a translucent brown appearance centrally and a more yellowish keratotic periphery. Frank pus formation is not as obvious in these areas as about the nails.

On the genitals (usually male; genital acropustular eruptions are rare in females) and perianally, the predominant aspect is a pustular erythematosquamous eruption with peripheral undermining. Around some of the pustules or lakes of pus there is bright erythema.

DIFFERENTIAL DIAGNOSIS

To make a definitive diagnosis on morphology alone is very difficult.

If there is a family or personal history of psoriasis, if other characteristic psoriasis lesions are present on the elbows or scalp, and if the pattern of an accompanying arthritis is reasonably compatible with so-called psoriatic arthritis, then pustular psoriasis should be the diagnosis. (See also "Psoriasis" in Chapter 6.) Generalized pustular psoriasis also may have pustular lesions on the palms and soles.

If there is a penile discharge (or discharge from a prostate massage) from which gonococcus can be grown, then gonorrheal keratoderma blennorrhagica may be the diagnosis. In these cases, the seropurulent keratoses may be bigger and thicker and more numerous. Arthritis may also be present.

Reiter's disease usually presents more exudative lesions, with more marked involvement of the mucosa. Heaped-up ostraceous crusty scales may be present on many areas (e.g. elbows, knees, ankles, backs of hands) as well as the palms and soles. Arthralgias with urethral and conjunctival discharges should also be present.

Acrodermatitis enteropathica is characterized by psoriasiform or impetiginous skin lesions on the acral areas and around natural orifices along with alopecia and diarrhea. Stomatitis, glossitis, blepharitis, retardation of growth, and susceptibility to infection may also be present.

There is no morphological certainty separating these conditions one from another. I have seen a patient who at one time had an attack of generalized pustular psoriasis, the next time Reiter's disease with conjunctival discharge, arthralgia, and gonococci in the urethral discharge. Two years later he developed another attack of generalized pustular psoriasis. It seems as if the disseminated persistent pustular eruptions are a reaction pattern that can be stimulated to occur by different known and unknown causes.

Septicemic or Pyemic States

Now rare, these states appear in patients as deep-seated epidermal-dermal pustules. The amount of pus varies, and some cases present more as purpura, e.g. gonococcemia. The eruption, being blood borne, is widely disseminated. Other systemic findings confirm the diagnosis.

Miscellaneous

Many eczemas and dermatitides may develop secondary pyoderma. Pompholyx, atopic dermatitis, and vesiculating tinea pedis are three examples. Usually marked erythema, edema, pain and tenderness, and frank pustules or pyogenic crusts may be seen. At times, especially with pedal blistering epidermophytosis, in addition to the local findings, an ascending lymphangitis and lymphadenitis with fever may be present. Sometimes, especially on the hands, it may be difficult to determine clinically the difference between a flare of the underlying eruption and a secondary pyoderma. Deep fissuring, swelling, tenderness, and lack of response to usual therapy should make the clinician suspicious.

Many chronic infectious diseases may at times cause discharges of purulent material or have actual pustules. The papulocrusted variety of secondary syphilis consists of an extensive eruption irregularly scattered on trunk, limbs, face, and scalp.

It consists of round lenticular crusts, which are brownish yellow, swollen, slightly adherent, sometimes exuberant, ostraceous, or rupial. The crusts cover a papule with a smooth moist surface, not an ulceration as one might expect. Malignant syphilides of the ecthymatous type begin, before undergoing ulceration, as a large papule with an epidermis raised by pus, which hardens into a crust. Under the crust and at its periphery, the ulceration develops and progresses. Circinate scarring tuberculocrusted ulcerative syphilitic granuloma may have some pus formation. Bomb-explosion-arranged lesions may be seen. Various forms of tuberculosis ulcers, vegetating tuberculosis, and papulonecrotic tuberculides may at times have a pustular element. Tuberculosis sinuses may also discharge pus. Rarely glanders, anthrax, cutaneous diphtheria (desert sore), and some deep mycoses such as sporotrichosis, blastomycosis, and cervicofacial actinomycosis occasionally have a pustular element. The peripheral lesion about candidiasis may be pustular.

Some drug erythemas, especially those from iodides and bromides, may present with a vegetating pustular eruption.

There is a variety of dermatitis herpetiformis which at times has a definite pustular element. Generalized pustular psoriasis has already been mentioned.

Subcorneal pustular dermatosis (Sneddon-Wilkinson disease) is a widespread, minute, pustular eruption occurring in arcs and clusters especially on the torso, particularly groins, axillae, and sides of elderly men. There is an erythematous flare in the early stages. Within a few days the pustules dry up, leaving a superficial leafy scale or crust. The pustules tend to form groups in annular or gyrate shape, forming a serpiginous outline. The pustules may be large (1 cm), and the fluid in them may be translucent at the top and turbid at the bottom as in bullous impetigo. Faint brown pigmentation occurs. There are waves of pustules. The face and mucous membranes are not affected.

Acneform pustular eruptions on the extremities may be associated with ulcerative colitis and Behçet's disease.

Pustular porol closure eruptions of infants and children may present pustular eruptions in the form of miliaria pustulosa and multiple scattered intradermal pea-sized papules, which on puncture reveal a small amount of creamy pus (miliary coccal abscess of little children).

Anthrax starts as a bulla with an intense inflammatory reaction. Rapidly the bulla breaks, exposing a black eschar. This is surrounded by groups of small vesicles or pustules which can be found in a peripheral erythematous zone. Swelling and edema are quite marked. Regional adenitis is common. In some cases, gangrene occurs, the regional lymph nodes break down, and death may occur.

Superficial and intermediate mycoses (such as kerion and mucocutaneous candidiasis) may have a pustular element.

Helusi Behçet, 1889–1948, Turkish Dermatologist, Istanbul

Darrell Sheldon Wilkinson, 1919–   English Dermatologist, High Wycombe

Some viral infections such as herpes simplex and zoster may have a pustular phase.

Impetigo herpetiformis is a pustular psoriasis-like eruption with fever, which occurs in pregnant women, especially on the medial thighs. I have never made this diagnosis.

Miscellaneous conditions, which may have a pustular element are some protozoal diseases (e.g. amebiasis), tar folliculitis, some foreign body granulomas, pustular acne, and the secondary formation of pus in some ulcers.

Erythema neonatorum allergicum, infantile acropustulosa, transient neonatal pustular melanosis, and neonatal acne may have a prominent pustular element. Miliara pustulosa should also be mentioned.

Erosive pustular dermatosis of the scalp occurs in elderly women and presents as chronic, extensive, pustular, crusted, and occasionally eroded lesions. Scarring alopecia is a common sequela.[6]

Folliculitis decalvans is a scarring pustular scalp eruption of unknown etiology.

References

1. Darier J. Textbook of dermatology. Pollitzer S, trans. Philadelphia:Lea & Febiger, 1920.
2. Jackson R. Non-bacterial pus-forming diseases of the skin. Can Med Assoc J 1974; 111:801–806.
3. Siemens HW. General diagnosis and therapy of skin diseases. Wiener K, trans. Chicago:University of Chicago Press, 1958.
4. Mitchell JH. Streptococcic dermatoses of the ears. JAMA 1937; 108:361–366.
5. Hubler WR. Lingual lesions of generalized pustular psoriasis. J Am Acad Dermatol 1984; 11:1069–1076.
6. Pye RJ, Peachey RDG, Burton JL. Erosive pustular dermatosis of the scalp. Br J Dermatol 1979; 100:559–566.

CHAPTER 11
Papules

A small (less than 1.0 cm) solid persistent elevation above skin level and caused by an increase in number and size of cells and cell products rather than an accumulation of liquid.

Overview

A papule is a small, solid elevation usually above skin level, caused by an increase in number and size of cells and cell products rather than accumulation of liquid. Exceptionally, small papules may be imbedded so deeply in the skin that they protrude scarcely at all and can only be palpated. If they are almost level with the surface of the skin, they may at first glance appear as a spot, but on palpation prove to be papular. This is seen in the lupus vulgaris papule. Papules may be very flat, especially on the palms and soles. Papules may have clearly demarcated edges; they may be constricted at the base; or they may even be pedunculated and pendulous if the stem is long enough. They may be elongated (filiform papule), with or without a horny tip.[1]

Other types of lesions may, on superficial examination, give the impression of being papules. This sometimes occurs if a wheal remains very small and does not grow peripherally. Small erythemas may also appear to be slightly elevated, e.g. the papular erythemas of erythema multiforme.

Papules may be so small that they are just perceptible. The largest ones may reach the size of a lentil (0.5–1.0 cm in diameter). Papules may be red (inflammatory) or pale (anemic) brown, white, or simply normal skin color. Some cellular infiltrates have a color of their own, which becomes apparent only after the accompanying erythema is eliminated by glass pressure.

Papules are extremely multiform. Their shape depends in part on the level of the underlying cellular infiltrate in the skin. It is possible to draw conclusions as to the depth of the cellular infiltrate from the appearance of the papule [Fig. 11.1]. One can distinguish superficial epidermal and deeper cutaneous papules. Superficial papules are plateau like with sharp edges. Deep-seated ones are hemispherical with indistinct borders. These differences can be understood from pathological findings. If the increase in cells is located mainly in the horny layer, the

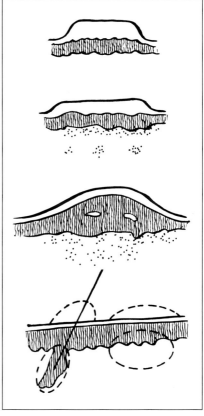

Figure 11.1 Schematic diagrammatic representation of shapes of papules. *Top to bottom:* Epidermal; epidermal-dermal or lichenoid; epidermal-dermal or eczematoid; and follicular and non-follicular. Redrawn after Siemens.[1]

*Portions of the Overview have been taken and modified from Siemens[1] (pp. 57–71).

keratohyaline layer, and the rete of the epidermis, as seen in verrucae planae, then the border of the pathological process is clearly visible and appears sharply delineated. However, if the accumulation of cells lies in the dermis, as is seen in the papule of secondary syphilis, then the entire thickness of the epidermis is lifted, the center more than the periphery, and the edges appear less distinct, forming a flat, hemispheric prominence.

If the infiltrate is localized about a follicle, it follows the follicle vertically downward into the depths of the skin. These follicular infiltrates may also push themselves steeply above the surface. Therefore, follicular papules are mostly cone-shaped or pointed. The follicular location of a disease can also be recognized from the pointed follicular opening or hair in the center. A dark plug or a light, pointed, even filiform scale in the center may take the place of the hair (keratosis pilaris, lichen planopilaris). If all follicles in a skin area appear to be papular, the follicular character manifests itself by the strikingly regular arrangement of the lesions, especially the equal distance between them. This picture resembles "goose flesh", where the follicles are forced to a more erect, protruding position by contraction of their attached arrector pili smooth muscles. One could call these physiological swellings "pseudopapules". The different picture of a nonfollicular arrangement is shown by the quite irregular positions of the squamous papules in eczema. In spite of all these characteristics, the decision as to whether an eruption is follicular or nonfollicular may still be difficult in some cases. Histologic examination may help decide the issue.

There are two types of papules which play an important part in practical diagnosis, namely the lichenoid papule and the eczematoid papule. The lichenoid papule is the characteristic primary lesion of lichen planus but is encountered in a great variety of papular rashes (lichenoid eczema, lichenoid tuberculids, lichenoid syphilids, lichenoid trichophytids). It is a superficial epidermocutaneous papule. The increase in cells takes place in the horny layer (hyperkeratosis), in the keratohyaline layer beneath (hypergranulosis), and in the other layers of the epidermis (acanthosis). The dermal cellular infiltrate, however, fills at most only the papillae and a narrow subpapillary zone. It then ends rather abruptly, leaving the deeper layers of the dermis almost free. Infiltration of the upper dermis is accompanied by exudation of fluid from the vessels. This edema of the cutis is also very superficial, involving mostly the papillae, which swell and become mushroom-shaped.

In correlation with its histologic structure, the lichen planus papule has the following clinical characteristics: its surface is smooth and of a waxy glossiness, since it consists mainly of a compact, thickened horny layer. This is the reason why the lichen planus papule is rarely excoriated by scratching. As the papules increase in size, the granular layer, which is thickened in some places, becomes visible as delicate, spider-web, star- or drop-shaped bluish or milky-white figures (Wickham's striae). These striae become more visible after the horny layer is cleared with a droplet of oil. The shape of the lichen planus papule is plateau-like. From above, it does not appear round but polygonal or mosaic-like, because its borders follow the surface relief of the skin. Quite frequently the lichen planus papule has small extensions which may make it star-shaped. The characteristic flat and polygonal form is best observed in the smallest papules, especially if tangential lighting is used to make the smooth surface appear shiny. Often, in order to make the diagnosis, it is necessary to look for and find these small early papules. In contrast to the eczematoid papule, the lichenoid papule has no tendency to evolve into advanced type of lesions such as blisters, pustules, or erosions.

The eczematoid papule, i.e. the primary lesion of eczema, is located a little deeper than the lichenoid papule. The horny layer is not greatly thickened, but there usually is parakeratosis with absence of the keratohyaline layer. The increased cellularity in this type of papule is situated in the deeper layers of the epidermis and also in the cutis. The infiltrate in the cutis does not end suddenly below the papillae but continues as a perivascular infiltrate into the depths. The accompanying edema is also much more extensive and is not confined to the papillae, but spreads through the epidermis and cutis. In the epidermis the marked accumulation of fluid separates the cells, forming small, liquid-filled cavities (spongiosis) which may coalesce into a larger cavity and convert the papule into a vesicle. Because of the succulence and the loosening of the epidermis, and also the desquamation and thinning of the horny layer, the eczematoid papule, in contrast to the lichenoid papule, is easily scratched open. Its center may become eroded or may be entirely shelled out by the scratching nail. Finally, it is replaced by a pinhead-sized, round erosion with or without a crust ("eczema pore"). Thus the clinical differences between eczematoid and lichenoid papules can well be explained by the differences in their histologic structures. The eczematoid papule is hemispheric, and only exceptionally conical and pointed, if it happens to be follicular. Usually, it has an indistinct edge, so that the border line of the papule cannot be exactly defined. The whole structure is less clear-cut than is the lichenoid papule, and its surface is not glossy. Its clinical course is marked by a tendency to develop into a vesicle because of spongiosis. In contrast to the stability of the lichenoid papule, the eczematoid papule runs a typical course, the stages of which are erythema, papule, vesicle, erosion, crust, scale. In most eczemas, one notices several stages existing simultaneously; sometimes one can find the entire development of the lesion from erythema to scale recorded on the skin.

In papules of somewhat larger circumference, which also extend a little deeper, a dome-shaped form becomes especially marked (papular secondary syphilis, xanthomas) [Fig. 11.2]. Some papules are depressed in the center, or they have in the center a small dull area or a larger area with a irregular depression (molluscum contagiosum).

Papules may be so close together that they no longer form separate prominences, but instead a common plateau, a papule overgrown in width. In this case the skin is infiltrated horizontally, in width rather than in depth. This occurs frequently with

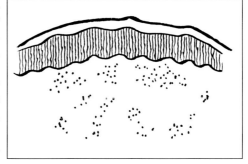

Figure 11.2 The shape of a dermal papule. Redrawn after Siemens.[1]

lichenoid papules, hence this condition of the skin has been called lichenification. There may be small papules visible on the periphery, or groups of discrete papules can be found in the vicinity, which indicate that the skin change developed by the crowding together and confluence of papules. If lichenification has been produced by dense grouping of papules, it must, like the lichenoid papule itself, consist of increased amounts of cells, either with or without inflammatory exudate. The thickening is easy to detect by raising a fold which feels thicker in the lichenified area than in a symmetric or otherwise comparable site. The very typical change of surface relief makes it possible to see the plaque-like infiltration of the skin. The finer furrows of the skin surface are smoothed out by the infiltrate and exudate, which causes the few remaining ones to become deeper. In other words, the surface relief becomes coarsened and reminiscent of shagreen* leather. If the edge of the lichenified area is distinct, it can be noticed that the level of the changed skin is higher than that of the normal surrounding skin. If the transition to normal skin is a gradual one, the difference between the levels can, of course, not be so clearly noticed, and the coarsened skin relief gradually fades into the delicate, hardly visible furrows of the normal skin. If the entire skin is lichenified (as in some erythrodermas) so that there are no borders at all, one should compare it with the skin of a normal person. The lichenification may be very fine or coarse. The papules may become so large and the edges so rounded that they resemble the convolutions of the brain (hypertrophic lichenification). If the thickening of the skin of the face causes deep, cut-like furrows with bulging infiltrated skin between, one speaks of leontiasis ("lion's skin"). Because of the disappearance of the small furrows, lichenified skin is smoother and glossier, particularly if itching causes the patient to rub it constantly. In other cases it is more dull and looks dusty from being covered with fine scales. Sometimes there are larger scales, or even more coherent horny masses, suggestive of the verrucous change of confluent viral warts. There may be point- to pinhead-sized erosions on the altered skin, indicating the excoriation of individual papules or vesicles. The color of the lichenified skin area may be red, due to the inflammatory hyperemia, but it is more frequently pale and somewhat grayish. After a process of long duration, brown hyperpigmentation or, rarely, hypopigmentation or depigmentation develops. The surrounding skin may also be a hyperpigmented brown color.[1]

In many cases, rubbing or scratching play a big role in the production of lichenification, but I doubt that all lichenification is caused by external friction. For example, must all of the skin be rubbed to produce the lichenification of erythroderma?

Acanthosis and infiltration are not the only causes of a more pronounced accentuation and coarsening of the skin's surface relief. It may also be brought about by other processes, e.g. a thickening of the horny layer (ichthyosis). Especially on the fingers, ichthyosis may resemble lichenification very closely and may be confused with it. In cutis hyperelastica (rubber skin) and in old age, wrinkles may produce a distinct pattern, particularly in the face. The highest degree of coarsening of the skin's relief is encountered in cutis rhomboidalis nuchae. This condition is produced by sun-induced degenerative changes in the cutis. In none of these conditions are papules the preceding lesion.

---

*Leather with a rough, granular surface, frequently dyed green.

The papule of prurigo is a variant of the eczematoid papule described previously. The prurigo papule is a more or less dome-shaped, rarely pointed (follicular) eminence with indistinct borders. It is not very striking and may be easily overlooked, especially because its color is frequently normal, though it may be reddish or brownish. Its presence can be recognized easily, as a rule, by the point- to pinhead-sized, roundish erosions or bloody crusts which mark the location of excoriated papules. If a disseminated rash consists of excoriated papules resembling prurigo paules, it is called pruriginous. Pruriginous, therefore, means "papulo-erosive", and this expression is usually used to designate eruptions of a kind which, in their morphology, resemble the excoriated papular phase of atopic dermatitis and not the plaque-like circumscribed unexcoriated lichenification of lichen simplex chronicus. If the prurigo papule is not eroded, its surface, like that of the papule of chronic eczema, is sometimes smooth and almost glossy, but is more commonly covered with fine scales and dull. These clinical characteristics give clear indication that the histologic structure of the prurigo papule is the same as that of the eczematoid papule except for the more marked acanthosis and the tendency to lack vesiculation.

Eczematoid as well as prurigo papules may, by apposition of groups of closely packed foci of infiltration, grow into larger papules, which may then form larger than pea-sized hemispheric prominences. This kind of lesion may have a smooth or excoriated surface. Its relief may be coarsened, but more frequently it is dull from scale formation, or it is pitted and even verrucous. These large groups of papules which sometimes are closely grouped together and sometimes spaced more widely apart are called nodular or obtuse papules, or prurigo nodularis. They can be considered as circumscribed large papular areas of lichenification. They are either pale, skin-colored, or brown and horny. They have the disagreeable property of being very resistant to treatment and, peculiarly, much more resistant than areas of lichenifications.[1]

Accumulation of scale on a macule does not make a papule—it makes an erythematosquame or a scaly macule. Because you can feel the scale on a macule it is not a papule.

Papular Dermatoses

Lichen Planus

The eruptive lesion of lichen planus* is a small (1 to 2 mm) flattened polygonal papule, sometimes slightly depressed or umbilicated in the center, with a smooth or shining surface. The length of the sides is not necessarily the same; this produces at times rather lopsided lesions. Not all the papules are polygonal (Fig. 11.3). Some, especially the small and early ones, are circular; others have one straight side with the remaining periphery being annular. The papules have a dry and firm consistency and their color varies from a yellowish pink to a dusky or purplish red to a normal skin color. Most of the time they are purplish red. The presence of white or grayish opaline streaks and dots makes, on the surface of the papules, a network of streaks or stars on a pink background (the sign of the net, or Wickham's striae). These are visible

*Portions of this description have been taken and modified from Siemens[1] (pp. 131,132).

only on well-developed papules which may be isolated or grouped in plaques. If the papules are moistened with oil or water, the horny layer is made transparent, and the net can be seen more easily.

The incipient papules are punctiform, pink, and glistening; they enlarge in a few days or weeks. Full-grown papules may remain isolated in discrete eruptions, but they often become more numerous and confluent in plaques of variable size. The shape is round, oval, or irregular, usually thicker on the borders than in the middle. They are of a dusky red or brownish color. Annular lesions are common. Lichen planus papules may develop in lines, presumably from scratching (Koebner phenomonon).

Their surface is covered with fine, very adherent, often scarcely visible scales, but the fingernail passing over the surface will show a scaly line. The papules constituting the plaque are sometimes recognizable, especially on the borders. Extensive plaques, when there is complete confluence, are cut in squares by lozenge-shaped or polygonal designs having a smooth and glistening surface, producing a mosaic appearance. On the surrounding skin, isolated papules and other groupings may be seen.

The plaques and papules may become colored varying shades of brown, and sometimes there is a brown areola. The most common localization is on the anterior surface of the wrists, the forearms, and the legs, but it is also seen on the flanks, lumbar region, genital regions, buccal mucosa, neck, inner aspect thighs, and palmar and plantar regions. It is rare on the face and hairy scalp.[1]

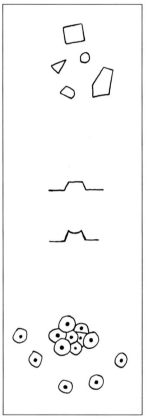

Figure 11.3 *Upper:* Plane view of lichen planus papules. *Middle:* Cross section of lichen planus papules. *Lower:* Plane view of lichen sclerosus et atrophicus.

The eruption may be universal and produce an erythroderma. Scratching may cause lichenification, which may mask the typical eruption.

DIFFERENTIAL DIAGNOSIS

The differential diagnosis of lichen planus varies considerably, depending on the region involved and the type of lichen planus. Common lichen planus should be distinguished from the following.

Lichen planus-like keratoses are usually solitary, irritated and located on sun-damaged skin of the upper torso and forearms.

Lichenoid drug eruptions are of two types: those due to contact with color-film developers and those due to the systemic administration of gold or the anti-malarials such as quinacrine or chloroquine. The list of drugs which rarely can cause lichenoid eruptions is very long. Rarely, these eruptions may be indistinguishable from lichen planus. Some pityriasis rosea-like drug eruptions may develop into lichen planus-like eruptions.

Color developer (C-D2) contact lichen planus starts on the dorsa of the fingers, hands, and forearms and may spread to other areas, including the V of the neck and the penis. It starts as an eczematous dermatitis which slowly subsides, becoming more and more papular, lichenified, and lichen planus-like.

Lichen nitidus is an eruption of small (1 mm) flat, glistening, skin-colored, sometimes slightly dusky isolated dermal papules, which never become confluent, and localize on the torso and penis. It is common in the prepubertal child, while lichen planus is a disease of adults.

Lichen amyloidosus occurs on the shins and consists of a palm-sized cluster of round, purplish, mainly dermal papules. The papules are not confluent, not polygonal, and not scaly.

Lichen scrofulosorum is a papular, pinhead-sized, often follicular eruption. The papules are flattened, polygonal, pale yellow or dusky red color, of soft consistency, with a smooth glistening surface. These papules are arranged in plaques, rings, or semicircles. The flanks and loin are the usual localizations. In some cases the eruption is definitely follicular, with spinous lesions. Also, it may blend into the papulosquamous and papulonecrotic tuberculids.

Lichenoid syphilis presents as follicular squamous, 2 to 5 mm papules of a dusky red color, and crowned with a dry scale, which is enclosed in the follicular orifices and not easily removed. Arciform lesions may be present. A principal feature is the degree of dermal infiltration, i.e. the papules are epidermal-dermal papules. Alopecia, mucous patches, and other stigmata of syphilis may be present. Other types of lesions may be present. The eruption tends to be more disseminated than lichen planus.

Lichenified papular psoriasis has a deep red color, has a mica-like scale, and shows circular lesions. Pitting and subungual keratoses may be seen on the nails.

Lichen simplex chronicus has hemispherical papules, less glistening, and has no white streaks. The papules commonly form plaques. The lesions are less clearly defined. They have no appreciable scale.

Lichenified atopic dermatitis, especially flexural, and particularly in children, may present as a papular eruption. The papules are flattish and whitish yellow in color. They are confluent, but the plaques so formed are not as clearly defined as the plaques of lichen planus. The occurrence of the papules in areas where the normal skin lines are accentuated is usually easily seen.

Certain varieties of lichenified eczema may resemble lichen planus.

Flat-topped purplish papules may occur over the skin area in association with the changes of chronic venous stasis. They are firm, not itchy, and disappear with support or relief of stasis.

Verrucae planae are small epidermic papules, not more than 3 mm in diameter, flattened, and barely protuberant. They are round or polygonal, and sharply circumscribed; the color of normal skin with grayish or brownish hue. The surface is finely dotted. There is no scale. Linear lesions are common. Sometimes plaques are formed of confluent papules, but peripheral papules or other isolated papules are usually seen. This is usually a childhood disease. The sites of predilection are the face, forearms, and dorsa of the hands.

Infantile papular acrodermatitis (one type of Gianotti-Crosti syndrome) presents in young children as a symmetrical lichenoid purpuric eruption occurring almost exclusively on the extensor surfaces of the extremities. Occasional lesions may be seen on the ears, cheeks, and buttocks. The papules are flat-topped, 2 to 5 mm across, and lichenoid, but without the irregular linear borders of lichen planus and with no Wickham's striae. There is little or no scale. Mucosal involvement is rare or nonexistent. As time passes, the eruption becomes more confluent and the lichenoid character decreases in significance.

Frictional lichenoid eruption consists of skin-colored, discrete, nondescript 1 to 3 mm papules on the dorsa of the hands, the elbows, and the knees. It occurs in children, primarily in the summer.

Two rare conditions of doubtful existence which have been described as resembling or being a variety of lichen planus are lichen ruber moniliformis and lichen planus erythematosus.

Lichen aureus is mentioned in the pigmented purpuric eruptions.

Lichen Planus of Mucous Membranes

Lichen planus occurs on the buccal mucosa, usually opposite the interdental cleft. In some cases, the dorsum of the tongue, the inner aspect of the upper and lower lip, and the soft palate are involved. In some cases. only mucosal lesions are present. The eruption consists of superficial, grayish white to purplish lesions in the form of minute puncta, linear streaks, circles, and reticulated or solid areas. Mostly the lesions are smooth, but sometimes there is a slight roughness. The lesions do not peel off. Rarely, superficial erosions, bullous lesions, and deep chronic ulcers are present. Even more rarely seen is the development of hard epithelial carcinoma.

DIFFERENTIAL DIAGNOSIS

This condition must be distinguished from leukoplakia. Leukoplakia is, as the name implies, basically a white plaque with more or less infiltration. Dotted, circular, or reticulated areas are not seen. Leukoplakia is white; lichen planus has a purplish hue. Leukoplakia is common in the commissures and lower alveolar ridge areas; lichen planus is rare in these areas. Keratoses and epithelial carcinoma formation are not uncommon.

Another purplish erosive oral mucosal eruption is discoid lupus erythematosus. In this condition the lesions are more localized, usually erosive, and often show some

Agostino Crosti, 1896– Italian Dermatologist

Fernando Gianotti, 1920– Italian Dermatologist

telangiectases and atrophy. The hard palate and buccal mucosa are favorite locations. A raised erythematous border with central depression (or atrophy) may be present. Thrush presents as a superficially erosive eruption with varying sized areas of white peeling beneath which a velvety moist surface is seen. The white sponge nevus of Cannon is a fixed white linear plaque on the buccal mucosa.

Lichen planus of the red lip (usually the lower) presents a similar picture to that on the oral mucosa, except that erosions are rare.

DIFFERENTIAL DIAGNOSIS

Lichen planus of the lips must be distinguished from discoid lupus erythematosus, which usually shows more scaling, some atrophy, and frequently involvement of the adjacent lip skin with the usual features of cutaneous discoid lupus erythematosus, sometimes with a raised erythematous border. Other white scaly lesions to be included in the differential diagnosis are solar cheilitis and, rarely, psoriasis. Solar cheilitis is a scaly, fissured, wrinkled lesion, sometimes with interspersed small keratotic spots that appear on areas of the lower lip exposed to the sun. Lichen planus of the conjunctiva and nasal mucosa is very rare.

Lichen planus of the male and female genital mucosa and semimucosa presents many features similar to that of the oral mucosa. However, the lesions are whiter and erosions are uncommon. On the semimucosa, characteristic lichen planus papules are seen. Also, circinate and annular forms are common, especially on the penis.

DIFFERENTIAL DIAGNOSIS

The differential diagnosis includes white lesions of genitalia and is discussed fully under "Lichen Sclerosus et Atrophicus".

Linear Lichen Planus

This type of lichen planus occurs most frequently on the extremities of children and usually follows the linear pattern of a linear epidermal nevus, i.e. they are not related to the course of blood or lymph vessels, nerves, or Voight's lines, but follow the lines of Blaschko. It should be distinguished from Koebnerization, where the linear lesions are rarely over 2 cm in length.

DIFFERENTIAL DIAGNOSIS

The differential diagnosis of these lesions includes linear psoriasis (which has the characteristic psoriatic lesions), linear epidermal nevus (which is more brownish and warty, is persistent, and does not have the previously described lichen planus papules), and lichen striatus. Lichen striatus is a short-lived (about 6 months) linear eruption composed of small papulovesicles at the beginning, which become pink discrete lichenoid papules that coalesce into small plaques. The papules are not violaceous, not umbilicated, and show no Wickham's striae.

Alfred Blaschko, 1858–1922, Berlin Dermatologist

A. Bruce Cannon, 1885–1950, U.S. Dermatologist, New York

Christian August Voight, 1809–1890, Austrian Anatomist, Vienna

Hypertrophic (Verrucous) Lichen Planus (Lichen Planus Obtusus)

Hypertrophic lichen planus consists of pea- to coin-sized pinkish or red warty protuberances, usually covered with very adherent, brownish, chalky, horny masses. Most frequently they are grouped, or even confluent, forming plaques in a roughly outlined network. Surfaces may have an alveolar appearance, produced by numerous corneal cones dipping into the cutaneous pores. Areas of brown pigmentation may be interspersed between the hypertrophic plaques. The anterior portion of the legs is the site of predilection.

Palmar and Plantar Lichen Planus

In these areas, the papules of lichen planus are sometimes horny, pointed, and wartlike; sometimes sharply demarcated red and scaly spots; and sometimes bullous. Sometimes partial keratodermas may be present.

Bullous Lichen Planus

Rarely, bullous lichen planus appears as 1 to 2 cm noninflammatory bullae in a widespread distribution, usually excluding the mucosae. In rare cases, small vesicles occur at the tops of lichen planus papules. Usually, typical lichen planus papules are also seen, although these may not develop until later in the course of the disease.

Lichen Planus of the Eyelids

Lichen planus of the eyelids can exist in three forms: (1) the ordinary lilac-colored, slightly delled, shiny papules; (2) papules arranged to form annular lesions, as are frequently seen on the glans penis; or (3) sepia brown, retiform pigmentations simulating erythema ab igne, and similar to the brown staining seen in certain patients with lichen planus in the late stages of regression.

Lichen Planus of the Nails

The earliest changes are longitudinal striations or ridging. As the early ridging becomes more pronounced, the nail plate is often reduced to two paperlike leaflets with the cuticle growing forward as a pannus and attaching itself to the nail plate (ptergium). Rarely, complete shedding of the nail plate with scarring and obliteration of the nail fold may occur. These changes are usually seen in extensive long-standing disease. They are probably not specific for lichen planus.

Follicular Lichen Planus

Lichen planopilaris is a patchy, noninflammatory cicatricial alopecia of the scalp, a follicular spinous eruption on the scalp, trunk, or extremities, and often a cicatricial alopecia of the axillary or pubic region. The areas of alopecia may not show the lesions of lichen planus. Typical lesions of lichen planus may also be seen on the glabrous skin or mucous membranes. In children, horny filiform papules may be distributed on the torso and extremities without alopecia (for lichen spinulosus, see Chapter 20).

Atrophic or Sclerotic Lichen Planus
On two occasions I have seen areas of atrophy of the epidermis and upper dermis arising in areas adjacent to typical lichen planus papules, with other typical lichen planus elsewhere without atrophy or scarring. Both lesions have been on the forearms. In both cases the scarring lesions had been there for many years and had remained persistent even though the other lichen planus lesions had come and gone. There were no mucosal lesions.

Destructive Lichen Planus
Cicatricial alopecia of the scalp, bullae, and ulceration of the toes and soles of the feet along with permanent loss of the toenails, in addition to chronic, painful, and crippling ulcerations of the plantar surfaces, have also been reported as occurring with typical lichen planus elsewhere and with the histology of lichen planus.

Lichen planus subtropicum is a variant of lichen planus in which numerous round or oval sharply marginated macules on the forehead, dorsa of the hands, and forearms. Eventually the eruption becomes papular. The emphasis on localization to sun-exposed areas is a particular feature of this condition.

Lichen planus-like keratoses are mentioned under "Solar (Actinic) Keratoses" in Chapter 15.

Lichen Nitidus

The basic lesion found in lichen nitidus is a 1 mm, discrete, flat-topped, dome-shaped, or occasionally umbilicated papule. Fine radiations traverse the surface of many papules from near the summit to just beyond the periphery. The dome-shaped papules are tense and glistening, and very rarely, with a hand lens, a tiny vesicle is visible on the tip. The lesions are usually disseminated, never coalesce, and show no grouping, although sometimes they tend to pack together. Many of the lesions may be follicular. Linear lesions are not common.

The shaft of the penis is usually involved. Other areas of involvement are the flexor wrists and abdomen. The eruption is more common in children and young adults.

DIFFERENTIAL DIAGNOSIS
The differential diagnosis of lichen nitidus includes small lesions of lichen planus, verrucae planae, and rarely, tuberculous and syphilitic lichenoid eruptions. Lichenoid drug eruptions should also be considered. In most cases, the diagnosis is not difficult.

Rarely, lichen nitidus and lichen planus occur together. Linear lichen nitidus can occur.

Lichen Sclerosus et Atrophicus

The basic lesion of lichen sclerosus et atrophicus is an irregular, often polygonal, flat-topped papule, white or yellowish in color, with each papule having a central dell or even follicular plugging (see Fig. 11.1). The lesions become confluent in the center, but about the periphery, isolated papules can still be seen. In the confluent areas (plaques), individual lesions can still be seen. There are almost never oral mucosal lesions. The skin and semimucosa about the anus, on the median raphe of the perineum, and about the vagina, labia minora, clitoris, ill-defined areas in the vestibule and introitus, and the inner aspects of the labia majora are the sites of predilection. The lesions often form a figure-8 about these structures. The lateral aspects of the labia majora are seldom affected. Many lesions may be level with the surrounding skin but of a firm consistency. In the past, this has been called kraurosis vulvae.

In children, guttate lichen sclerosus et atrophicus may occur, in which there are many separate individual lesions with almost no plaque formation and no localization to the pressure areas. Sometimes, white atrophic areas may be present in the perianal area.

Later the lesions become atrophic; there is a central keratotic plug with delling, and an ivory or yellowish parchment-like wrinkling, telangiectatic blood vessels, and occasionally bullae. The bullae are most common on the atrophic vulvar tissues. Some frank hemorrhage occurs from the telangiectatic blood vessels in the atrophic and sclerotic vulvae, sometimes forming hemorrhagic bullae. Also, leakage of red blood cells occurs from the telangiectatic blood vessels (so-called telangiectatic purpura). On the vulva, there may be a secondary lichenified/verrucous change, perhaps due to persistent rubbing or scratching.

In the female patient (in whom the disease is more common), lesions often are located in areas of pressure, e.g. beneath the breasts, on vulvar areas, genitocrural fold, and on the shoulder beneath the brassiere strap. In male patients, the nape of the neck appears to be a favorite location. In children, face and neck lesions are seen. These lesions are to be distinguished from morphea, which is rare on the face and rare in children.

Occasionally the disease may be widespread and almost generalized in the female patient. In these cases, interestingly enough, the vulvar and perianal tissues may be uninvolved.

Very rarely, keratoses and carcinoma may develop on vulvar and other lesions.

The analogous condition in male patients is called balanitis xerotica obliterans. It produces white, smooth, parchment plaques with telangiectatic blood vessels, erosions, and hemorrhage or serous subepidermal bullae. These are located on the glans, sulcus, and adjacent foreskin. This chronic atrophic sclerosing process produces gradual narrowing of the urethral meatus. Regions undergoing this process also can have superimposed areas of a whitish verrucous change. These are not warts. Only rarely does this condition occur on the torso in males.

DIFFERENTIAL DIAGNOSIS

The differential diagnosis of lichen sclerosus et atrophicus can be divided into two groups of diseases. One is sclerotic spotted atrophies occurring on the skin. The rare condition atrophic lichen planus has at some times and in some places, the purplish polygonal flat-topped papules. Follicular lichen planus may show follicular atrophy with alopecia on the scalp and groin. Also, the purplish reticulated pattern on the mucosae of the mouth and vulva is quite characteristic. Guttate morphea consists of small white plaques of sclerosis and atrophy. However, this is not basically a follicular papular eruption, and there is no delling. Most cases of so-called guttate morphea are lichen sclerosus et atrophicus. Circumscribed scleroderma lesions are larger sclerotic plaques, somewhat erythematous in the beginning, with a lilac tinge at the periphery. There are no satellite follicular lesions. This condition does not occur on the semimucosa or in the mouth. Very rarely, both morphea and lichen sclerosus et atrophicus may be present.

The second group of diseases to be considered in the differential diagnosis of lichen sclerosus et atrophicus is that of white lesions of the genital mucosa. On the vulva, leukoplakia (or leukokeratosis or cancer-in-situ) is basically a hyperkeratotic condition with no atrophy, sclerosis, telangiectatic blood vessels, or delled peripheral papules. This involves basically the mucosa or semimucosa, but not the skin, which is almost always involved in lichen sclerosus et atrophicus.

Lichen simplex chronicus in the genital area is essentially a hypertrophic process with red velvety enlargement of the clitoris and labia, excoriations, and thickening and wrinkling of the affected parts. Browning is frequently present. The eruption is poorly defined and usually involves both the semimucosal areas and the adjacent skin. Macerations may make the surface look white.

Radiation sequelae present in patients as a yellowish atrophic sclerotic telangiectatic eruption, usually sharply demarcated. Keratoses may occasionally be seen. The total treated area is involved, albeit to a different degree. Radiation sequelae from grenz ray treatments present only as a mottled telangiectasia with no other visible change.

Extramammary Paget's disease is basically an erosive disease, sharply marginated, that bleeds easily. Papules and nodules, and hard enlarged regional lymph nodes are sometimes present.

Senile atrophy of the vulva does not extend onto the adjacent skin and presents with some atrophy of the epidermis and looseness of the underlying tissues. There are no delled papules, sclerosis, or telangiectasia.

Other lichenified dermatoses may become white due to maceration. Bullous lichen sclerosus et atrophicus can be confused with mucous membrane pemphigoid.

Other lesions of the glans penis which at times may have whitish aspects include erythroplasia of Queyrat, a red velvety process; lichen planus, a purplish papular flat-topped eruption frequently forming nickel-sized (2.0 cm diameter) annular lesions; psoriasis, a sharply marginated red scaly eruption; Zoon's erythroplasia; and, I suppose, fixed drug eruptions (in their subsiding phase).

Auguste Queyrat, 1872– French Dermatologist, Ricord Hospital, Paris

Johannes Jacobus Zoon, 1902–1958, Dutch Dermatologist, Utrecht

Chronic graft-versus-host disease in its early phase is a lichen planus-like eruption involving the buccal mucosae and palms, with an associated erythroderma early. Later, the lesions become poikilodermatous and sclerodermiform often with large chronic ulcers. Fever, diarrhea, and hepatitis may also be present.

Atopic Dermatitis

Because atopic dermatitis[2,3] is a common disease with many and varied manifestations I have decided to deal with it in several ways—to wit, an overall description, a description by age,[4] a brief outline of some of the nonmorphological findings, a differential diagnosis, and finally an epitome (Table 20).[5]

Overall Description

Overall, the eruption (Besnier's prurigo, 1903; neurodermatitis of Brocq and Jacquet, 1891) is usually symmetrical and tends to be more severe and extensive on the upper half of the body, especially in adults. There is a brownish pigmentation of the upper and lower eyelids, making the eyes appear deeply set. A prominent lower lid fold, producing a groove, is present (Dennie-Morgan sign). In the postauricular crease, there may be faint, ill-defined, erythema and scaling.

The most marked skin changes occur on the flexural aspect of the elbows, the flexor wrists, the popliteal fossae, and the dorsa of the ankles. The eyelids, forehead and scalp, anterior chest, front and sides of neck, and dorsa of fingers and toes are also often involved. These changes include the following.

1. Ill-defined erythematous dome-shaped to flat-topped brown or reddish-brown papules of 1 to 2 mm in diameter. These become confluent in many areas and patients present with lichenoid plaques with indefinite or moderately sharp borders and outlying discrete scattered papules.
2. Numerous scattered areas of crusted excoriations and erosions.
3. Coarse lichenification.
4. Large areas of brownish pigmentation, the margins fading into normal skin.
5. Small circular or oval 1 to 4 mm whitish areas of hypopigmentation. (See also "Pityriasis alba" in Chapters 6 and 17.)

There are also other areas of fine lichenification and excoriated papules, including the upper chest, abdomen, flexural aspect of the whole forearm, upper back, and buttocks. In some patients, side lighting is necessary to see the extent of this fine lichenification. Loss of hair from rubbing is a feature, especially on the scalp and eyebrows. The nails may show buffing and actual v-shaped wearing away of the distal central portions. Considerable debris may also be present under the nails.

On the face, the rubbing may produce various-sized, purplish, faintly lichenified plaques with poorly defined borders with little or no scaling. Other involved areas tend to show more effects of scratching (e.g. excoriations) than rubbing. The lips and oral commissures are commonly involved.

Atopic erythroderma is described in Chapter 7.

C. C. Dennie, U.S. Dermatologist

D. B. Morgan, U.S. Dermatologist

Sequelae include mottled areas of light brown and whitish color with no definite atrophy especially notable on lower sides and front of neck. This has been called the "dirty neck" sign. Scars are usually small and round, showing the pattern and distribution of neurotic excoriations. Surprisingly, though, in many patients, areas severely involved in childhood, such as the elbow flexures, will show no sequelae in adulthood.

The cardinal lesion of true eczema, the pathognomonic intraepidermal vesicle, does not constitute a feature of the primary process of atopic dermatitis beyond infancy except for the frequently associated lesions of nummular eczema and pompholyx.

In some patients, the underlying atopic dermatitis may be masked by the tremendous overlay of traumatic lesions, so that excoriations, scratch marks, rubbed areas, and others may seem to be the only lesions.

When the scalp is involved, poorly demarcated scaly excoriated crusted areas are present, sometimes with loss of hair from scratching.

Xerosis, ichthyosis, and keratosis pilaris are common features. Sometimes the xerosis is very marked, and the distinction between an irritated and traumatized xerosis and mild atopic dermatitis may be difficult to make. There is an accentuation of the skin lines of the palms (palmar hyperlinearity). In adult patients with marked keratosis pilaris, and prominent follicular orifices, the papules of atopic dermatitis may be, at times, mainly follicular, i.e. somewhat elongated with a central excoriated depression on the top. Sometimes hair can be seen coming through this top. Other nonfollicular, less elevated papules, lichenification, and brown pigmentation are seen as well. In children, irregular follicular and nonfollicular papules arranged in varying sized clumps may be seen on the torso. Rarely are they linear. These clumps are more common in black children. In the Caucasian race, a central hypopigmented area as seen in pityriasis alba may be present.

Rarely, lesions of nummular eczema may be present on the torso and limbs. There is no sweating in the lesions of atopic dermatitis, but sweating increases the pruritus.

White "dermatographism"* is present in all extensive cases and in some without much evidence of disease. Following stroking, after an initial erythema, a linear, 1 to 2 cm, blanched streak lasting 4 to 5 minutes develops. A well-recognized consequence of this phenomenon is the typical pale well-rubbed face of atopic dermatitis patients.

Localization of a fissured dermatitis in the skin at the juncture of the ear lobule and side of the head is very suggestive of atopic dermatitis.

Involvement of the hand and foot presents at times as an eczematous dermatitis on palms and on the sides of the fingers and toes (see Chapter 5, "Localized Varieties"). Recurrent superadded pyoderma seems to be common in some patients, rare in others. Some patients (especially in the postpubertal age group) show very extensive, superadded, excoriations similar to that seen in neurotic excoriation. Lichenification occurs more rapidly and extensively in asiatics.

Lichenified plaques commonly occur on the anatomical snuff box and on the adjacent dorsum and lateral aspect of the wrist. The dorsa of the fingers can also be

---

*Because there is no hive formation, dermatographism is not the correct word. Blanching following stroking is a more accurate description.

involved. The dorsum of the foot is a frequent location. When seen alone these lesions look like lichen simplex chronicus. The semimucosae and adjacent skin of the lips and perianal area may show a lichenified, fissured, excoriated eruption. Recurrent blepharitis and conjunctivitis are common.

Some enlargement of lymph nodes is a feature of many patients with atopic dermatitis especially in the inguinal, axillary, and cervical areas. Atopic dermatitis at times may exhibit large oozing areas, sometimes with peripheral undermining and with enlarged tender lymph nodes. This is atopic dermatitis with secondary pyoderma. There may be almost no frank pustulation and no laudable pus. In fact, edema, erythema, and oozing may be the only signs. The creases of the neck, behind the ears, beneath the ear lobes, and on the wrists are favorite sites. In association with these manifestations, there may be an irregularly defined, scattered, excoriated, papulovesicular eruption. Both the large oozing areas and the papulovesicular id are strangers to uncomplicated atopic dermatitis. One should also consider a super-imposed eczematous dermatitis and a superimposed blistering viral infection due to herpes simplex. The viral infections are more pock-like.

Rarely, ichthyosis linearis circumflexa (Netherton's syndrome) may also be present.

Description by Age

MORPHOLOGICAL FINDINGS: INFANCY

Infantile Atopic Eczema or Infantile Atopic Dermatitis

This form occurs in infants (to the age of 2). The eruption is that of the classic so-called "infantile eczema". It generally has its onset as early as the first few months of life, but rarely before the second month. It usually consists of an erythematous, papular, sometimes papulovesicular, weeping, oozing or crusting eruption starting principally on the cheeks and later extending over the face and then to other parts of the body, in particular the outer [lateral] portions of the forearms, wrist and legs in the form of disseminated patches, frequently nummular. When the hairy scalp is involved with an accumulation of scaling, with erythema, sometimes present from birth, the changes are often referred to as "cradle cap". Acrocyanosis is common in infants with severe, extensive disease.

Those infants with atopic dermatitis who do not "outgrow" their eruption before the end of the second year (and this is the minority) carry over to the next phase of the disease.[4]

MORPHOLOGICAL FINDINGS: CHILDHOOD

Atopic Dermatitis of Childhood

The "second" phase of atopic dermatitis may be a continuation of the first, may have its onset a year or two after termination of the first or may appear as the first dermatosis in the patient's life (i.e. after the age of 2). In this second phase the dermatosis commonly assumes one of two forms. The first is the papular or prurigo form which consists mainly of succulent, elevated papules with a crusting, scratched central top. In this prurigo type the favored locations are the extensor surfaces of the extremities. The second is the lichenoid

Earl Weldon Netherton, 1893– U.S. Dermatologist

variety which consists of small, discrete, rather flat-topped, brown or reddish brown papules, becoming confluent in many areas and presenting lichenified plaques with indefinite or moderately sharp borders and outlying discrete, scattered papules. The flexor areas, particularly those of the cubital and popliteal spaces, are favored locations in the lichenoid type. In both of these childhood types, the tendency to oozing and crusting is less than in the infantile type. The course of the disease following the second phase is like that of the first; i.e. it may disappear (around the ages of 10 to 12 years) never to return again, it may recur after a free period of several years, or it may continue from the second phase into the "third" without interruption.[4]

MORPHOLOGICAL FINDINGS: ADULT

Atopic Dermatitis in the Adolescent and Adult

The "third" or adolescent phase of this disease features the papule and lichenification rather than vesicles and prurigo lesions. The lesions are usually drier and thicker than in younger patients; there is a greater tendency to confluence of the individual papules and to formation of larger lichenified plaques. The favored locations of the adolescent and adult form are the flexures, including the popliteal and cubital spaces, neck and eyelids.

General Comments

Other forms frequently encountered include combinations of all or any of the aforementioned types, which can appear in patients of any age. Moreover, the dermatosis may affect any part of the skin and may even become generalized. In addition to the typical sites, it is not unusual to find localizations on one or more of the following areas: scalp, back of neck, upper portions of the chest and back, pubic and inguinal areas and dorsa of the fingers, hands, toes and feet. One or more of these sites may be affected without other areas being involved. Thus, what appears to be just a chronic or chronic recurrent "eczema" of the hands or feet, or of the eyelids, etc., may actually be a partial or localized form of atopic dermatitis.

Because the eruption is so intensely pruritic, irritation from scratching or unsuitable medications is not at all uncommon. Hence many patients, when first seen, present superficial skin irritations and minor infections superimposed on the originally dry lesions. Considering the chronicity of the dermatosis and the tremendous amounts of pruritus, scratching and rubbing which occur, superimposed severe pyodermas are relatively infrequent. This is in contrast to certain virus infections such as herpes simplex, verrucae and mollusca.

In infants, it is the rule to find the eruption acutely inflamed and oozing and presenting minute pinhead-sized closely agminated, delicate superficial vesicles. Thus the clinical appearance of some of the lesions of atopic dermatitis is often similar to, and sometimes identical with, that of acute, subacute, or chronic eczematous dermatitis. It is certain, however, that in the characteristic atopic dermatitis of adults, the essential process is not a direct eczematous one. For the cardinal lesion of true eczema—the pathognomonic intraepidermal vesicle—does not constitute a feature of the primary process of atopic dermatitis in the ages beyond infancy. Whereas the infantile form of atopic dermatitis clinically presents very minute grossly visible vesicles,* these are rare or unknown in older patients.

It is our opinion that after infancy the primary lesion of atopic dermatitis is an edematous and inflammatory process situated beneath the epidermis in the superficial cutis. Any epidermal changes observed are secondary in the adult forms; and in view of the properties peculiar to infantile skin, it seems possible that the epidermal changes in infants are also, in most instances, secondary.

The small lichenoid papule and the plaques formed by the juxtaposition and coalescence of such papules may be considered primary in atopic dermatitis; and the oozing, weeping, crusting,superficial infection, the thickening of the epidermis, the pigmentation and the chronic torpid lichenifications are secondary.[4]

Non-morphological Features

Atopic dermatitis (along with hives, dermatitis herpetiformis, insect bites, and scabies) is one of the truly pruritic skin diseases. Often, a personal or family history of asthma, allergic rhinitis, and atopic dermatitis exists. Physical and environmental factors such as irritation from wool and occasionally petrolatum-containing salves, aggravation in cold, dry winter or hot, humid summers are factors in atopic dermatitis. Another environmental finding is the increased incidence of the disease in newly immigrated persons of black or asiatic origin when compared to the incidence in their native country. In children, there is an association with attention deficit disorder and hyperactivity. Keratoconus and anterior subcapsular cataracts have been reported in severe cases, but they must be very rare.

Laboratory abnormalities include peripheral eosinophilia, elevated IgE, many positive intradermal skin tests, and positive reaction to patch-testing with nickel sulfate.

DIFFERENTIAL DIAGNOSIS

In a full-blown eruption of atopic dermatitis, the main differential diagnosis is pollenosis—contact dermatitis from the airborne oily fraction of certain pollens. In cases of pollenosis, there is no history of atopy. The eruption is limited mainly to those areas exposed to the outside and is worse in the summer and fall. For example, limb flexural involvement is minimal. Interestingly, an eczematous hand eruption has been reported in pollenosis. The degree of lichenification may be very severe.

In scabies, the basic lesion is a burrow usually most easily seen on the sides of the fingers. The other secondary papulo-vesicular id lesions are symmetrically located on many parts of the body; tend to be located more on the extensor surfaces than in the creases; and are rare on the neck where atopic dermatitis is common.

---

* In this connection it is significant that many dermatoses which are essentially nonvesicular in adults, commonly assume a vesicular or bullous character in infants and young children; e.g. the bullous syphilids of pemphigoid type, vesicular or bullous scabies, bullous insect bites, bullous impetigo, etc. This suggests that the superficial layers of the infant's skin may be more permeable to substances coming from below or from above than are those layers in the skin of an adult and the infant's skin thus tends more strongly to the formation of superficial vesicles. In view of this generally increased tendency to vesiculation and weeping on the part of the infantile skin, as well as in consideration of many immunologic and clinical facts, it is probable that the vesiculation, weeping and crusting seen in the infantile forms is not a fundamental difference between the disease process in infants and adults but a difference in the reaction patterns of infantile and older skin.

Dermatitis herpetiformis occasionally should be considered. Some lichenified lesions of atopic dermatitis closely resemble lichen simplex chronicus.

Certain eczematous eruptions as, for example, on the eyelids, are hard to distinguish from atopic dermatitis especially if there is much lichenification. At times, only the natural evolution of the disease, other cutaneous findings, or other nonmorphological findings confirm the diagnosis.

Table 20A: **Atopic Dermatitis: Findings Common to Childhood and Adult Stages**

1. Symmetry.
2. More extensive and severe on the upper half of the body, especially in adults. Can be erythrodermic.
3. Orbital darkening.
4. Accentuated infra-orbital skin fold (Dennie-Morgan line).
5. Flexural papular and lichenoid eruption.
6. Flexural areas of coarse lichenification.
7. Brownish pigmentation in and about lesions.
8. Hypopigmentation alone (pityriasis alba) or at periphery of active lesions.
9. Fine lichenification and excoriated papules on torso and on nonflexural areas of extremities.
10. Loss of hair from rubbing, particularly on eyebrows and scalp.
11. Nail buffing with V-shaped nicking at tip, and debris under distal end.
12. Purplish, faintly lichenified plaques with poorly defined borders on face—may also have facial pallor from white dermographism.
13. Traumatic lesions—excoriations, effects of rubbing, picking.
14. Variegated pale and brown spottiness in areas of burnt-out disease, particularly on flexures and V of chest.
15. Xerosis—ichthyosis—palmar hyperlinearity—keratosis pilaris.
16. Follicular accentuation of papules (particularly in blacks).
17. White dermographism.
18. Fissured dermatitis at juncture of ear lobule and scalp.
19. Tendency to eczematous "dyshidrotic" dermatitis on hands and feet; rarely nummular lesions on torso and extremities.
20. Tendency to marked lichenification in asiatics and blacks.
21. Tendency to cutaneous infections, because of impaired cell- mediated immunity, to the following: Staphylococcus aureus
    Streptococcus pyogenes
    Herpes simplex
    Human papilloma virus
    Molluscum contagiosum.
22. Lichenified fissured nipple dermatitis.
23. Cheilitis with lichenification especially at corners of oral commissure. Loss of sharpness of border of red lip.
24. Localized areas resembling lichen simplex chronicus.
25. Recurrent blepharitis and conjunctivitis.
26. Nickel sulfate dermatitis on ear lobes.
27. Prurigo nodularis lesions.

Infacy Findings

1. Oozing cheeks.
2. Nummular eczema on lateral portion of extremities.
3. Scaling, erythema and oozing on scalp.
4. Acrocyanosis.
5. Restless, scratching.

Table 20B: Atopic Dermatitis: Non-Morphological Findings

---

1. Pruritus.
2. Personal or family history of atopy (asthma, allergic rhinitis, atopic dermatitis).
3. Onset, at age 2–6 months.
4. Chronic or chronically relapsing dermatitis.
5. Sweating increases pruritus.
6. Aggravation on contact with wool.
7. Worse in cold dry winter and hot humid summer.
8. Environmental factors as displayed by occurrence in immigrated dark-skinned population (and oriental).

Laboratory Findings
1. Many positive, immediate, intradermal skin tests.
2. Peripheral eosinophilia.
3. Elevated IgE.

Nonskin Findings
1. Multiple pea- to grape-sized lymph nodes in neck, axilla and inguinal areas.
2. Attention deficient disorder with hyperactivity in children.
3. Keratoconus.
4. Anterior subcapular cataract.
5. Asthma.
6. Seasonal rhinitis (hay fever).

Table 20C: Atopic Dermatitis: Diagnostic Guidelines

This rather simplistic, but practical and apparently reproducible list of criteria for the diagnosis of atopic dermatitis has recently been proposed.[5]
Must have:
1. History of involvement of the skin creases such as folds of elbows, behind the knees, fronts of ankles or around the neck (including cheeks in children under 10).
2. A personal history of asthma or hay fever (or history of atopic disease in a first-degree relative in children under 4).
3. A history of a general dry skin in the last year.
4. Visible flexural dermatitis (or dermatitis involving the cheeks/forehead and outer limbs in children under 4).
5. Onset under the age of 2 (not used if child is under 4).

Lichen Simplex Chronicus of Vidal

The sites of predilection are the nape of the neck, upper medial thighs, genitals and intergluteal fold, lateral surface of the legs, popliteal and axillary spaces, elbows, knees, and posterior aspect of the forearms.

At the onset, there is only intermittent itching; later it assumes the character of distinct, especially nocturnal, crises lasting a few minutes, with furious scratching followed by a voluptuous sensation of relaxation.

Each individual lesion is generally oval, palm-sized, and has three zones. The peripheral zone is 2 to 3 cm wide, imperfectly outlined, brownish and barely thickened. Isolated peripheral papules may be present (Fig. 11.4). In the middle zone

Emile Vidal, 1825–1893, Dermatologist, St. Louis, Paris

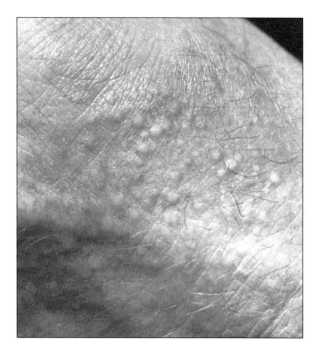

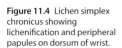
Figure 11.4 Lichen simplex chronicus showing lichenification and peripheral papules on dorsum of wrist.

appear lenticular and hemispherical prurigo papules, with an excoriated or shining surface towards the center. The central zone is an infiltrated, brown or hypopigmented plaque, lichenized to the highest degree with a scaly or macerated epidermis. Excoriated papules and some scaling may be present. In certain races (e.g. Chinese), lichen simplex chronicus is more frequently seen. Also, eczematous reactions in these races commonly show an increased amount of lichenification.

For lichen simplex chronicus of the genital mucosa, see "differential diagnosis" for white lesions of genital mucosa on page 174; for lichen simplex chronicus of intertriginous areas, see "Intertrigo" in Chapter 1. See also "Nuchal Scaly Eczemas" in Chapter 6. For lichen simplex chronicus of the palms and soles, see Chapter 15.

Traumatic Lichenification

There are many aspects to the clinical diagnosis of self-induced traumatic lichenification. As indicated before, easily diagnosable skin conditions (e.g. psoriasis), can be so altered by rubbing that the typical clinical features are all but obliterated. Also, a host of lichenified plaques, large and small, can be produced on normal skin by external trauma, including occupational marks, which are not included in this handbook.

Of the external traumas, a few examples will be given. The lichenified periungual tissues following biting, rubbing, and chewing of these parts may be quite striking.

The inferior and lateral periungual tissues are usually involved. The lichenification is fairly sharply marginated and often is surprisingly heaped up. Thumb sucking, lower lip sucking, picking and rubbing of the nuchal area all can produce lichenified areas. Some will be linear. Most will show other evidence of trauma (such as excoriations and crusting).

There are many variations of traumatic lichenification. A useful reference as to what occurs in the mentally challenged is by Butterworth (see also "Self-inflicted Lesions" in Chapter 14).6

In localized lichenified eruptions, always consider trauma as the possible cause.

Lichen Striatus

The eruption of lichen striatus consists of grouped, linear erythematous papulovesicles or papules. At first, the eruption tends to be vesicular; later, it is more papular, hyperkeratotic, and may show varying degrees of browning. The papules are of the eczematous type at the blistering phase; later, they are of the lichenoid type.

Eruption of lichen striatus is common below the age of puberty, usually extending for at least one-third the length of an extremity, and usually lasting about 6 months.

The linear arrangement does not follow vascular, nervous, or lymphatic tissue; it follows Blaschko's lines.

DIFFERENTIAL DIAGNOSIS

Linear papular psoriasis has the characteristic silvery, salmon-colored, scaled, sharply marginated papule.

Linear lichen planus has angular flat-topped purplish papules.

Linear verrucae planae presents with small, flat-topped, skin-colored or slightly brownish papules. The extent of the linear nature is not so extensive, rarely longer than 2 inches (5 cm).

In linear lichen simplex chronicus, the brown papules form a lichenified plaque, often of a brown color and often with evidence of rubbing or scratching.

Nevus unius lateris commonly presents a difficult problem in differential diagnosis, particularly in the late papular and hyperkeratotic stage. Nevus unius lateris tends to be more keratotic and the linear streaks are usually less complete. It is, of course, lifelong, but may not be present at birth.

Axillary Dermatitis of Fox-Fordyce

Skin-colored to slightly brown, dome-shaped, follicular papules are seen in each axilla, and sometimes in the anogenital area or around the breasts. The central area tends to have more of the papules, and toward the periphery, the number decreases and the papules are somewhat smaller. The papules are partially lined up in the normal skin axillary creases. Hair is frequently absent. Excoriations may be present. At times the eruption has a waxy or yellowish hue. The condition is seen mainly in women after puberty.

John Addison Fordyce, 1858–1925, U.S. Dermatologist, Columbia, N.Y.C.

Tilbury William Fox, 1836–1879, English Dermatologist

The differential diagnosis of Fox-Fordyce disease includes lichen simplex chronicus. In lichen simplex chronicus condition, the papules are more confluent and less discrete, the border is more brown and poorly defined. Other areas are commonly involved.

Zirconium (foreign body) deodorant granuloma presents as a small papular semitranslucent eruption which is nonfollicular.

Hutchinson's Summer Prurigo (Prurigo Aestivale, Actinic Prurigo)

The eruption involves the face, dorsa of the hands and forearms and, rarely, the light-exposed areas of the legs. On the limbs, the eruption consists of small scattered excoriated papules with lichenification and white pitted scars. On the face, the eruption consists of weeping, excoriated, and crusting lesions. Excoriated plaques or small edematous papules on the nose, eyes, and cheeks are frequent.

Papular Photodermatitis in North American Indians (Birt)

In infants, on the sun-exposed areas, especially the cheeks, an acute eczematous eruption is seen with erythema, edema, exudation, and crusting. Vesicles and bullae are not clinically evident. The lesions on the arms and legs are always papular and prurigo-like, crusted, and leave faint depigmented scars. As the patients become older, the lesions become more papular, prurigo-like, and plaque-like, all with excoriations. Secondary impetigo may occur.

A cheilitis consisting of an edematous, denuded area partially covered with a yellowish-brown crust may be seen, either in connection with the above described facial or extremity lesions or alone.

This condition is probably the same as prurigo aestivalis or actinic prurigo. (See classification of "Causes of Abnormal Reactions to the Sunlight" in Chapter 1.)

Hodgkin's Prurigo

Some patients with Hodgkin's disease show a widespread eruption consisting of more or less dome-shaped papules with indistinct borders. The papules are up to 0.5 cm in diameter and are skin-colored or brownish red. Point- to pinhead-sized round erosions, or bloody crusts, are often present. The lesions are located mainly on the extremities, and to a lesser degree on the torso.

Lymphomatoid Papulosis

The basic lesion is a papuloangiomatous or hemorrhagic papule with a central scale, slight crust or necrosis. They are up to 1 cm in diameter. Most lesions produce a superficial atrophic scar, sometimes with considerable dirty brown pigmentation. Upon presentation, lesions are in all stages and tend to occur in clusters. Each lesion lasts from 1 to 2 months. The torso and proximal extremities are the sites of predilection. The face and scalp are rarely involved.

Thomas Hodgkin, 1798–1866, English Physician, Guy's Hospital, London

The main differential diagnosis of lymphomatoid papulosis is pityriasis lichenoides, where the lesions are less papular, less angiomatous, and more scaly. In contradistinction to pityriasis lichenoides, lymphomatoid papulosis usually occurs in patients over 25 years of age, lasts for years, and is more common in women.

Macaulay has coined the term "rhythmic paradoxical eruptions" for that group of diseases which includes acute parapsoriasis, lymphomatoid papulosis, and mycosis fungoides, because they may wax and wane despite rather ominous histopathological findings.

Miscellaneous Lichenified and Papular Dermatoses

There is a group of diseases that may present at certain stages and at certain times with a large degree of papulation and/or lichenification. Most of these diseases are covered in detail elsewhere. They are mentioned here, as they should be considered in the differential diagnosis of many papular eruptions, particularly lichen simplex chronicus.

Eczema, especially in the subsiding or chronic phase, may be surprisingly lichenified. Certain areas, e.g. palms, perianal area, and ankles, seem to lichenify quicker and more extensively than others. Also, in these areas all the stages of eczema may not be present, e.g. oozing, crusting, and minute vesiculation, so it may be very difficult to distinguish these lichenified eczemas from basically papular eruptions. Usually, however, careful search will reveal that lichenified eczemas are multilesional, while the papular eruptions are not.

There is a group of conditions that presents with a mainly small or micropapular eruption. This includes papular contact dermatitis (as from nickel sulfate or from colored sheets), certain types of atopic dermatitis, and dermatitis from fiberglass. The morphology of the sheet eczema, nickel sulfate eczema, and atopic dermatitis have already been covered. Fiberglass dermatitis presents as a mainly follicular eruption on the medial aspects of the extremities or on other areas exposed to the fibers. Excoriations may be present.

Psoriasis, when occurring in isolated areas and following much scratching and rubbing, may present as a primarily papular and lichenified eruption. The scale gets rubbed off, there may be excoriations at various stages, the lesion may be brown-colored, and the border may be indistinct. The legs (lateral aspect) and forearms are favorite locations for this type of lichenified psoriasis. Search for other lesions, especially in the nails, is the easiest way to make a diagnosis. Protection of the traumatized lesion from rubbing and scratching will allow the more characteristic psoriasis scale and color to develop.

Pityriasis lichenoides is a widespread papulo-erythematosquamous condition occurring usually on the torso and having large areas of a reticulated papular and often lichenoid eruption with little or no scale. Evidence of scratching or rubbing is rarely seen.

W. L. Macauly, U.S. Dermatologist

Lichenoid trichophytosis is an unusual transient follicular lichenoid eruption occurring on the torso of patients who have an acute inflammatory ringworm elsewhere. The eruption is diffuse, poorly demarcated and presents as small skin-colored follicular papules. Sometimes, side lighting or palpation are necessary to appreciate the presence of these lesions.

Papular dermatitis herpetiformis presents as 2 to 3 mm juicy dermal-epidermal papules, most of which have been traumatized. Frequently an erythematous component is concomitant, and of course at times vesicles and bullae (or the remains thereof) may also be present. Also, brown pigmentation, symmetry, and grouping may be features.

The distinction between insect bite papules, dermatitis herpetiformis, and neurotic excoriations has been discussed under "Papular Urticaria" in Chapter 2.

Schistosome dermatitis ("swimmer's itch") due to cercarial penetration of the skin presents as pea-sized excoriated papules on those parts of the body exposed to infected water. The lesions are randomly distributed, usually on the legs and thighs. There may be some associated wealing in these lesions.

Solar eruptions presenting solely as papules or plaques are unusual. They have been described in Chapter 1 and in Chapter 5 as solar induced eruptions.

Reactive perforating collagenosis is a trauma-induced scattered papular eruption, each lesion having a central keratin plug that fills a central depression. The face and the dorsa of fingers are common locations. These lesions are not follicular, but may be confused with other follicular papular lesions with a central umbilicated core. They are common and widespread in patients receiving hemodialysis. Clinically and histologically they can resemble prurigo nodularis or keratoacanthomata. They have been called follicular hyperkeratoses. Follicular hyperkeratoses morphologically includes elastosis perforans serpiginosa, Kyrle's disease, and reactive perforating collagenosis (see also Chapter 2.).

Frictional lichenoid dermatitis occurs in children on the backs of the hands, fingers, elbows, and knees. Most of these children probably have an atopic diathesis.

Transient acantholytic dermatosis consists of discrete, pruritic, edematous papules and papulovesicles mainly on the chest, upper abdomen, back and thighs of elderly males. Occasionally the lesions are clustered in a haphazard manner and some may be crusted.

Papular Granulomas

It is just as hard to define granulomas when referring to papular lesions as it is when referring to nodular lesions. My concept of the clinical and histological features of a granuloma is in the "Overview" to Chapter 12.

Joseph Kyrle, 1880–1926, Austrian Dermatologist, Vienna

Granulomas of Eyelid Margins

The patient with granulomas of the eyelid margins may show up with 2 to 3 mm, reddish, rather pointed papules located, at the outer edge of the eyelid margins. They are randomly located but are more common on the lower than the upper eyelid. There may also be small, more inflammatory papules or styes. The exact nature of these granulomas is not obvious to me. I would classify them as being a peculiar granulation response to some insult on the sebaceous glands on the eyelid margin.

DIFFERENTIAL DIAGNOSIS

At times, if solitary, these lesions can be mistaken for small molluscum contagiosum or basal cell carcinomas. The molluscum contagiosum tends to have a central dell and the lesion is less pointed. The basal cell carcinoma has a firmer consistency, may show telangiectasis, and may show ulceration and destruction of the eyelid margin.

Cactus Granuloma

Cactus granuloma presents as clusters of up to fifty flesh-colored, domed, 2 to 4 mm papules with a central black dot located mainly on the extremities. There is often a large amount of wealing associated with these lesions.

For other foreign body granuloma, see Chapter 12.

Papular Sarcoidosis

The patient presents with scattered light brown or brown red, partially translucent, shotty dermal papules, the central portion of which do not fade completely on pressure. Some of the papules have formed clusters, semicircles, or circles. The central cleared portion may give the impression of atrophy. Other lesions are isolated and distinct. There is no epidermal change. The eruption may be very widespread or localized. Ichthyosiform sarcoidosis has been reported in blacks, where biopsy of an acquired ichthyosis revealed a sarcoidal reaction in the dermis. The plaque, nodular, nodal, and other varieties of sarcoidosis are described elsewhere (see Chapter 12).

Granuloma Annulare

A firm, slightly pink or skin-colored, smooth papule the size of a small pea develops rather rapidly in granuloma annulare. By eccentric growth, or by accession of other papules, this becomes transformed into a ring, usually about 2 mm in height. This ring may stay the size of a dime (1.8 cm) or enlarge to become the size of a silver dollar (3.5 cm), or larger. The circles may become incomplete or arcuate in the resolving phase. There is no epidermal change, although the center may appear slightly atrophic. The lesions are frequently multiple, with several on the sites of predilection, which are the dorsa of the feet, dorsa of the hands, fingers, elbows, knees, and nape of neck. Rarely, the eruption may be almost generalized in a photodermatitic pattern. Rarely, larger nodular lesions are present. On the scalp, the lesions are dermal and hypodermal. Occasionally, a dark purple lichen planus-like color may be present in and following after the lesions. This is particularly true of larger, older, and incomplete lesions, and of lesions on the dorsa of the feet.

Rarely a central perforation occurs, when the necrobiosis is high in the dermis. This is called perforating granuloma annulare.

DIFFERENTIAL DIAGNOSIS

The differential diagnosis of granuloma annulare includes the following:

In papular sarcoidosis, the lesions are more deeply dermal and shotty; have a darker brown or brown red color, and diascopy does not make the lesion totally disappear. Also, in papular sarcoidosis, the ring formation may be present but is not so constant.

Larger lesions may be confused with rheumatic nodules especially on the scalp in children, erythema elevatum diutinum and nodular sarcoidosis.

Annular papular eruptions include granuloma annulare, annular sarcoid, and annular lichen planus. The latter, of course, has flat-topped purplish epidermal papules that have coalesced into a ring. Mycosis fungoides may present as arcuate or circular rings of reddish or reddish brown dermal plaques or infiltrate. Other erythematosquamous patches or plaques and tumors may be present. There is no scarring. Actinic granuloma (giant cell elastotic granuloma) is an annular or arcuate lesion occurring most often on the temples. The peripheral edge shows scaliness and slight dermal infiltration. The central area suggests atrophy. Sometimes, a grass-fire-type papular basal cell carcinoma simulates actinic granuloma.

A group of scarring annular papular eruptions includes various forms of syphilis, tuberculosis, and necrobiosis lipoidica.

Papular Syphilis

Because florid secondary syphilis is now unusual, it is only of historical interest to review all of the characteristic morphological patterns it may produce. Any student of morphology should at some time or other consult the morphological bible of syphilis by Stokes, Beerman, and Ingraham.[7] Not only the morphology of syphilis, but also much about the morphology of skin diseases that have been confused with syphilis can be learned. For example, in the 62 pages on the differential diagnosis of early cutaneous syphilis, there are numerous excellent photographs and no less than 55 tables outlining the morphological differences between syphilis and conditions that may mimic it. Although there may be a variety of constitutional signs and symptoms of systemic organ involvement in secondary syphilis, in most cases the clinical diagnosis is made (or suspected) on the basis of skin (Fig.11.5) and/or mucous membrane lesions. General diagnostic features of secondary syphilitic eruptions are listed in Table 21.

The diagnosis of papular syphilides is usually easy. Lichen planus, psoriasis, and parapsoriasis differ from these syphilides by the features of their own lesions. The

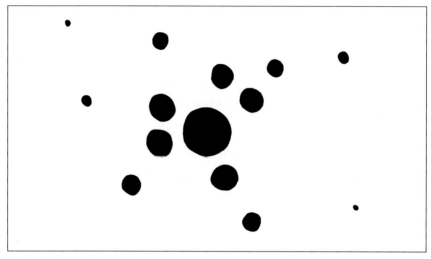

Figure 11.5 Shape of bomb-explosion syphilides.

Table 21: **General Diagnostic Features of Secondary Syphilitic Eruptions**
1. Symptomless, multiple, disseminated, discrete lesions with an annular or bomb-explosion arrangement. The annular "nickel and dime" lesions on the face, chin, and genitalia are especially frequent in blacks.
2. Macular, papular, papulonodular, follicular, erythematopapulosquamous, and pustular lesions. Symmetry is a feature. Cooked ham macules on the palms and soles are strongly indicative of secondary syphilis. A greasy scaly infiltrated hair line eruption is sometimes seen (corona veneris).
3. Vesicles and bullae are not seen except in infants.
4. Non-scarring moth-eaten alopecia of the scalp hair and loss of eyelashes and eyebrows.
5. Eroded moist papules on the mucocutaneous junctions and in intertriginous areas. The flexural or genital lesions may become erosive.
6. Eroded whitish erosions on the mucosal surfaces.
7. Lymphadenopathy with moderately enlarged, nontender discrete lymph nodes.
8. Constitutional signs and symptoms include malaise, low grade fever, arthralgia, iritis, periostitis, and meningeal irritation.
9. In late relapsing secondary syphilis, the lesions are less numerous, less symmetrical, arciform, and scarring.

papules of the diffuse and circumscribed prurigos are distinguished by the very active pruritus by which they are accompanied.

Papulonecrotic tuberculides may give rise to serious diagnostic difficulties. Although they chiefly affect the limbs, the development of papulonecrotic tuberculides is successive and usually slow, and they become hollowed out by ulceration and leave a cicatrix. In a given case, however, the decision may have to be based upon the coexistence of other specific manifestations of syphilis and serodiagnostic tests. The diagnosis of posterosive syphiloids in the newborn is still more difficult. The presence of other manifestations of congenital syphilis and the clinical and serological findings in the parents must be considered.

The follicular syphilides often leave persistent brown macules. The differential diagnosis of follicular syphilides is keratosis pilaris, follicular eczematides, pityriasis rubra pilaris, acne, papulonecrotic tuberculides, and others. The differential diagnosis from lichen scrofulosorum may be much more difficult.

In general, the general diagnostic features of mucocutaneous syphilis in neonates and young infants are similar to adults with secondary eruptions (see Table 21) except there is a greater tendency to form florid mucocutaneous lesions, particularly in the nose and pharynx ("the snuffles"). There is also an occasional tendency to form frank bullous lesions.

Papular Tuberculides (Lichenoid Tuberculides)

Lichenoid tuberculides present the following appearance. An eruption of small papules, of the average size of a pinhead, slightly prominent, flattened, polygonal, pale yellow or more rarely dusky red color, of rather soft consistency, with a surface that is smooth and glistening or more commonly is covered by a slightly adherent scaly layer arises. These papules are almost invariably grouped in more or less numerous nummular plaques or in patches. The interpapular areas remain normal. The eruptions usually occur on the trunk, especially the flanks and loins, but may spread to the limbs and, exceptionally, to the face.

Lichen scrofulosorum is observed at all ages, but occurs by predilection in children and young adults suffering from tuberculosis elsewhere.

DIFFERENTIAL DIAGNOSIS

The differential diagnosis of lichen scrofulosorum is difficult. In view of its habitual polymorphism, it is advisable to examine not only one eruptive group but the eruption as a whole, thereby guarding against confusion with the follicular eczematides, follicular lichen planus, and pityriasis rubra pilaris.

The differential diagnosis from the follicular lichenoid syphilides is sometimes almost impossible, even with biopsy. Serological tests for syphilis are of great help in these cases.

Insect Bite Granuloma

This rather puzzling dermal, papular, reddish blue-brown eruption usually exists on the torso, but can occur anywhere. They are isolated lesions, up to a dozen in number. As in papular urticaria, there may be twin lesions. Lymphocytoma cutis benigna, granuloma faciale and sarcoidosis should be considered in the differential diagnosis. Scabetic nodules usually occur on and about the genitalia and the genital regions.

Papular Facial Eruptions

For many years there have been many attempts to classify and diagnose micropapular eruptions involving the face. All may show varying degrees of papulation and sometimes plaque formation. There also may be an apple jelly appearance to the center of the lesion when diascopy is performed. Below are listed a few of the useful clinical differential points.

DIFFERENTIAL DIAGNOSIS

Rosacea usually has associated erythema, telangiectatic blood vessels, and pustule formation. Also, a flushing tendency is often present. As well, there may be rhinophymatous changes.

Tuberculids such as rosacea-like tuberculid of Lewandowsky, lupus miliaris disseminatus faciei, and acnitis may have apple jelly papule formation. The lesions tend to be more monomorphous and are not pustular or erythematous as is rosacea. Central necrosis and scarring may be prominent. The degree of infiltration may be marked. Also, other nonrosacea areas are commonly involved, for instance the neck, the underside of the chin, the forehead, and even other parts of the body. Also, the central facial area including the nose may be spared.

Sarcoidosis may involve the face as a primarily papular eruption, although usually some conglomeration of papules occurs, forming plaques.

Leprosy usually presents as an eruption of nodules and plaques, sometimes annular, with loss of eyebrows, enlarged ear lobes, wrinkled forehead, deformed, thickened, and enlarged nose, and lobulation of the lips and chin. Thickened palpable cutaneous nerves, loss of sensation and dyschromias may be present.

Granuloma faciale presents as brownish red, diascopy positive, dermal papulonodular, circular plaques, usually located on the face and scalp.

Lymphocytoma cutis presents with purplish red dermal papulonodules. The lesions may be widely disseminated, but facial and scalp lesions also occur.

In blacks, acne vulgaris, peri-oral dermatitis, occlusive effects from the use of petrolatum, follicular eczema, and dermatosis papulosa nigra must be considered in the differential diagnosis of papular facial eruptions.

Papular Tumors

Because this section contains so many entities it is useful for the student to emphasize color in the differential diagnosis.

Black or Brown Papulonodules

From a practical point of view, the number of black or brown nodular tumors is small and consists of almost the same diseases as the black or brown papular tumors, so I have decided to consider them together (see Table 22). Descriptions of some of these conditions appear elsewhere in more detail. They are included here in somewhat shortened form.

Pigmented basal cell carcinoma of the "common" variety is a firm, rather deep-seated papule, often with a grayish translucent (or pearly) character. Ulceration is not necessarily present. The lesion may have scale or crusted scale. The pigment is of a black or black brown color. It is usually unevenly distributed, some areas showing scattered black dots, other areas showing a totally black color, and still others showing only the more typical translucent gray color. Sometimes the redness from the numerous telangiectatic blood vessels adds another component to the color hue. Occasionally,

Table 22: **Brown or Brown-Black Papular Tumors**
Pigmented basal cell carcinoma
Malignant melanoma
Pigmented nevus
Hematoma
Thrombosed angioma
Pigmented dermatofirbroma
Blue nevus
Foreign body
Benign juvenile melanoma (Spitz)
Seborrheic keratosis
Dermatosis papulosa nigra
Urticaria pigmentosa
Pedunculated papilloepitheliomata

there is a halo of brown or black pigmentation. Brown or brownish areas occur frequently in the micropapular border of the superficial multicentric variety; occasionally, the central areas are pigmented as well. Rarely, the lesion may present as a freckle with no perceptible papular border.

Malignant melanoma usually presents as a pitch black, elevated, friable, glistening papule or nodule. Sometimes the central portion has a red angiomatous element with a black halo around the base. Sometimes a bluish cast is present. At times the pre-existing lesion can be seen, e.g. Hutchinson freckle or junctional or compound nevus. There may be a halo of black or dark brown pigment. Ulceration and evidence of bleeding are unusual except in large lesions of long standing. Small (2 to 3 mm) satellite maculopapules may be present. When less than 1.0 cm, clinical distinction from pigmented basal cell carcinoma may be impossible (See Table 23). See also "Malignant Melanoma" in Chapter 12.

Table 23: Comparative Features of Pigmented Basal Cell Carcinoma, Versus Papular Malignant Melanoma Under 1.0 cm		
	Pigmented Basal Cell Carcinoma	Papular Malignant Melanoma
Speckled Uneven Pigmentation	+++	+
Translucent/Pearly*	+++	0
Telangiectasias	++	0
Angiomatous	++	++
Ulceration	+	0
*Pearly refers both to color and firm consistency	0 = absent; + = rare or unusual; ++ = occasional (sometimes); +++ = common	

Sophie Spitz, 1910–1956, U.S. Pathologist

Pigmented nevi are soft, hairy, nonulcerated papulonodules of varying shape and size. Their color varies from skin color to brown or rarely black. Usually the color is distributed evenly throughout, although occasionally there may be some variation or a few black dotted areas. A halo of brown pigmentation is not unusual.

Small fresh hematomas are small, round, black, or deep purple papules with a flattish surface. They occur at sites of trauma, e.g. fingertips, subungual areas, heels, and in devitalized tissues, such as skin over arthritic joints. There is no ulceration. Paring usually reveals clotted blood.

Thrombosis and/or hemorrhage formation in a pre-existing angioma may produce a black lesion. In most hemorrhages, the yellowish-green-brown hues of degenerating hemosiderin may appear.

Pigmented dermatofibromas are small subepidermal areas (up to 1 cm) of fibrosis that present as a firm thickening with varying degrees of elevation of the overlying epidermis. The overlying epidermis is attached to the fibrosis and cannot be wrinkled as can the adjacent normal epidermis. The lesions are round or oval shaped, most commonly on the shins, thighs, and forearms. Frequently, they are multiple. Color varies from skin-colored to light brown, frequently with a reddish brown cast. Occasionally, they are dark brown or black throughout. Pigmentation is not clearly demarcated and tends to become diffuse at the borders as it blends in with the normal skin color. Ulceration is very rare.

Blue nevi are bluish, greenish or black papulonodular tumors. They are usually located deep in the dermis, hence causing a dome-shaped or flattish papule. The pigment may be very intense. The dorsa of the hands and feet, buttocks, scalp, and forehead are common locations, but blue nevi may occur elsewhere. They have a firm consistency and do not ulcerate.

A foreign body (as in a gun shot wound) may present a dermal or hypodermal tumor with some brownish or bluish pigmentation visible. Usually, scarring is present.

Spitz tumor (benign juvenile melanoma) is a reddish, rapidly growing, pigmented nevus, usually located on the face of the prepubertal child. A certain degree of brown color may also be present. Telangiectatic blood vessels are often visible on the surface.

Seborrheic keratosis is a localized thickening of the epidermis and hence is classified as a keratosis rather than a papule or nodule. The fissuring or pitted surface, the stuck-on character, and the verrucous nature of the lesion should make the diagnosis easy, even if the lesion is pitch black, as they often are. They may also have a yellow-brown or gray-brown color. At times, there is some black or brown peripheral pigment spread suggesting an active compound or junctional melanocytic nevus.

Dermatosis papulosa nigra consists of 1 to 2 mm, round or oval, black papules disseminated mainly on the cheeks of blacks. The lesions are sharply bordered, have a smooth dotted surface, and sometimes have a slight undercutting at the periphery, i.e. they are slightly pedunculated.

Urticaria pigmentosa may exist as widespread light brown papules or nodules, which urticate or produce bullae on firm rubbing. The nodular form is frequently solitary. This is basically a childhood disease.

Pedunculated brown papilloepitheliomata (acrochordons, skin tags) on the neck, axillae, and groin also should be considered.

Malignant Papular Tumors

While most of the malignant tumors are described and classified in Chapter 12, it must be realized that at some stage they are papules.

Papular Basal Cell Carcinoma

The common "nonulcerated" basal cell carcinoma appears first as a round, firm, rather deep-seated papule with telangiectasia. At times, especially in the central portion of the face, the lesion may present as a nonulcerative depression about which can be seen, when the skin is put on tension, and felt as a rather sharply demarcated pearly* infiltrate, morphologically resembling a plaque. Sometimes dots of black and brown pigment are present. Occasionally, lesions appear to have a bluish gray cystic aspect. However, incision of this cystic nodule produces little fluid.

Two clinical types are basically papular; these are the superficial multicentric and the grass-fire.

DIFFERENTIAL DIAGNOSIS

On the eyelid margin, these lesions must be distinguished from the cyst of the gland of Moll. Papular basal cell carcinoma should also be distinguished from a pigmented nevus, which is more skin-colored, often hairy, and of a soft consistency. Facial neuromas should be considered in the differential diagnosis as well. At times, a thick adherent scale may suggest a heaped-up solar keratosis or cutaneous horn. Removal of this scale-crust reveals an ulcer.

Small acneform granulomas, when solitary and persistent, also have to be considered in the differential diagnosis. Usually they are less firm, less clearly demarcated and may contain some yellowish material.

Small squamous cell carcinomas and keratoacanthomas may present as dome-shaped papules. These lesions tend to occur exclusively on sun-exposed areas, or areas of prior damage (except for keratoacanthomas, which are common on the moustache area). They are firmer in consistency and have less telangiectasia than basal cell carcinoma. Also, they tend to be more exophytic. They do not contain brown or black pigment; and they are ulcerated only when large.

Rarely, secondary papular metastatic deposits mimic other primary papular tumors. However, the lack of epidermal change over the deposit, the deep dermal or hypodermal location, and their multiplicity usually suggest the diagnosis. Also, secondary deposits are unusual on the sun-exposed areas.

*Both a color (translucent gray) and a consistency (firm, sharply marginated).

Chondrodermatitis nodularis chronica helicis ("painful nodule of the ear") is a globular or ovoid papule raised above the surrounding inflamed red skin with a 1 to 2 mm central erosion-ulcer with a covering scab. It is from pressure and so it is found most often on the upper pole of the helix of the external ear. Occasionally, the lesions are multiple. It occurs more often in elderly men, particularly those with thin, skinny pinnas. In former times, they were found in religious sisters from continual pressure of tight-fitting wimples. As well, such lesions were often seen following the wearing of heavy earphones in telephone operators.

Apart from the pain and the redness, the lack of a pearly consistency or color makes them easy to distinguish from basal cell carcinomas.

Superficial Multicentric Basal Cell Carcinoma

With the superficial multicentric type, the basic lesion is a mainly round, superficial patch or plaque, varying size from 1 to 10 cm, occurring usually on the torso (but also on the face, neck, thighs, and arms). The border consists of an irregular dotted thread-like 1 mm edge, which is slightly raised and often shows brown pigmentation. While the overall shape of the border is arcuate, small microarcuate irregularities are often present (Fig. 11.6). The center is flat, erythematous, and may have an overlying, white, nondescript scale. In many cases, there is no scale. Telangiectases are often present, as are numerous 1 mm crusted areas and erosions. The central area may show pseudoatrophy. The central area may also show an irregularly black or brown pigmentation. Occasionally, elevated papular tumors or succulent hemorrhagic papular tumors are present in one area of the tumor.

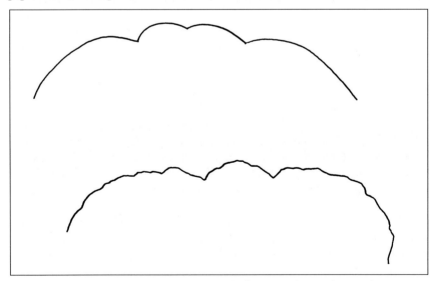

Figure 11.6 Shape of border of superficial multicentric basal cell carcinoma *(lower)* and Bowen's disease *(upper)*. Sharply demarcated, but irregular borders are characteristic of superficial primary cutaneous carcinomas.

DIFFERENTIAL DIAGNOSIS

Bowen's disease is a plaque of slightly elevated orange-brown tissue of softer consistency than the adjacent skin. Its border is arcuate with none of the microarcuate irregularities seen in superficial multicentric basal cell carcinoma (see Fig. 11.6). The lesions are of varying size and occur on the torso and extremities, usually on areas not exposed to the sun. The lesion is the same throughout. It may have a scaly or eroded surface. Rarely, one area may show a firm angiomatous 1 to 2 cm tumor. Very rarely, the border shows black or brown pigmentation, in long standing cases, it can be verrucous.

Carcinoma in situ of the hairy and semimucosal surfaces of the vulva are described here. These lesions are characterized by plaque formation with erosions, scaling, brown pigmentation, and sharply demarcated lesions. They may or may not be clinically multicentric.

Paget's disease (see Chapter 5 "Nipples and Areola") is mentioned again because occurring as it does on the female breast, and especially near or touching the nipple and areola, it may be very difficult to distinguish between Paget's disease, Bowen's disease, superficial basal cell carcinoma and, rarely, nonpigmented "pagetoid" melanoma. Florid papillomatosis of nipple ducts may present as small recurrent erosions of the nipple.

Extramammary Paget's disease is a sharply marginated, sometimes arcuate, red, superficially eroded plaque with some induration. The degree of induration and the amount of erosion vary. Sometimes the plaque has a white macerated surface. The sites of predilection are the vulvar area (skin and mucosa), perineum, perianal area, and the axillae.

Solar keratosis, as the name implies, is a keratosis with whitish to gray colored thick scale, which is firm, adherent, and on removal causes bleeding from torn capillaries. These lesions do not have an arcuate border, are rarely pigmented black or brown, and usually occur on the sun-exposed areas. Although the lesions are rarely over 1 cm, occasionally very large lesions (up to 4 cm) may be seen on the dorsa of the hands, the forehead, or the cheeks.

Lichenoid solar keratosis is a flat-topped red, just slightly papular, usually solitary keratosis up to 5 cm in diameter. When on the back, it is almost impossible to to differentiate from a superficial multicentric basal cell carcinoma. The same can be said for the atrophic solar keratosis.

Arsenical keratoses are smaller keratoses, and usually associated with discrete keratoses on the palms and soles. It should be noted that a common sequelae of trivalent arsenic ingestion are multiple superficial basal cell carcinomas on the torso.

Several benign lichenified or scaly conditions such as psoriasis, lichenified eczema, and lichen simplex chronicus occasionally present a problem in differential diagnosis. These lesions rarely have the persistence of the above described tumors.

Table 24: Persistent Localized Papular and Scaly Erythematous Lesions

Superficial multicentric basal cell carcinoma
Bowen's disease
Carcinoma in situ–vulva and peri-anal area
Paget's disease
Extramammary Paget's disease
Solar keratosis, especially lichenoid or atrophic variety
Arsenical keratosis
Radiation keratosis
Psoriasis
Lichenified eczema
Lichen simplex chronicus
Discoid lupus erythematosus

I wish to stress the difficulty in clinically distinguishing between the causes of localized persistent scaly lesions particularly on sun-damaged skin (Table 24). The superficial multicentric basal cell carcinoma, the solar keratoses and the isolated facial plaque of discoid lupus erythematosus continue to defy easy diagnosis. A biopsy may be necessary.

Grass-Fire Basal Cell Carcinoma

The grass-fire type of basal cell carcinoma ("flat cicatricial rodent ulcer") consists of a rather large area with a raised papular border (up to 5 mm in width and height) and a central white sclerotic area. The border is pearly, telangiectatic, and in a few areas, small ulcerations may be seen. No black or brown pigmentation is present. The border is often not complete, and areas can be found where no definite papulation is seen. The central area occasionally shows a few scattered papular tumors. The temple is a favorite site.

Pigmented Nevi (Melanocytic Nevi)

These are dome-shaped elevated papules that may be skin-colored to brown to black, with lanugo or large black hairs. They are sharply marginated, usually round, and of a consistency only slightly more dense than the surrounding skin. The surface may be smooth or verrucous. Occasionally they are pedunculated. Sometimes the papule is just palpable and the prominent feature is the thick black hair. On the face, a few telangiectatic vessels may be present on the surface. Rarely, pigmented nevi may be eruptive following a severe bullous disorder.

On the face, particularly in those patients with acne or with a greasy skin, acne pustules or papules or granulomata may develop in hairy facial pigmented nevi. These lesions present as inflamed, tender papules from which occasionally a bead of pus can be expressed.

In children, nevi may be macular. They can be distinguished from freckles by their more irregular and larger shape and by their persistence. Also, the brown black pigment is dot-like, and reticulated. The lateral margin merges gradually into the surrounding skin.

Nevi with a white halo up to 1 cm in diameter are called halo nevi. They are usually on the torso and may be multiple. Sometimes only the white circle may be present. The white halo is of uniform width. Young adults and teenagers are the usually affected age group. There may be associated vitiligo. A circular area of non-specific dermatitis around melanocytic nevi has been called halo dermatitis.

Spitz nevi (benign juvenile melanoma) are red, rapidly growing papules with occasionally some telangiectatic blood vessels, usually on the face of the prepubertal child. Rarely, multiple lesions may be present. Four types of multiple lesions have been described: disseminated, grouped on normal skin, grouped on hyperpigmented skin, grouped on hypopigmented skin.[8]

Target-like (or cockade) pigmented nevi consist of central, 2 to 4 mm, brownish black papules surrounded by a number of small pinpoint-sized pigmented papules or macules arranged in a circle at a distance of 4 to 5 mm from the central lesion. Within this circle, the skin is slightly brownish.

Fibrous papules of the nose are small (2 to 5 mm) dome-shaped, sessile, skin-colored or red papules mainly on the alae. They may represent fibrotic, angiomatous resolving pigmented nevi or angiofibromas.

Penile pearly papules are 1 to 3 mm pedunculated firm papules sometimes with a purplish hue. They are located on the coronal margin and sulcus. Sometimes they are quite white.

Bathing suit nevi (giant congenital nevi) are very large, extensive, confluent papular plaques of a brown to black color, usually furrowed on the surface and often containing black coarse hair, and covering as indicated the bathing suit area (the bathing suit of the 1920s). The term cape nevus is used to describe lesions covering the cape area of the upper back. In most cases the back is more involved than the anterior portion of the chest.

In addition to the huge primary lesion, there may be hundreds of other papular, hairy, brown or brown black lesions on all areas, including such rather unusual sites as the palms, soles, and scalp. In some cases, these present only as macular brown lesions, sometimes with coarse black hair. Sometimes the lesions present bizarre shapes: some are rectangular, others have a linear component, and so on. These lesions tend to be ovoid with varying degrees of light brown, dark brown, or black coloration. The borders are not map-like, and do not have a café au lait color. In some cases, there is a looseness of the skin in the nevus so that it can be picked up and appears relatively inelastic, like the skin of a cat.

Rarely, there is pigment regression and partial spontaneous resolution of giant congenital nevi. This change is most obvious on the mid and lower back.[9]

Small congenital pigmented nevi are usually over 2.0 cm in their longest axis, ovoid and contain thick black hairs. They are evenly pigmented in varying degrees of brown or black.

The suggested morphology of dysplastic or atypical nevi is listed in Table 25.

Table 25: **Morphology of Atypical or Dysplastic Nevi**
1. There are many more nevi than the normal adult average of 27. Sometimes there may be as many as 200 to 300.
2. Many are over 1.0 cm in diameter, an unusual size for a normal nevus.
3. Many have irregular, notched borders. Many are not oval or round, as are normal nevi.
4. The irregularities in their red, brown, or black color are noteworthy. The peripheral accentuation or cockade formation have been called "fried egg" appearance.
5. Location of many of these lesions is characteristically on the sun-exposed areas of the upper extremities, chest and back. A smaller number are present on such atypical areas as the frontotemporal area of the scalp, the breasts, the buttocks, the ankles and dorsa of the feet and toes, all areas in which moles are only rarely found.

In any particular case, any one or all of the five features may be predominant. In some patients, a certain pattern of difference is noted, e.g. almost all or many of the moles in some patients have a "fried egg" appearance.

The clinical selection of which nevus should be biopsied is difficult. Obvious changes such as bleeding, crusting, rapid changes in shape, color or size, make for an easy decision. What is more difficult is to make a decision on the first visit when there are multiple, variegated lesions on the back. One criterion which has been suggested is the "ugly ducking" nevus. As mentioned above, many times the pattern of variation from normal is present in many, if not all of the atypical nevi. The "ugly duckling" concept suggests that if all the nevi show, for example, a large, flat, red-brown profile, or a "fried-egg" arrangement, then a small, black, flat lesion in such a patient might by considered worthy of biopsy. "The 'ugly duckling' nevus is the nevus that does not resemble its brother nevi".[10]

Some have questioned the validity of separating dysplastic or atypical moles from regular moles is open to question because clinically dysplastic moles may be histologically normal and clinically normal moles may be histologically dysplastic.

Some correlation can be made between the clinical and histological types of nevi.[10]

Junctional nevi, usually in children and on the palms and soles in adults, have a dark color and tend to be flat or just slightly elevated.

Compound nevi, as in young adults, are more protuberant and have a lighter brown and often have more than one color.

Intradermal nevi, as on the faces of older adults are often even more protuberant, are apt to be skin-colored and have large hairs in them.

Nevus spilus (speckled lentiginous nevus) is a pale brown pigmented patch studded with darker brown or black tiny to medium-sized papules. These papules have a pigmented nevus-type appearance.

Blue Papular Tumors

The blue nevus of Jadassohn-Tiéche is an intradermal papule with a blue or blue green color, which is usually circular or ovoid, and has a sharply marked border.

Josef Jadassohn, 1863–1936, German Dermatologist, Bern and Breslau

Max Tiéche, Swiss Dermatologist, Zurich

Average size is from 0.5 to 1 cm. The surface is dome-shaped and smooth. The color is really quite distinctive and involves varying shades of blue, blue-green, blue-brown, and blue-black. The degree of elevation varies, and in some lesions appears macular.

Table 26: **Blue Papular Tumors**
Blue Nevus
Blue and true (combined) nevus
Malignat melanoma
Cellular blue nevus
Osteomas on face, colored with tetracycline

The dorsa of the feet, hands, forearms, and buttocks are favorite sites.

Malignant melanoma may have a bluish tinge, but in almost all cases, the black or brown features overwhelm the blue color. They often have many colors of black or brown as well. The pigmentation is not so regular as it is in a blue nevus.

Cellular blue nevus is a deep-seated (hypodermal-dermal) blue black lesion, often occurring on the buttock.

Blue, 2 mm, firm, tetracycline-stained osteomas may be seen scattered over the cheeks in patients who have had severe scarring acne.

Table 26 lists the varieties of blue papular tumors.

Papular Angiomatous Tumors

A pyogenic granuloma is a soft, pea-sized papule, bright red in color, with a smooth or slightly irregular glistening surface. The lesion has the appearance of being strangulated at the base, and normal epidermis can be seen to cover the lower 1 to 2 mm of the stalk where it is attached. The rest of the lesion is obviously devoid of covering epidermis. Evidence of recent hemorrhage is commonly present. The lesions are most common on the hands and fingers but may develop on an underlying pre-existing telangiectasis (usually congenital such as a port wine stain or angioma). Rarely, recurrent satellite lesions appear following removal.

Beside the common pyogenic granuloma, other lesions on the palms and soles may develop a moat or gutter at their base. Examples are eccrine poroma and palmar and digital fibrokeratoma.

Proud flesh (as around in-growing toe nails) shows the same basic tissue as in pyogenic granulomas, but the mushroom shape is often absent. Ulcers of long standing, or slow-healing wounds are common sites for proud flesh.

In a few patients with severe solar dystrophy, erosive red areas may develop to look like angiomatous basal cell carcinomas, but these are in fact proud flesh. I have seen the same phenomenon

Table 27: **Papular Angiomatous Tumors**
Pyogenic granuloma
Proud flesh
Erosive angiomas on severe solar bald scalp dystophy
Kaposi's sarcoma
Bacillary angiomatosus
Amelanotic melanoma
Basal and squamous cell carcinoma
Angiosarcoma
Spitz nevus
Aggressive angiomatosis
Pregnancy angioma
Lyphangioma circumscription and lymphangiectases
Senile angioma
Caviar tongue
Gingival hypertrophy
Angiokeratoma

develop in scars following electrodesiccation and curettage on solar dystrophic skin, and be mistaken for recurrent basal cell carcinomas. The sun-damaged bald pate is a favorite location for this to occur.

Table 27 provides a list of papular angiomatous tumors.

DIFFERENTIAL DIAGNOSIS

The differential diagnosis of pyogenic granuloma should include the following:

Classic Kaposi's sarcoma usually shows multiple, usually nonulcerated, non-pedunculated, more deep-seated and firm angiomatous papules, frequently located about the ankles and feet. Evidence of bleeding is not present. The lesions may have a purplish hue. As time goes by, the lesions may become nodular (over 1 cm, and situated more deeply in the dermis) and more frequently ulcerated. Kaposi's sarcoma is to be differentiated particularly from recurrent pyogenic granuloma with satellites.

In some cases, the lesions are widespread, sharply marginated purplish spots, plaques, and lightly infiltrated papules. These can be widely disseminated, but are more numerous and larger on the lower extremities, especially on the feet and ankles.

In epidemic Kaposi's sarcoma great variations in color (from pink to black) and morphology (from nondescript erythematous macules to follicular papules to varying sized red papules to large fungating masses) occur.[12] Occasionally, acro-angiodermatitis may have have an angiomatous element.

Bacillary angiomatosis lesions in AIDS are accumulations of blood vessels at the dermal or hypodermal level. The lesions are commonly multiple, and depending on their depth and size, may resemble cherry angioma, pyogenic granuloma, or angiosarcoma.

Newly described (1991) skin disorders found in patients with HIV disease are:
- hairy leukoplakia
- ecthymatous varicella-zoster infection
- multiple resistant facial molluscum contagiosum
- bacillary angiomatosis
- epidemic Kaposi's sarcoma

Amelanotic melanoma may present as an ulcerated angiomatous lesion. Some dots of brown or black pigment are occasionally present in the periphery. It should be pointed out that amelanotic does not mean achromic, i.e. without color or white; it means that these lesions are skin-colored or reddish or purplish. Ulceration and evidence of recent bleeding, and the presence of semitranslucent gelatinous-appearing tumor tissue are more common characteristics of the larger or nodular lesion. Pressure on an angioma may cause the lesion to flatten; this will not happen with a malignant melanoma.

Rarely, other tumors with an angiomatous component (e.g. squamous cell carcinoma about the nail, the early lesions of angiosarcoma of the head and neck, angiomatous adult or childhood pigmented nevi, or angiomatous basal cell carcinoma on the helix or thigh) may be confused with pyogenic granuloma.

Aggressive angiomatosis shows numerous (up to 15) 3 to 4 mm angiomatous

Tokuya Kimura, 1871– Japanese Pathologist, Tokyo

papules scattered here and there, in and behind the ears, and in the scalp. The papules are fairly deep and purplish red. The lesions vary in size and bleed easily. Recurrences or new lesions often appear. Angiolymphoid hyperplasia with eosinophilia is a similar condition as are pseudo-pyogenic granuloma, Kimura's disease and histocytoid hemangioma.

Rarely, the telangiectases of pregnancy may be papular, or even nodular.

Remember to include lymphangioma circumscriptum and lymphangiectases in the differential diagnosis, as they may contain blood-filled cysts and angiomatous lesions. The basic lesion of clear dilated cystic lymphatics can usually be found.

Senile angiomas are punctiform or lenticular, 1 to 3 cm, carmine angiomas, often developing in large numbers on the trunk and limbs of individuals past 40 years of age. They are not compressible.

A thrombosed capillary angioma is a solitary, soft, dark blue or black papule, often with the surrounding coloration of a bruise. Prior to thrombosis, it has a red strawberry-like surface. This should be distinguished from the neonatal strawberry hemangioma. Caviar tongue is the name given to numerous 2 to 3 mm purplish dark blue dilated venous lakes usually located on the side of the tongue.

Angiomatous gingival hypertrophy, as produced by phenytoin, can produce a hyperplasia of the gingivae that circumscribes the necks of the individual teeth. It is quite firm, mucosa colored, with little tendency to bleed. As it increases in size, the surface may become finely lobulated, finally producing a large tissue fold partially obstructing the tooth from view and possibly interfering with occlusion.

The hyperplasia of the gums in pregnancy, and their tendency to bleed readily, are not really a true hyperplasia. There is enlargement of the gingival tissues. A localized area of inflammatory hyperplasia may present as a deep purple mass 2 to 10 mm in diameter, usually arising from a gingival papilla between two adjacent teeth. Ulceration may occur.

Angiokeratoma (of Mibelli) is composed of multiple, discrete, dark red, 2 to 4 mm, angiomatous papules the surfaces of which are hyperkeratotic and verrucous. Pressure obliterates the red color. The lesions are located mainly on the dorsal surface of the fingers.

Angiokeratoma of the scrotum (angiokeratoma of Fordyce) consists of numerous, small, spherical, dark purple papules from 1 to 3 mm in diameter, which appear to rest on the skin rather than be embedded in it. The surface is thickened and horny. Pressure obliterates most of the red color.

Rare cases of angiokeratoma circumscriptum and angiokeratoma corporis diffusum (Fabry's disease) have been described by Fabry. Other rare angiokeratomas may be present on the scrotum, penis, and tips of toes. Not all angiokeratomas have a keratotic horny surface; some appear just as papular angiomas. Other types of telangiectatic, lymphatic, or papular angiomas may develop a keratotic surface.

Johannes Fabry, 1860–1930, German Dermatologist
Vittorio Mibelli, 1860–1910, Italian Dermatologist, Parma

Leukemia Cutis

The basic lesion in leukemia cuits is a purple-, violet-, or plum-colored papule located primarily in the mid and lower dermis. This can be determined, because the papules have gently sloping edges and a mainly dome-shaped contour with no epidermal change. The papules have a slightly oval shape and tend to be situated along the lines of tension. There is quite a variation in size and color. The early lesion is a just palpable dermal papule of a light brown or skin color. The largest, most palpable, most purple lesions are located on the anterior mid torso; smaller and less purple colored lesions are located on the sides of the neck and tops of shoulders.

DIFFERENTIAL DIAGNOSIS

This condition is to be distinguished from mycosis fungoides, where the lesions are larger, usually ulcerated, and rarely have a distinct purplish color; there are also arcuate lesions with central healing and some areas will show psoriasiform plaques. Kaposi's sarcoma lesions are redder or browner, rarely as widely disseminated, and usually having an acral distribution.

In other cases, the purplish masses are nodules or nodes and are located on the nose, cheeks, ears, and gingival mucosa. These, along with their differential diagnosis, are discussed under nodes and nodules.

Papilloepitheliomata (Skin Tags, Polyps, Acrochordon)

These are multiple (often innumerable), flabby, light or dark brown, usually small (1 to 2 mm) pedunculated tumors. They occur on the sides of the neck, in the axillae, and in

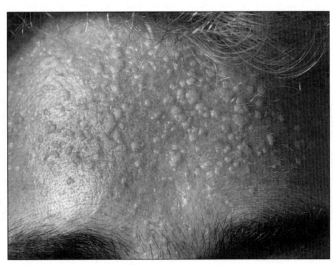

Figure 11.7 Verrucae planae on the forehead.

the genital regions. Occasionally, pea-sized or grape-sized lesions are seen. They may occur during pregnancy. If many are present along with café au lait spots, suspect neurofibromatosis. Some of these have the histological features of seborrheic keratoses.

Flat Warts (Verrucae Planae)

The warts designated by this name appear as an eruption of small epidermal papules, not more than 3 mm in diameter, flattened, and barely protuberant (Fig. 11.7). They have rounded or irregularly polygonal contours, are sharply circumscribed, have the color of the normal skin or show a yellowish, grayish, or brownish tint. In blacks, they have a dark brown or black color. Their surface is finely puckered or slightly scaly. The papules often occur in lines, usually from scratching. Confluent plaques may occur.

These warts are seen especially on the face, specifically the cheeks, temples, forehead, and chin, and vary in number from a few to several hundred. They may also occupy the back of the hands, sometimes in association with common warts, but are less common on the forearms. They usually occur in children. They also can be seen in women who shave their legs.

DIFFERENTIAL DIAGNOSIS

Epidermodysplasia verruciformis is morphologically indistinguishable from disseminated flat warts. The lesions of bowenoid papulosis are located on the glans penis and vulva. They are quite brown.

Molluscum Contagiosum

These papules are small, firm, hemispherical, prominent elevations of a pearly or skin color, umbilicated in their centers. Pinpoint- to pea-sized, they are usually multiple. Occasionally, secondary staphylococcal pyoderma occurs. Often, healed erythematous erosions can be seen at the site of lesions removed by scratching. Sometimes a half-dollar sized (2.7 cm diameter) area of scaly eczema surrounds one or several, but not all, of the papules. This eczema may also occur on the skin in apposition to a molluscum lesion. The condition occurs most often in children and young adults. After being squeezed out, the molluscum "body" is seen to have a translucent pinkish color and to be of a firm rubbery consistency. Brisk capillary bleeding occurs from the erosion once the body is removed. Rarely, multiple eruptive molluscum contagiosa lesions occur in pre-existing diseases such as atopic dermatitis, psoriatic erythroderma, or burn scars, or in immunosuppressed patients. A linear arrangement may also be seen. Spraying with a refrigerant clearly shows the central delling.

DIFFERENTIAL DIAGNOSIS

Solitary large molluscum, particularly on the eyelids, may be confused with keratoacanthoma or may have a yellowish hue like a solitary sebaceous adenoma. Solitary lesions can resemble a nonulcerated basal cell carcinoma.

Accessory Tragi

These are solitary, lifelong, sessile, soft, skin-colored papules about 3 to 5 mm in width and up to 1 cm in length. Baby hairs may be present on the surface. they are usually located in the preauricular area, usually just above or below the tragus.

Supernumerary digits may occur in all shapes and forms. They should be distinguished from acquired digital fibrokeratomas.

Adnexal Tumors

Senile Sebaceous Hyperplasia (Adenoma)

These are small (up to 3 mm diameter) yellow or orange papules, translucent, circular, and usually with umbilication. They are seen around and past middle life on the forehead and cheeks, often in patients with clinically oily skin. They may have fine peripheral telangiectatic blood vessels.

Rarely, an extensive hyperplasia of sebaceous glands occurs, producing leonine facies. There is also a variety called premature sebaceous gland hyperplasia which occurs on the face and chest in adolescents.

Nevus Sebaceous

Before puberty, this may be present as a thin yellowish plaque; after puberty, as a linear, corn-yellowish cluster of papules, usually occurring on the head and neck. An average size is 3 by 1 cm. The size of the papules may vary, with the larger ones being together at one end or in the center, and the smaller papules occurring at the periphery and occasionally appearing as satellites. In some cases, a prominent pore may be present in the center of some of the papules. These lesions follow the lines of Blaschko. Basal cell carcinoma can arise on these lesions. It is best considered as a sebaceous variety of epidermal nevus (nevus unius lateris).

Adenoma Sebaceum (Angiofibromas)

The lesions of adenoma sebaceum are pinhead- to bean-sized, firm, fibrous papules varying in color from yellowish white to deep brownish red.[13] Many lesions are the color of the normal skin, often with the surface vascularized by the presence of minute capillaries. The lesions are usually discrete, but confluence sometimes occurs, with the formation of plaques, often verrucous, especially on the forehead. Transverse grooves may cross these plaques. Sometimes the lesions are polypoid. They are situated chiefly on the face, over the cheeks, chin, forehead, and particularly in the furrows beside the nose. The circumoral area is frequently free of lesions. They do not occur below the clavicle. Symmetry is a definite feature. Histologically, these papules consist of excess sebaceous glands, excess fibrous tissue, and excess capillary tissue, in varying degrees and combinations.

Many other cutaneous findings are present in the full-blown case of tuberous sclerosis. These include various types of fibromas in the scalp, axillae, groin, mouth, and periungual and subungual areas. Shagreen (a type of processed leather) plaque (the collagenous plaque) usually is located on the sacral area. In these plaques, the pilosebaceous orifices are prominent. Some of the fibromas resemble cutaneous tags or papilloepitheliomata. The nail plate may show longitudinal linear depressions or grooves from the fibromas.

Various kinds of pigmented, hairy, and vascular nevi may also be present. Café au lait spots may be present on the torso. Also, white macules on the trunk may occur, varying in size from a few millimeters to several centimeters. They are linear, oval configurations, with one end round and the other pointed and serrated, like a mountain ash leaflet. Wood's light examination is helpful in identifying these lesions.

Mental retardation and seizures may also occur.

Trichoepithelioma (Epithelioma Adenoides Cysticum, Brooke's Tumor)
With Brooke's tumor, the central portion of the patient's face is studded with pearly colored, firm, round papules up to 8 mm in diameter. In many central areas, the lesions are confluent and no normal skin can be seen. The lesions are symmetrically located and extend onto the forehead, eyelids, and chin, with the most dense areas being on the sides of the nose. A considerable degree of telangiectasis is present over and about the papules. Laterally, the size and number of the papules decreases, so that almost none are present in the preauricular area. A few papules are present on the scalp and upper back. Milia may be present in the lesion.

Syringoma
Syringoma are yellowish or skin-colored, pinhead- to split-pea-sized, well-demarcated, ovoid papules that occur mainly in the central portion of the face (including the forehead, lower eyelids, infra-ocular area and paranasal area), and on the anterior sides of the neck. Rarely, they occur on the central chest and upper back. There is a close resemblance to perifollicular fibromata. The papules are dermal with a sloping smooth surface. They tend to run along the lines of cleavage of the skin on the neck. Only rarely are the majority of lesions not on the face.

A familial eruptive form often seen in young girls which can be very extensive and even involve such areas as the umbilicus. Other rare varieties are the linear, vulvar, acral and milia-like on the eyelid.

Neurofibromatosis (Von Recklinghausen's disease)
This condition is characterized by: (1) a frequent extensive freckling in each axilla (Crowe's sign), groin and often on the torso as well; (2) map-like, café au lait colored, pigmented often ovoid patches from 2 to 10 cm in diameter, located most frequently on the torso; (3) cutaneous papules and nodules of varying size, shape, and location; (4) mental retardation, seizures, and skull and facial deformities; and (5) Lisch nodules which are raised brown hamartomas on the iris.

Henry Ambrose Grundy Brooke, 1854–1919, British Dermatologist, Manchester

R. S. Crowe, British Physician

K. Lisch, 1907– Austrian Ophthalmologist

Friedrich Daniel Von Recklinghausen, 1833–1910, German Pathologist

The size of neurofibromas varies from 0.5 to 4 cm; the shape is mostly circular, although some are pendulous. They are located mainly above the level of the skin, but a few are obviously in the hypoderm. Some resemble the shapes of nipples. Consistency varies from firm to flabby. Most have a peculiar rubbery, thick, gelatinous consistency. These often have a bluish cast. Some can be pushed in, as a hernia (button-hole sign), but this also can be found in polypoid intradermal nevi. Occasionally the tumors are segmental. Some enormous, almost elephantiasis-like abnormalities of the extremities are occasionally seen. These may be associated with underlying bony abnormalities.

Facial Neuroma

The typical lesion of facial neuroma is a solitary, painless, flesh colored, dome-shaped papule or papulonodule, usually appearing in the central portion of the face, especially on the chin.[14] On palpation it is firm, yet not stony hard. It is clearly dermal and well demarcated. The overlying skin, which is smooth and somewhat pearly, is stretched from the underlying dermal swelling. The skin markings are obliterated. Telangiectases may be present. Terminal hair is usually not present. Average size is 5 mm. The lesion appears in adults only. When cut into, the lesion shells out like a white pea. The tissue is of a rubbery consistency.

DIFFERENTIAL DIAGNOSIS

Intradermal pigmented nevi, which often show terminal hairs, may have some brown pigmentation, show no loss of normal skin markings, and tend to be softer in consistency.

Basal cell carcinomas, which contain more telangiectatic blood vessels, have a more definite pearly color and consistency, and may show some central delling or ulceration.

Solitary neurofibroma, which is softer and may show herniation, should be included in the differential diagnosis.

Other adnexal tumors such as eccrine spiradenoma and leiomyoma must be considered.

Leiomyomas

Generally, with leiomyomas, a young patient presents with numerous, slowly growing tumors, usually on an extremity. The lesion may be dermal-papular or dermal nodular in nature. They appear to cluster, and some have an arciform or linear appearance. They are of a reddish brown color, with occasional telangiectases. There is an "apple jelly" or translucent brown appearance on diascopy. Tenderness may be a feature.

Fordyce's Condition

Fordyce's condition is a chronic condition characterized by discrete, 1 to 2 mm, yellowish or light-colored, milium-like maculo-papules, located just beneath the epithelium. They appear on the vermilion borders of the lips, on the inner side of the lips, and on the oral mucosa, particularly extending posteriorly from the oral commissures.

Sometimes plaques and bands are formed by coalescence of lesions. They are best seen by stretching the mucous membrane. The condition is usually symmetrical.

Multicentric Reticulohistiocytosis of the Skin and Synovia

The cutaneous lesions of multicentric reticulohistiocytosis consist of up to 200 small, firm papules, mainly on the hands and ears. These papules are oval or circular, 2 to 6 mm in diameter, deeply set in the skin, but apparently not attached to underlying structures. On the fingers, many arise at the bases of the fingernails and about the distal interphalangeal joints. Fewer appear on the palmar surfaces of the fingers and on the palms. The ears are studded with papules, especially on the upper half and especially on the posterior surface. Rarely, lesions may be seen on the forearms and elbows, scalp, forehead, neck, nose, and nasal septum.

A rheumatoid type of arthritis, moderately severe, is usually present in the hands, but occasionally in the wrists, elbows, shoulders, spine, and jaw. An enlarged thyroid gland may also be present.

DIFFERENTIAL DIAGNOSIS

The differential diagnosis consists of benign tumors of the synovia and tendon sheath, xanthomatoses, and the skin lesions of histiocytosis X.

Histiocytosis X (Langerhans Cell Histiocytosis)

LETTERER-SIWE DISEASE

The basic lesion is a brown scaly papule that occurs in crops and becomes confluent on the face, neck, and trunk. Vesicles or pustules may develop, followed by erosion. The consecutive stages may be infiltrated dermal papules, vesicles, ulceration, crusting, and scarring. Many of the papules show hemorrhage. Rarely, only purpura is present.

Also rarely, the accumulation of scales and crusts resembles a scaly dermatitis, e.g. seborrhea, but of course the basic papular nature, the hemorrhage, and the scarring exclude most banal dermatoses.

The gingiva may be inflamed and show necrosis. Oral and perianal ulceration with petechiae and hemorrhages may also be present.

HAND-SCHÜLLER-CHRISTIAN DISEASE

The basic lesion of this disease is a flesh-colored or brown petechial erythematous papule, which rarely has a yellowish hue. They do not appear in crops and are not as confluent as the papular eruption of Letterer-Siwe disease. Scarring may occur. A feature is a mixed scale-crust simulating an erythematosquamous eruption. Rarely, large nodular lesions occur.

Henry Asbury Christian, 1876–1951, U.S. Internist, Boston

Alfred Hand, 1868–1949, U.S. Pediatrician, Philadelphia

Paul Langerhans, 1847–1888, German Pathologist

Erich Letterer, 1895–1982, German Pathologist

Artur Schüller, 1874–1958, Austrian Neurologist, Vienna

Sturre Augst Siwe, 1897–1966, Pediatrician in Sweden

Ulcerative hemorrhagic lesions with loosening of the teeth occurs in the mouth. Oral, genital, and perianal ulcerations may be the presenting complaint.

Eosinophilic Granuloma of Bone

Only rarely is the skin involved in eosinophilic granuloma of bone. The presenting feature can be a persistent ulcerative granuloma of the palate and oropharyngeal tissues or of the perianal and perivulvar tissues.

DIFFERENTIAL DIAGNOSIS

Very rarely, xanthomatous lesions are seen in patients with histiocytosis X, as are lesions of nevoxanthoendothelioma (juvenile xanthogranuloma).

The differential diagnosis consists of eruptive histiocytoma, reticulohistiocytoma cutis, nevoxanthoendothelioma and the various xanthomatous eruptions.

Variations in the clinical and histological findings of Letterer-Siwe disease, Hand-Schüller-Christian disease and eosinophilic granuloma of bone suggest that each disease is not a clearly defined entity.

Connective Tissue Nevi

Connective tissue nevi are slightly raised, pale or yellow papules, often centered about hair follicles that tend to group in irregular patterns. The trunk is the most common location. Shagreen plaques of tuberous sclerosis are an example. Many may also show a peau d'orange appearance; also seen in pretibial myxedema, scleroderma, and cancerous infiltration of the skin of the breast.

Miscellaneous Rare Benign and Malignant Papulonodular Tumors

There are numerous rare papulonodular tumors (Table 28) without distinguishing features. These rare tumors can only be diagnosed by biopsy, unless one is very skilled, very lucky, or both.

In this group of rare tumors, the malignant ones may grow rapidly, be ulcerated, and metastasize.

The syndrome of multiple sebaceous gland neoplasms in association with an underlying colonic carcinoma should perhaps be mentioned here. The lesions are numerous (up to 50), are disseminated over the upper torso and face, and may present as adenoma sebaceous type lesions, as 2 to 4 mm papules, or as larger (up to 2 cm) erythematous infiltrates.

Papular Deposits

Amyloidosis: Localized

Lichen amyloidosus is characterized by papules, plaques, and pigmentation. It usually occurs on the lower legs, but may appear in other areas and, rarely, all over.

The papules are 2 to 3 mm in size, firm, and have a flattish top with slightly sloping edges. They are sharply marginated. There is no scale. They have a reddish or reddish

Table 28: Rare Benign and Malignant Papulonodular Tumors

Benign

Apocrine myoepithelioma

Atypical fibroxanthoma

Clear cell myoepithelioma

Eccrine poroma is a solitary, reddish, dome-shaped papule, usually occurring on the soles

Eccrine spiradenoma

Folliculoma is a solitary lesion, usually on the face, and consists of a small, whitish pearly papule with a central core

Glomus tumor

Mixed tumor of skin (chondroid syringoma)

Pseudorecidives are firm, sometimes angiomatous, elevated, papulonodules occurring in the center of an irradiated area where the ionizing radiation was given for skin cancer, usually basal or squamous cell carcinoma; usually solitary and appear 4 to 8 weeks after therapy has been finished, and usually disappear spontaneously in 3 to 4 months; residual tumor must, of course, be considered in the differential diagnosis

Sebaceous epithelioma

Solitary neurilemmoma

Solitary neuroma

Solitary reticulohistiocytoma

Nevus lipomatosus superficialis — flesh-colored or yellowish papules or plaques on the sacral area

Clear cell acanthoma

Warty dyskeratoma

Piezogenic pedal papules — soft skin-colored papules on the non-weight bearing portion of the heel that appear on standing

Soft fibrous round papules about which the lines of the palmar or plantar skin go; also called acquired fibrokeratoma

Perifollicular fibroma and trichodiscoma

Helical and anti-helical papules (see "Solar Dystrophy" in Chapter 18)

Trichofolliculoma

Malignant

Carcinoma of apocrine sweat glands

Carcinoma of eccrine sweat glands

Carcinoma of sebaceous glands

brown color. The papules may form small plaques, but usually there are areas of normal skin between the papules and plaques. The border is reasonably well demarcated, with the papules less numerous and smaller toward the periphery.

There is much browning, both of the papules and of the intervening and adjacent skin. A degree of purple color is often present.

Macular amyloid is a dyschromia.

DIFFERENTIAL DIAGNOSIS

The differential diagnosis includes lichen planus, in which the papules are more lichenoid (flat-topped with straight edges), more purplish and polygonal, and have some scale and occasionally (on the legs), Wickham's striae. Also to be considered is lichen simplex chronicus, with less clear definition of the papules, lesions less well defined, and more brown coloration. The lateral aspect of the lower leg is the site of predilection. Excoriations or the effects of rubbing are often seen.

Amyloidosis: Systemic

Macroglossia is present. The tongue is thick and indurated, movements are limited, and speech is muffled. The papillae are obliterated; the tongue, smooth and diffusely reddened, may be studded with red or yellowish papules and nodules, both dorsally and on the ventral and lateral surfaces (Fig. 11.8). The sides of the tongue may be indented by the teeth. Lesions may be present on the vermilion border of the lips at the oral commissures. Ecchymoses are common.

In systemic amyloidosis, the skin shows numerous translucent papules and plaques varying in size from 1 to 20 mm. They have a yellowish cast; but may be various shades of red due to the presence of purpuric hemorrhage (Fig. 11.9). The medial canthi, nasolabial folds, perioral regions, chin, neck, axillae, submammary areas, inguinal folds, and perianal area are common locations. Yellowish-brown bullae sometimes develop on normal shin or on waxy, brown, infiltrated plaques, especially on the pre-tibial areas.

In some cases, deposits of amyloid may present as a primarily macular eruption.

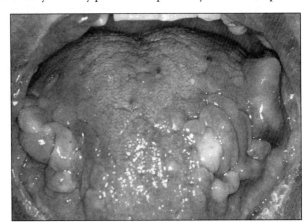

Figure 11.8 The tongue in systemic amyloidosis.

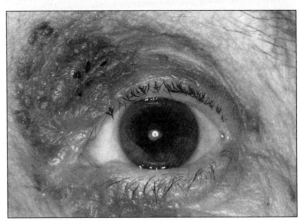

Figure 11.9 Plaques of amyloid on the eyelids.

Colloid Pseudomilia

Other names for colloid pseudomilia are colloid degeneration of the skin, hyaloma-colloid milia, elastosis colloidalis conglomerata, colloid milium, and miliary colloid degeneration of the cutis.

These lesions are translucent, soft, yellowish, waxy papules, ranging in size from pinhead- to pea-sized, disseminated or conglomerated, on light-exposed areas, especially on the upper one-third of the face around the orbits, but also on the dorsa of the hands and forearms, the helixes of the ear, and the neck. A rare type, with nodules and plaques up to 5 cm in diameter and usually with telangiectasia, is present on the facial skin.

Tophi

The seat of election of gouty tophi is on the external ears, especially the upper portion of the helix. These concretions, from one or two to about ten in number, constitute small tumors from the size of a millet seed to that of a pea usually the color of normal skin or purplish, with an opaque white hue shining through it.

Occasionally, tophi are present on other areas such as the vicinity of gouty joints, over the olecranon or on the prepatellar bursa, or around the joints of the fingers and toes. These tophic concretions are intradermal or subcutaneous; at first small and multiple, they tend to become agglomerated and spread out. soft at first, they subsequently become extremely hard.

Sometimes tophi disappear spontaneously, sometimes abscesses develop, or sometimes the tight overlying skin opens without suppuration and discharges a white chalky substance.

Xanthomas

Plane xanthomas are plaques or papules, slightly raised, 1 to 5 cm or more in diameter, with a corn-yellow to whitish color. The neck, chest, buttocks, and creases of the palms may be involved. Xanthelasma occurs on the eyelids (medial canthus, upper and lower eyelids) as linear, diffuse, or solitary papules. The lateral canthus is rarely involved.

Xanthoma tuberosum are papular, plaque-like, nodular lesions with a predilection for the extensor surfaces and areas of trauma (elbows, knees, and heels). They may also occur around the axillae and perianal areas. This is a slowly progressive eruption, which starts with papules that become enlarged and confluent, forming large conglomerations separated by deep furrows. The color ranges from yellow to deep orange, although older lesions may be light or deep brown. These conglomerations are usually soft, unless they become fibrosed. The epidermis covering these lesions may be normal or keratotic. The lesions rarely ulcerate. The oral mucosa is not involved.

When the tendon sheaths are involved, coalescence of nodules and nodes occurs, forming hazelnut- to egg-sized tumors that are knobby and quite firm or fibrotic. Rarely, the lesions may be very widespread and have many of the characteristics of plane xanthoma.

When numerous small papular lesions appear suddenly and have the distribution of xanthoma tuberosum, the clinical picture has been called xanthoma diabeticorum or xanthoma eruptivum. The oral mucosa may be involved. Occasionally the lesions may be perifollicular. They tend to have a reddish-yellow hue.

Xanthoma disseminatum presents with papular or nodular lesions, with the sites of predilection being the flexor (not the extensor) surfaces. The neck, groin, antecubital fossa, and mucous membranes are often involved.

Mixed forms do occur, and the clinical patterns may not be as clear-cut as described above. Occasionally a solitary xanthoma may be found, usually in the upper extremity without systemic disease. Xanthelasma is almost never associated with a lipidemia.

DIFFERENTIAL DIAGNOSIS

Numerous conditions present in papular or nodular lesions with a yellowish cast. Some are solitary, others are widespread.

Nevoxanthoendothelioma presents rather deep-seated papules or nodules, alone or in groups, in the infant or young child. The face, upper torso, or arms are frequent sites. The lesions have a yellowish-red color.

Some epidermal inclusion cysts on the eyelids may have a yellowish color. Incision with a fine eye knife will reveal the diagnosis.

Some adnexal tumors, especially syringoma, may have a yellowish hue. However, these are separate, ovoid-shaped dermal papules, often present on other areas of the face or neck.

Dermatofibromas on the shins and elsewhere may show a yellowish color. These are indurated lesions with a flattish surface and with much upper dermal fibrosis.

Urticaria pigmentosa may occasionally have a yellowish hue, but the urtication is easily produced on rubbing.

Many conditions may have a yellowish cast, but other findings usually make a diagnosis obvious. These may include Letterer-Siwe disease, eosinophilic granuloma of bone and skin, solar degeneration of the skin, pseudoxanthoma elasticum, multiple ganglioneuromas (reticulohistiocytosis), lipoid proteinosis, rheumatoid nodules, colloid pseudomilia and gouty tophi.

Pseudoxanthoma Elasticum

The lesions of pseudoxanthoma elasticum are asymptomatic, discrete, yellow to orange, pinhead- to pea-sized papules, which assume a linear arrangement or which manage to form plaques of various sizes. The flexural folds often become lax or stretched. The neck and axillae are favorite sites, but lesions also may occur on the antecubital and popliteal spaces and the groin. Symmetry is a striking feature. One could argue that this is not a true deposit. It is included here for convenience.

DIFFERENTIAL DIAGNOSIS

The differential diagnosis includes solar elastosis of the neck, xanthoma disseminatum, colloid milia, amyloidosis and cutis laxa.

Lipoid Proteinosis (Hyalinosis Cutis et Mucosae)

Papular and nodular, keratotic verrucous, and fibrous sclerosing lesions are present on the face, extremities, and mucous membranes, including the larynx and pharynx. The eyelid margins are a favorite site of lesions. The tongue has a firm, almost wood-like consistency and is bound to the floor of the mouth. The mucous membrane of the lips exhibits white plaques. Hypertrophic plaques are present on the elbows and knees. Verrucous lesions are frequently present on the fingers and feet. The lesions are of normal skin color. The patient has a hoarse voice.

Lichen Myxedematosus

This is a widespread eruption of asymptomatic, soft, pale red or yellowish, waxy papules, usually 2 to 3 mm in diameter. They may be densely packed, but are not patterned in their arrangement. Scleromyxedema shows the same type of papule, but the skin has a diffuse, moveable thickening. Sometimes a peau d'orange picture is seen; sometimes the lichenification is most pronounced; and sometimes the lesions are nodular. Varying degrees of red or red- brown erythema may be present.

Pretibial myxedema is discussed in Chapter 19.

Other focal papular mucinoses are listed in Table 29.

Table 29: **Focal Papular Mucinoses**						
Disease	Age	Regions	Lesions	Paraprotein	Thyroid Disease	Resolution
Lichen myxedematosus	Adults	Face, arms, axillae	Multiple	Yes	No	No
Cutaneous focal mucinosis	Adults	All	Single	No	No	No
Self-healing juvenile cutaneous mucinosis	Adolescents	Head, abdomen, thighs	Multiple	No	No	Spontaneous
Cutaneous mucinosis	Infant	Upper Limbs	Multiple	No	No	No
Mucinosis with thyroid disease	Adults	All	Multiple	Occasional	Yes	No
Acral persistent papular mucinosis	Adults	Forearms	Multiple	No	No	No

References

1. Siemens HW. General diagnosis and therapy of skin diseases. Weiner K, trans. Chicago:University of Chicago Press, 1958.
2. Hanafin JM, Rajka G. Diagnostic features of atopic dermatitis. Acta Dermatol Venereol 1980; 92(Suppl).:44–47.
3. Sehgal VN, Jain S. Atopic dermatitis: clinical criteria. Int J Dermatol 1993; 32:628–634.
4. Sulzberger MB, Wolf J, Witten VH, Kopf AW. Dermatology diagnosis & treatment. 2nd Ed. Chicago:Year Book Publisher, 1961; 197–199.
5. Williams HC, Burney PGJ, Pembroke AC, Hay RJ. U.K. working party report. Br J Dermatol 1994; 131:411.
6. Butterworth T, Strean LP. Behavioural disorders of interest to dermatologists. Arch Dermatol 1963; 88:859–867.
7. Stokes JH, Beerman H, Ingraham NR Jr. Modern clinical syphilology—Diagnosis, treatment, case study. 3rd Ed. Philadelphia:WB Saunders, 1944.
8. Prose NS, Heilman E, Felman YM, Tanzer F, Silber J. Multiple benign juvenile melanoma. J Am Acad Dermatol 1983; 9:263–242.
9. Hogan DJ, Murphy F, Bremner RM. Spontaneous resolution of a giant melanocytic nevus. Ped Derm 1988; 5:170–173.
10. Grob JJ, Boner Andi JJ. The ugly duckling sign; identification of the common characteristics of nevi in an individual as a basis for melanoma screening. Arch Dermatol 1998; 134:103-104.
11. Jackson R. Origin and development of malignant melanoma of the skin. Can Med Assoc J 1968; 99:1–10.
12. Fisher BK, Warner LE. Cutaneous manifestations of the acquired immunodeficiency syndrome. Int J Dermatol 1987; 26:615–630.
13. Butterworth T, Wilson M. Dermatologic aspects of tuberous sclerosis. Arch Dermatol Syph 1941; 43:1–41.
14. Reed RJ, Fine RM, Meltzer HD. Palisaded, encapsulated neuromas of the skin. Arch Dermatol 1972; 106:865–870.

CHAPTER 12
Nodules

> A persistent large (over 1.0 cm) epidermal-dermal, dermal,
> or dermal-hypodermal papule with well-defined borders.
> It is a solid lesion with a prominent vertical dimension.

Overview

Solid, well-defined eminences on or in the skin that are too big to be called papules (larger than a lentil, pea, or almond) are called nodules. The nodule is simply a large epidermal-dermal, dermal, or dermal-hypodermal papule with well-defined borders. In one case, namely in the nodular hypertrophy of sebaceous glands and connective tissue of the nose, one speaks of a phyma (bulb).[1]

Epidermal nodules, such as keratoacanthoma, should be distinguished from lichenification and plaque formation. The latter two are surface lesions with the lesion being much more spread out and with only a small depth component. The epidermal nodule on the other hand can have as much depth component as breadth. At times, the concept of nodule and plaque can be combined, as in nodular plaques on the legs.

Granuloma

Clinically, nodular granuloma has the following meaning: a deeply situated dermal and/or hypodermal papulonodular lesion or lesions. Each lesion is solid, well circumscribed, more or less prominent, of slow development, and painless. Some of the granules are small seed-sized, some pea-sized, and some grape-sized. They often occur in annular or arcuate conglomerations, although at the periphery isolated smaller single lesions may be seen. Because of their deep location, the papulonodules have smooth sloping surfaces. Most have a reddish brown semitranslucent appearance; a few are skin-colored. Pressure with a glass slide removes the erythema, but not the cellular infiltrate, which shows as a brown opaque color, the apple jelly papule or nodule.

Breakdown of the papulonodules may result in the formation of ulcers (with crusts), scarring, and sinus formation. Scarring may occur without ulceration. The number of lesions is usually small (up to ten), but solitary lesions or up to 50 may be present. In most cases, the cause of a granuloma*2 cannot be determined from its living gross morphology.

Historically, the term granuloma has been applied to such nodular eruptions as tuberculosis, syphilis, leprosy, the deep mycoses, sarcoidosis, and foreign body granulomas. I have included the granulomatous diseases as a type of nodular eruption, but there are many nodular lesions that are not granulomas.

Curiously, many diseases called granulomas have none or very few of the above described clinical characteristics. Admittedly, some have histological granulomas. Some of these are granuloma fungoides, pyogenic granuloma, granulation tissue (proud flesh), cheilitis granulomatosa, monilial granuloma, Wegener's granulomatosis, granulomatosis disciformis chronica et progressiva, granuloma faciale, eosinophilic granuloma, and insect bite granuloma.

*For an interpretation of the histological concepts of term granuloma see Section IV, Granulomatous inflammation and proliferation, pp. 217–219, in Reference 2. The basic histological findings are a chronic, focal, inflammatory reaction with epitheloid and giant cells. Necrosis, atrophy, ulceration and sclerosis are also often present.

Portions of the Overview have been taken and modified from Siemens[1] (p. 72).

The description and differential diagnosis of these various clinical diseases is discussed under the appropriate morphological heading.

Nodular Granulomas

Nodular Syphilis

The general diagnostic features of late cutaneous syphilitic eruptions and late congenital syphilis are listed in Tables 30 and 31.

Nodular tertiary syphilides begins as a single lesion or as a small group of granulomas that spread out and multiply at the periphery and can involve an area of from 2 to 12 cm. This peripheral spread results in a kidney-shaped arcuate or circinate border. Complete circles are rare. There may be one or two, or even three, imperfectly formed arcuate borders. The border usually contains a few isolated granulomas. As the lesion progresses outwards, the central portion flattens, fades, and undergoes sclerotic changes forming scars without ulceration. The central scar is depressed, sclerotic, or interspersed with stellate scars and streaks; its color is earthy rather than white, and mottled with purplish or brownish shades.

When a syphilitic granuloma commences in an arcuate or circinate form, the central area may present nonscarred normal skin, although scars will develop in the peripheral arcuate area. The reappearance of granulomas in the scar is rare in tertiary syphilis; it is common in nodular granulomatous tuberculosis.

A scaly form occurs where there are grayish, abundant adherent scales with more or less infiltration. It is distinguished from psoriasis by its scarring, its lack of mica scaling, and the solitary or small number of lesions.

When these granulomas become eroded or ulcerated, they form the ulcerating granulomas, and these are considered under ulcers. It will be obvious that in some cases features of both may be present.

Table 30: **General Diagnostic Features of Late Cutaneous Syphilitic Eruptions**

1. Indolent, deeply infiltrated, destructive, asymmetric, commonly gimped, punched out ulcers and noncontractile scarring. Few or solitary lesions.
2. Sharply marginated, scalloped, arciform and serpiginous outline, slowly progressive with healing at the center or at one border and extension at the other. The scar retains the arciform pattern of the original lesion.
3. The lesions may be psoriasiform (as on the palms), verrucous (on the nose), or ulcerative (as on the legs and face).
4. Persistent brown hyperpigmentation.
5. Sclerosis with leukoplakia on the tongue.
6. Possible perforation of the hard palate.
7. Charcot's degeneration of joints (tabetic arthropathy) and malum perforans.

Table 31: **General Diagnostic Features of Late Congenital Syphilis**

1. Not mucocutaneous (unless by involvement of underlying bone and cartilage) except for rhagades.
2. Prominent frontal bosses, syphilitic saddle nose, wing type scapulae, saber shin, Clutton's joints.
3. Notched screwdriver central upper incisors, interstitial keratitis, eighth nerve deafness, (Hutchinson's triad), palatine perforation, mulberry molars.

Jean Martin Charcot, 1825–1893, French Neurologist, La Salpêtrière
Henry Hugh Clutton, 1850–1909, British Surgeon, London

Nodular Tuberculosis (Lupus Vulgaris)

Tuberculous granulomas are rounded tubercles, pea-sized, sometimes elevated, sometimes level with the skin. Their color is yellowish brown, the surface varies from smooth to scaly to erosions to crusting or even ulceration. They are soft, compressible, and velvety, and are easily penetrated with a sharp instrument. On diascopy, after the blood has been driven out, the granuloma is seen to be a translucent deep yellow color comparable to barley sugar or apple jelly, distinctly outlined from the creamy white surface of normal skin. Some are surprisingly erythematosquamous in appearance.

Resolution with scarring is frequently seen. The scar tissue tends to intermingle with the granulomas, usually in the center of the lesion. The scar is white, smooth, pearly, and flexible. Tuberculous granulomas may be present in the scar.

Necrosis and ulceration may occur as part of this process. Ulcerating tuberculous granulomas are discussed in Chapter 14.

On exposed areas, such as elbows, knees and backs of hands, a swimming pool granuloma due to the chromogenic strains of mycobacteria should be considered as a possible cause.

Most human or animal type tuberculosis occurs on the face.

In some cultures, the habit of sitting on the sputum-laden ground explains nodular tuberculosis seen on the buttocks.

Nodular Leprosy

The granulomas of leprosy vary in size from that of a small pea to a large almond; they are hemispherical in shape; and their elevation is variable. The color of the lesions is a dull pink, purplish, or brownish. The nodule's surface is smooth, usually hairless, and they are of a firm consistency. The nodules are anesthetic to pricks or burns. They may become confluent in lobulated tumors or as prominent protruding plaques. As with other granulomas, they heal leaving a scar. Ulceration may occur. The face and limbs are favorite locations.

In addition to a compatible cutaneous lesion, the diagnosis of leprosy should be based on the presence of one or more of the following:
1. definite localized anesthesia,
2. (clinically or histologically) thickenings of the superficial cutaneous nerves, and
3. the presence of acid-fast bacilli.

Mycotic Granuloma

There are at least nine deep mycoses: paracoccidioidomycosis, chromomycosis, blastomycosis, coccidioidomycosis, cryptococcosis, histoplasmosis, sporotrichosis, actinomycosis, and Madura foot. There are three basic reaction patterns in which the skin may be involved. These are the primary cutaneous infection (the cutaneous chancriform syndrome), the allergic cutaneous manifestations of systemic disease

Madura (a town in Southern India)

(such as erythema nodosum), and the specific cutaneous manifestations of disseminated infection. Because of the great variety of morphological groups and because of the clinical similarity of many of them, I have tried, in the Table 32, to summarize the salient morphological findings of the lesions that occur in the skin. Final diagnosis in all cases is made by laboratory studies, particularly fungal cultures.

Table 32: Mycotic Granuloma					
	Chancre	Granulomatous	Gumma*	Lymphangitic	Other
Chromomycosis		+ Nodular, tumorous, verrucous plaque, and cicatricial types; brown color			
Madura foot			+ Sinus formation; fistulae; elephantiasis; whitish granules may be extruded		
Actinomycosis	Rare		+ Face and neck		
Blastomycosis		+ Small pustular, verrucous, or vegetative papillomations; crusted scarring lesions; uncovered parts of the body; arcuate	++ Disseminated lesions	Rare	
Coccidioidomycosis		+May be vegetative and verrucous	+		
Cryptococcosis		+			Miliary
Paracoccidioido-mycosis		++ Mucocutaneous		+	
Histoplasmosis		+ Plaques; punched-out ulcers; vegetating			Oropharyngeal;
Sporotrichosis	+		++	+ Individual lesions may be verrucous	Oropharyngeal; miliary; limbs and head

*A nodal furunculoid lesion with softening, ulceration, sinus formation, and scarring.
+ = Major finding; ++ = Minor finding.

Nodular Sarcoid

These lesions are purplish or brownish-red elevations of hazelnut size, sometimes forming plaques. There are usually two or three lesions. Forehead, nose, shoulders, and elbows are favored sites. The plaque lesions may be large, but are freely moveable over the underlying structure. Diascopy reveals grayish yellow foci. Scar formation and ulceration are very unusual in the white race.

Annular or circinate lesions may occur with apparently normal skin in the center.

When the nodules are located in the hypoderm, more dome-shaped lesions are present. Color changes are less marked.

Lupus pernio and angiolupoid are names given to sarcoid nodules or plaques usually occurring on the face, especially the nose, cheeks, and ears. These lesions are quite bluish-red and often have numerous telangiectatic blood vessels. Lupus pernio of the digits of the fingers or toes may produce a thickening, irregularity, or loss of the nail plate.

The patient should be examined for lymph node enlargement, parotitis, and iritis as these are common systemic findings in systemic sarcoidosis. This is particularly common in blacks. Also, ulcerating, mutilating, and scarring may be seen, with destruction of the distal phalanges of the fingers.

Foreign Body Granuloma

The clinical findings in this condition depend on the foreign substance and the level at which it is injected or implanted. Many foreign bodies, if injected into the dermis, produce nodular granuloma in the exact sense of the word, with brownish-red dermal papules, ulceration, scarring, and rarely, an arcuate shape. Many substances, if injected into the hypoderm, produce nodal granulomas or gummas with subcutaneous nodules, scarring, and fistula formation.

The site gives a very important clue as to the causative foreign body.

Nodular granulomas in the axillae may be from zirconium, and in tattoos from the red mercuric chloride or chrome green dye. Papular granuloma may be seen on the beard area of the neck due to ingrowing hairs.

Nodal and nodular granulomas may be seen from silk sutures in surgical scars, in wounds from zinc beryllium silicate coated fluorescent lights, in war wounds where soil or glass-containing silica has been implanted into the dermis or hypodermis, by mineral oil injected to round out body contours, and by pieces of shrapnel from military shells. The granulomas in mastectomy scars are presumably foreign body granulomas.

See also Chapter 25 for "Hair granuloma sinuses".

Cutaneous Leishmaniasis

The basic lesion is an inflammatory, nontender, dermal nodular granuloma measuring up to 3 cm in diameter. It has a sloping erythematous border, which goes up to the central crusted area occupying about one-half the lesion. On removal of the crust, a turbid serous fluid is seen oozing from an ulcer with perpendicular eroded ragged margins and a light-red granular mammillated and papillomatous floor. Lymphangitis and lymphadenitis may be present. Slow scarring occurs. The scar is depressed, smooth, and colorless or of a dusky red hue with peripheral browning; frequently the scars are stellate.

The lesions are located on the exposed areas of the hands, face, and limbs and may be single or multiple. When multiple, they develop in succession and so are of different ages. In areas where leishmaniasis is endemic, many other morphological patterns, including verrucous, exudative, sarcoidal, and gummatous, can be seen.

Nodular Plaques on the Shins

There is a group of disorders occurring on the shins that requires some description.* Some of these conditions occur on other areas, where they may not present a problem in diagnosis.

DIFFERENTIAL DIAGNOSIS

Necrobiosis lipoidica (diabeticorum) is a brownish or brownish-yellow telangiectatic elevated dermal sclerosis with an atrophic epidermis. Scaling may or may not be present. Ulceration of varying size and extent may be present. There may be some peripheral ridging, but this is due mainly to the central atrophy and rarely involves all of every lesion. The lesions are commonly located on the shins, and consist of several, 4 to 5 cm plaques or one large long plaque. There may be a yellowish-brown translucent appearance on some parts of the border and in the central atrophic areas.

Granuloma annulare is a circular or arcuate papular eruption with peripheral ridging and no central atrophy or sclerosis. There may be some central browning. The lesions are usually small (up to 3 cm in diameter) and numerous (up to 20 lesions). There is no apple-jelly component. The small (0.5 cm primary or beginning lesion) is often present. Lesions are commonly present on the dorsa of the feet, knees, elbows, and hands. Ulcerations do not occur. Central umbilication on the sides of the fingers indicates perforating granuloma annulare.

Sarcoidosis may be an annular plaque-like eruption with an apple-jelly–like border. The lesions are of various sizes and various depths. There is usually no scarring or ulceration except in blacks.

Localized scleroderma (morphea) is a yellowish dermal sclerotic plaque with a peripheral violaceous hue. An indurated border is usually not present. The lesion is up to the size of a palm. It is rarely multiple, except in the linear or band-like form. Ulceration is rare.

Lichen sclerosus et atrophicus is a plaque of perifollicular papules which undergo atrophy and have no ridged border. At the periphery, small perifollicular papules (or white areas where they were) are often present, with central delling. Other lesions are commonly present.

Sclerotic radiodermatitis presents as a sharply demarcated area of yellowish sclerosis with telangiectatic blood vessels. Ulceration may be present. The area is depressed.

Also to be considered are rheumatoid nodes, late cutaneous tuberculosis and syphilis and, rarely, xanthomatous deposits. Rarely, other scleroses may be considered, such as that associated with stasis and following trauma.

Drug Granulomas

Rarely, classical granulomas (according to the definition in this text) are produced by iodides and bromides. They most resemble the dermal lesions of blastomycosis. The lesions are usually multiple and widely disseminated.

*Strictly speaking, this group of conditions are not all granulomas.

Other large fungating granulomas may occasionally be produced by other drugs, e.g. sulfathiazole, applied topically.

Nongranulomatous Nodular Dermatoses

Prurigo Nodularis

Although prurigo nodularis, like lichen simplex chronicus, has a large traumatic element in its cause, the two are rarely seen together.

The basic lesion of prurigo nodularis is a 1 to 1.5 cm elevated, sloping-sided nodule. Crusted or erosive portions are present on the top, especially in the central portion. The base of the erosion is clean and healing or healed. The borders of the erosion are sharp and sometimes angular or straight. In a few lesions, the surface is smooth and noneroded. There is little dermal infiltration, and the lesions are freely moveable. Some of the lesions have a light to dark brown color, both in the lesion and in the immediate surrounding skin. This is particularly so in the darker skinned races. The lesions are usually symmetrical. The lesions have no definite grouping. They are present mainly on the legs and forearms, but also scattered on the arms and thighs and on accessible sites on the torso. On the upper back and outer arms, many hypopigmented, 2 to 3 mm areas are present. These are scattered indiscriminately, with more being present at the base of the nape of the neck. These hypopigmented areas are from the occasionally associated neurotic excoriations.

Granuloma Annulare

This is not a true granuloma; the term is used here in a histological sense only. In general, granuloma annulare is a purely papular eruption. Only rarely are the lesions deep enough and large enough to be called nodules. On the scalp they may be subcutaneous, and both clinically and histologically may resemble rheumatic nodules or nodes.

Milker's Nodules

The mature lesion is a round, sharply demarcated, circular shaped epidermodermal nodule about 1 cm in diameter. The top of the lesion may be flat. The border is bright red. Incision reveals only a very small amount of serosanguinous fluid. At times there may be angiomatous component resembling pyogenic granuloma; hemorrhage with subsequent blackening may suggest malignant melanoma. Regional lymphadenitis and lymphangitis and toxic erythemas rarely occur. One or two lesions are present, usually on the hands and forearms.

Erythema Elevatum Diutinum

This disease is not an erythema, but a pea-sized to bean-sized pink to purplish papulonodular eruption. The site of involvement is the deep and middle dermis, and apart from stretching, the epidermis is normal. The nodules are clearly demarcated to begin with, but later they coalesce to form plaques, irregularly lobulated, infiltrated, and rarely, raised distinct tumors. The extensor surfaces of the joints of the limbs are the sites of predilection. There is no atrophy.

Juxta-Articular Nodes and Nodules

These nodules and nodes vary in size from 1 cm to 3 cm. They are found on the extensor surface of the forearm, over the olecranon, hand, knee, sacral region, and scalp. The lesions are discrete and firm, not attached to either the skin or the underlying periosteum, but frequently associated with the tendon sheath and the walls of the bursae. They enlarge slowly and persist for years. They are not painful.
Differential Diagnosis
The differential diagnosis includes the nodes and nodules seen in syphilis, the fibrous bands and nodes of acrodermatitis chronica atrophicans, gouty tophi, rheumatoid nodules or nodes (calcified or not), xanthoma tuberosum, and various types of synovial inflammations.

Nodular Tumors

Squamous Cell Carcinoma

The basic lesion is a moderately hard ovoid nodule, usually of a color close to that of the adjacent skin (Fig. 12.1). The tumor is sharply demarcated, with rather wide indurated borders, sometimes infiltrating into the underlying tissues. Particularly when small (under 1.0 cm), squamous cell carcinomas may have a pearly border, and with no central keratin formation or ulceration, it may be difficult to distinguish them from basal cell carcinomas, particularly in the nose. Ulceration frequently occurs in lesions over 2 cm diameter. At times, the ulcerative component may be the predominant feature (see Chapter 14, "Mucosal Ulcerations"). Occasional polypoid and verrucous lesions occur (epithelioma cuniculatum). Verrucous lesions are more common in the mouth, perianal, semimucosa, and glans penis. Very large lesions will have sloughing areas and may cause gross destruction of underlying tissues.

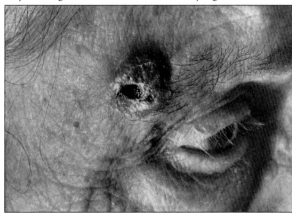

Figure 12.1 A nodule of squamous cell carcinoma.

Underlying conditions that may be present are skin damaged by habitual exposure to sun (95%), radiodermatitis, old burn scars, Bowen's disease, and more rarely, chronic discharging sinuses. The sites of predilection therefore are the locations of these pre-existing conditions. The lesion is rare on the mustache area. It is much more common in men. On the pinna of the ear, this tumor may present as sharply marginated ulcerative plaques extending over 2 to 3 cm.

On the scalp of elderly women, proliferating epidermoid cysts may closely mimic squamous cell carcinomas both clinically and histologically. On the face and bald pate of the elderly atypical fibroxanthoma may mimic squamous cell carcinoma.

Keratoacanthoma

The keratoacanthoma lesion starts as a firm, rounded, flesh-colored or reddish papule. Rapidly (within 4 to 6 weeks) it develops into a 1.0 cm nodule with a central core composed of firmly packed keratin (Fig. 12.2). At its largest size, the central keratin core occupies three-quarters of the surface. The wall is smooth, slopes to the top, and may contain an occasional telangiectatic blood vessel. The lesion sticks up above the skin level, and there is usually no spreading infiltration at the base. As the lesion heals, the central core is sloughed out and the border flattens. At this stage there is a shoulder where the overlying edge dips into the central core.

In large lesions, the border is definitely arcuate. This is particularly noticeable after the central core has sloughed out. Scar formation is not unusual. The lesions are usually solitary. When multiple, all stages may be present, including scars of resolved lesions. Very rarely, destruction of cartilage or bone may occur.

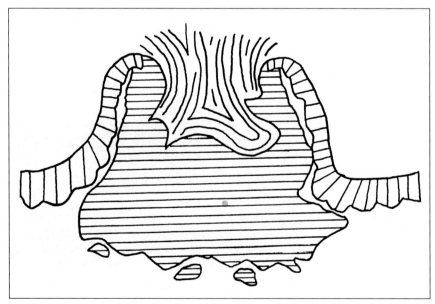

Figure 12.2 Illustration of keratoacanthoma showing shoulder of normal epidermis, cellular tumor, and central keratin core.

Keratoacanthoma usually occurs on the same areas as squamous cell carcinoma. The one exception is the mustache area, where keratoacanthoma is common and squamous cell carcinoma is extremely rare.

Occasionally, a large solitary molluscum contagiosum may be confused with keratoacanthoma, especially on the eyelids. Otherwise, the most common problem is distinguishing keratoacanthoma from the "button" type of squamous cell carcinoma.

In general, squamous cell carcinoma grows more slowly (about 1.0 cm a year) than keratoacanthoma and as the lesion gets bigger ulceration occurs—there is no central keratin core. Also there is more infiltration at the base and a squamous cell carcinoma will not disappear spontaneously (except in Ferguson-Smith syndrome).

Basal Cell Carcinoma

Of the many gross morphological variants of basal cell carcinoma[3] listed in Table 33, three are described in detail here.

The solid type is a firm, sharply demarcated, pearly or skin-colored nodule, usually with some infiltration of the base, although some can be mainly above the surface of the skin. Telangiectatic blood vessels may wander over the surface of the lesion. The lesions are usually hairless, although a few hairs may be seen at the border. Ulceration may be present. Some lesions may show varying degrees of irregular, usually dotted, light brown to black pigmentation. Some have a cystic aspect.

About 75 percent of basal cell carcinomas occur on the sun-exposed areas of the head and neck. The remainder occur on the upper lip, retroauricular crease, medial canthus, and occasionally on the torso and elsewhere. About one patient in four will have more than one lesion.

Table 33: Gross Morphological Variants of Basal Cell Carcinoma

Common
- Papulonodular or solid
- Cystic
- Superficial multicentric
- Ulcerative
- Angiomatous
- Recurrent

Fairly Common
- Rodent ulcer
- Black or brown (pigmented)
- Scaly infiltrative
- Following low-dose radiation
- Rhinophyma

Rare
- Horror[4]
- Fibrotic Premalignant fibroepithelioma of Pinkus
  - Self-healing (grass, flat cicatricial)
  - Morpheaform (sclerosing)
  - With irregular sclerosis
  - Basal cell carcinoma over dermatofibroma
  - Basal cell carcinoma in burn scar
  - Following treatment
  - Basal cell carcinoma in keloid or hypertrophic scar
- Intradermal
- Horn forming
- Children and young adults (perstans)
- Linear
- Adnexal
- Mucosal, palms, and soles
- Metastatic

J. Ferguson-Smith, 1888–1978, Scottish Dermatologist
Herman Pinkus, 1905–1985, U.S. Dermatologist

At times, solid nodular ulcerative basal cell carcinomas may present as bulging, angiomatous, friable, easily bleeding lesions. This is especially so on such nonfacial areas as the back, the helix of the ear, and the thigh.

The rodent ulcer type of basal cell carcinoma is an invasive, destructive, deeply burrowing, ulcerative nodular tumor. Portions of the lesion have the pearly border, the telangiectatic blood vessels, and the firm consistency of the so-called solid type of basal cell carcinoma. These lesions are usually 3 or more centimeters in diameter. The face is the most common location.

Admittedly, at times it may not be possible to differentiate between a large solid type with ulceration and the rodent ulcer. The main features of the rodent ulcer are the destructiveness, the deep burrowing nature and, of course, the ulceration.

Fibroepithelial tumor of Pinkus is a skin to pink-colored nodule forming a semipolypoid nodule, usually located in the small of the back. The lesion is sharply demarcated and of firm fibrous consistency. The lesion is ovoid in shape, with the long axis along the skin lines. All of the lesions I have seen have been on the lower back; one was in the intergluteal fold. There may be a few small erosions on the surface. Normal-appearing seborrheic keratoses may also be present, as may occasional patches of superficial multicentric basal cell carcinoma.

The nevoid basal cell carcinoma syndrome may have papular, nodular, sclerosing, superficial multicentric, or rodent ulcer varieties of basal cell carcinoma. Frequently, more than one type is present. The lesions are multiple (up to several hundred) and not necessarily on sun-exposed areas. They start in the teenage years as small "freckles" — particularly on the torso. Other visible stigmata are frontal bossing, hypertelorism, dentiginous cysts, palmar and plantar shortening of the fourth metacarpal and metatarsal, and numerous milia and small wens about the eyes.

Malignant Melanoma

There are 12 reasonably well-defined clinical varieties of malignant melanoma. In some cases, the morphology will show certain features in common.

1. The nodular malignant melanoma tumor produces bulk out of proportion to the surface area. This also includes the huge tumors and those showing a predominant degree of ulceration.

   The nodular type is an elevated round black nodule. The surface is smooth, frequently ulcerated and covered with a bloody crust. A translucent, bloody, black, gelatinous, eroded surface (commonly called frog spawn) is often present in large (over 2 cm) lesions. The border may show a peripheral erythematous halo, spreading black or brown pigment or satellite intradermal round papules. Huge lesions (10 by 10 cm) are rarely seen. They often have a smooth surface. Ulceration may or may not be present.

2. The superficial spreading malignant melanoma tumor produces little mass in relation to its surface area. It has an early peripherally spreading phase and a

later nodular phase. This group includes the so-called ringed melanoma and those showing central areas of sclerosis and whitening.

Peripheral or intrinsic dilated capillaries can often be seen with the hand lens. Earlier lesions may show a variegated bluish- red, bluish-black or bluish-brown color, an irregular nonulcerative surface, and an irregular notched border. They are more common in women. Some lesions are arcuate and some have a peripheral white halo.

Central hypopigmentation, scarring and healing may be present, forming the ringed malignant melanoma.

3. In the Hutchinson freckle (lentigo maligna) type, the pre-existing freckle of long duration, usually on the sun-exposed areas, is the main feature, with one or more papulonodular tumors of malignant melanoma. Scarring and healing are not present in the lentigo maligna melanoma.

In some cases, the pre-existing black brown freckle (see Chapter 17, "Melanin Increase") may be visible at the side or may form a black halo about the tumor. In lentigo maligna melanoma, the papulonodular tumor often is less black-brown and more red than the surrounding pre-existing freckle. This type usually occurs on the sun-exposed areas, especially on the face. Rarely, covered and even mucosal lesions occur. These are probably acral lentiginous melanomas.

4. The nonpigmented, i.e. not black, blue, or brown, malignant melanoma usually has a reddish color simulating a pyogenic granuloma (see "Nodular angiomatous tumors" in this chapter). Ulceration is common.

5. Acral lentiginous malignant melanoma consist of the volar and ungual types.

The volar lesions are noted for the diffuse spread of black- brown pigment beyond the central tumor which may or may not be pigmented black or brown. Quite often the central, more malignant, tumor is a bright angiomatous red color. In cases with limited peripheral spread and where the lesion is not black or brown, it may be impossible to differentiate the acral lentiginous malignant melanoma from a squamous cell carcinoma.

The nail melanomas (i.e.ungual, peri-ungual, subungual) are more common on the big toe and thumb, and are more common in blacks. Melanin streaking may represent any pigment-producing melanocytic lesion and is by no means always an indication of malignant melanoma. In darker skinned races, they are multiple and often of no consequence. The spread of black or brown pigment in the cuticle and adjacent peri-ungual tissues has been called Hutchinson's sign. Hutchinson likened it to staining produced by silver nitrate. This sign can also be seen with ungual hematomas.

6. Malignant melanoma of the various mucosal surfaces (oral, nasal, conjunctival, anal, vaginal) has, like the acral lentiginous lesions, the tendency for wide black pigment spread into tissues away from the primary tumor nodule.

7. The malignant melanoma may present with satellitosis which shows several or many perilesional, black, blue, dermal, 2 to 5 mm deposits. These deposits tend to cluster about the primary lesion, often in a bomb-explosion pattern (more and larger near the lesion; fewer and smaller, far away). Some of the deposits may present only as black or blue dots, a few may present as deep dermal or hypodermal papulonodules, some of the deposits may have perilesional spreading black pigment.
8. The pagetoid malignant melanoma presents as an erosive, sharply marginated, pink or red plaque, and usually suggests a diagnosis of extramammary Paget's disease (see Chapter 11, "Malignant Papular Tumors").
9. Rarely, malignant melanomas arise from a giant hairy bathing suit nevus or on a congenital or acquired pigmented nevus.
10. There also is a polypoid melanoma.
11. Ocular melanoma.
12. Rare melanomas from melanocyte cell rests in other organs.

Metastatic Carcinoma

Morphological types of metastatic carcinomas to the skin include carcinoma erysipeloides (inflammatory carcinoma) which is described in Chapter 1; papular, nodular, and nodal deposits are described in the appropriate chapters; carcinoma en cuirasse and telangiectatic carcinoma are described in Chapter 18. If one regards Paget's or extramammary Paget's as metastatic carcinoma, these conditions are discussed under malignant papular tumors or malignant erosions.

Malignant melanoma metastases seek the skin and subcutaneous tissue, and the lymph nodes. The deposits may be widely disseminated, but tend to be more numerous and larger close to the primary lesion. They may be nodal, intradermal, subcutaneous, or intra-lymphatic. The color will depend on the amount of melanin in the lesion and on the depth of the lesion. In some cases, extreme metastatic disease may be seen in the extremity on which the primary lesion occurred. These lesions may be strictly restricted to the lymphatic supply of the extremity. Bizarre patterns also occur, e.g. a primary site on the palm followed by scalp metastases appearing 8 years later with no other evidence of metastatic disease. Rarely, an irregularly shaped halo may be present about these lesions.

Carcinomas of the kidney and ureter may present on the scalp as metastatic disease in the form of innumerable 1 to 2 cm elevated skin-colored smooth nodules. Rarely, pulsating nodal masses may occur.

Carcinoma of the lungs may have dermatofibroma-like metastatic deposits on the upper torso area. Rarely, ulcerative keratoacanthoma-like lesions may be seen on the scalp and face (Fig. 12.3). Spread to the scalp is presumably by the vertebral vein system.[5]

I have also seen metastatic skin deposits from eccrine sweat gland carcinoma, prostate carcinoma, postmastectomy angiosarcoma, and various squamous cell carcinomas from the mucosae of the head and neck.

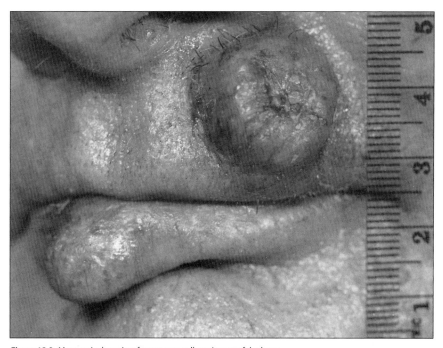

Figure 12.3 Metastatic deposits of squamous cell carcinoma of the lung.

There are many variations in the patterns of spread of metastatic deposits in the skin. Also, as a general rule, skin metastases indicate a widely disseminated and untreatable tumor.

Carcinoma of the breast may show a large nodular growth covering the entire anterior and lateral chest wall, extending into the axilla. The surface is grossly irregular and is formed by numerous firm red nodules varying from 5 mm to 5 cm in size, many of which have ulcerated. The surface shows areas of fresh bleeding, dark brown crusts, and thick yellow pus. The border is well defined and is surrounded by a margin of erythema about 5 mm in diameter. Deposits may be found on the skin of the contralateral chest and abdomen. These deposits consist of solitary nodules and clusters of firm reddish nodules from 1 to 8 cm. Associated venous distention is often present.

Peau d'orange (orange skin) on the breast is a thickening of the corium due to cancerous occlusion of deep dermal lymph vessels, the pits in the swollen skin being the exaggerated orifices of hair follicles. Both continuous permeation and embolic extension in dermal lymphatics are involved.

Nodular Angiomatous Tumors

There is a movement afoot to classify all blood vessel overgrowths as either hemangiomas or malformations.[6] The definition of the former includes all lesions that undergo a growth spurt and then disappear as opposed to malformations which do not change throughout life. The problem with this generalization is that while it is useful for lesions in infants and children, there are many exceptions to this definition. For example, nonchanging lifelong angiomas in adults are not rare (Fig. 12.4). For example, some of the growing angiomas in adults consist of small, rapidly dividing growing endothelial channels. Are these hemangiomas? For example, what of proud flesh and pyogenic granuloma? For example, what of the angiomatous element in some new growths? For example, what of the angiomas that arise from estrogen excess?

To start with, the reader should review the papular angiomatous tumors, including both varieties of Kaposi's hemorrhagic sarcoma, amelanotic melanoma, proud flesh, and the rare case of acquired angioma of pregnancy.

Figure 12.4 Lifelong angioma.

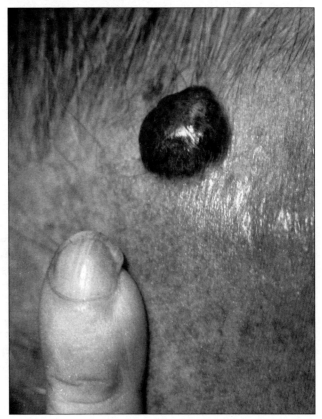

Capillary hemangioma of the strawberry type is a raised, bright red, soft, and usually lobulated tumor of varying size. It starts shortly after birth as a very small red macule or papule, and usually increases rapidly in size and height over the first 6 months of life. Then a grayish, irregular whitening appears on the surface, and occasionally, on large bulky lesions (over 3 cm in diameter) or in lesions in sites of trauma or in moist areas (vulva, axilla, neck, eyelid, lip, etc.) a superficial ulceration with some slight bleeding from the surface appears. The ulceration is central and heals with a scar.

This strawberry lesion may be situated on the top of a cavernous hemangioma (like an ice cream cone). Usually the strawberry portion occupies the central half to two-thirds of the total involved surface area. The changes that the strawberry portion undergoes in this situation are the same as described for the solitary strawberry lesion.

Interestingly, the spontaneous disappearance of the cavernous portion almost always occurs when there is a double or mixed lesion. If there is a large cavernous portion, scarring is more marked, and in hirsute areas such as the scalp, hair loss may occur. Ulceration and bleeding may be more marked in this double lesion.

In those rare, platelet-destroying, large, mixed, cavernous strawberry angiomas, hemorrhages and ecchymosis are present.

The cavernous hemangioma presents as a soft, doughy, rather poorly demarcated, dermal (and sometimes hypodermal) swelling. The overlying skin, as mentioned above, may show strawberry, or rarely flat, capillary markings. These lesions are not as apt to undergo spontaneous resolution. This is particularly so on the lips and perioral area. Large feeding veins can frequently be seen entering the tumors. Occasionally, this type of lesion may pulsate and is probably best classified as cirsoid aneurysm (or mixed arteriovenous hemangioma, i.e. it is a malformation). Occasionally, this type of lesion continues to increase in size throughout life. Both capillary and cavernous hemangiomas may have a verrucous surface, especially on the legs.

In the blue rubber-bleb nevus syndrome, cavernous hemangiomas may be very numerous and vary in size from 1 to 4 cm. They are dark blue to black, lobulated, sometimes pedunculated, and have a soft worm-like consistency. They can be partially or totally evacuated by squeezing, leaving a thin hernia-type sac which slowly refills. Hypodermal lesions of a similar consistency are also present. Associated areas of telangiectasia and eccrine sweating may be seen. The lesions may be painful. Bleeding from gastrointestinal lesions is not uncommon. Multiple glomangiomas should be considered in the differential diagnosis.

Mixtures of a telangiectatic capillary mark, strawberry hemangioma, and cavernous hemangioma are occasionally seen, especially in large (often facial) lesions. There are many congenital multisystem syndromes in which various types of hemangiomas may occur. Some of these are venous malformations.

Localized dilated veins (phlebectasias, e.g. varicocele) may be classified as a nodular angiomatous condition. If massive, they may be confused with cavernous hemangiomas, cirsoid, or arteriovenous aneurysms.

Angiosarcomas are purplish red, frequently ulcerated, and bleeding angiomatous nodules occasionally with papular-sized lesions, occurring on the head and neck of the elderly. Satellite lesions of the bomb-explosion type are common. Rapid growth is a feature of these lesions.

Postmastectomy lymphangiosarcoma of Stewart-Treves are angiosarcomas almost always occurring on the postradical surgical and postradiation lymphedematous upper extremity. These lesions consist of dark red angiomatous tumors (nodules and papules) on a purplish infiltrated base. There is usually a primary focus of tumors with many smaller satellite lesions. An ulcerated bleeding fungoid mass may develop.

Eroded nodular basal cell carcinomas may present with a red, friable, granular surface that bleeds easily. The helix of the ear, the torso, and the thigh are areas where I have seen such lesions. They can, of course, easily be confused with angiomatous nodular tumors.

Large lymphangiomas on the tongue and lips may present as basically angiomatous lesions. Usually some nonangiomatous portion may be visible.

There is a group of rare, vascular, nodular angiomatous tumors that can be diagnosed only by microscopic examination. These include angioleiomyoma, hemangioendothelioma, glomus tumors, and hemangiopericytoma.

Lymphocytoma Cutis

Lymphocytoma cutis may have alternate names such as lymphadenosis cutis benigna, Spiegler-Fendt's sarcoid, lymphocytic infiltration of the skin, cutaneous lymphoid hyperplasia, or a number of others.

The basic lesion is a purplish red, dermal papulonodule of quite firm consistency. The surface is dome-shaped, and there is no epidermal change. The lesions may become confluent, forming an elevated, irregular, nobby surface, forming smooth surface plaques of varying thickness, forming arcuate and circular patterns with central areas of partial or complete clearing, or forming large circular lesions with no central clearing. In some areas, there may be a lighter brown, semitranslucent, follicular appearance.

The lesions may be multiple or single. The face, especially the forehead and about the eyes, are common sites, although torso lesions may also be seen. The eruption is usually seen in the middle-aged. A slow progression is the rule, but some lesions may disappear.

Heinrich Fendt, 20th Cent, German Physician
Eduard Spiegler, 1860–1908, Austrian Dermatologist, Vienna
Robert D. Stewart,   English Dermatologist
N. Treves, 1894–1964, U.S. Surgeon

The differential diagnosis includes secondary deposits (as from carcinoma of the prostate), which may be very similar; but, of course, progression is the rule, either of the secondary deposit or the underlying tumor. Sarcoidosis papules or nodules tend to be more brownish red, and some of the lesions may be diascopy positive. Knobby lesions and arcuate lesions with central clearing are rarely seen (see "Granuloma annulare" earlier in this chapter, "Nodes of Rheumatic Fever" in Chapter 13, and "Necrobiosis lipoidica [diabeticorum]" earlier in this chapter under the heading "Nodular Plaques on the Shins"). Insect bites are usually scattered, solitary papulonodules, more often on the torso, not knobby, and not arcuate due to central clearing. The figurate erythemas may present with arcuate reddish lesions, but the color is much redder, less brownish, and less purplish, and the degree of induration is much less marked. Mycosis fungoides (see also parapsoriasis) presents usually with some lesion showing psoriasiform scale, eczematoid epidermal changes, or varying sizes of nodules, some of which are ulcerated. In the d'emblée type, varying sized (2 to 5 cm) ulcerative bulky exophytic tumors may be present. They are foul-smelling and may be very numerous. Leukemia cutis and lymphoma cutis present as a variety of purplish or red nodules and nodes, sometimes quite extensive. The florid patterns of tumor formation are now extremely rare because of
more effective radiotherapy and chemotherapy, so I have not spent much time or space in describing them.

Plaque-like photosensitivity eruptions are more purplish, less indurated, not knobby, and do not form arcuate lesions with central clearing. Lupus erythematosus of the erythematous type may show purplish-red swellings; however, the basic lesion is not really a papule, but erythema. Actinic reticuloid presents as a purplish dermal infiltrate on the sun-exposed areas of the head and neck.

Drug-induced pseudolymphomas, especially those produced by anticonvulsants of the hydantoin group should be considered in the differential diagnosis. Lymphadenopathy and organomegaly are often present in this condition.

Granuloma faciale presents as brownish red, diascopy positive, dermal, papulonodular, circular plaques, usually on the face or scalp. The lesions may be solitary, or up to six in number. They vary from 1 to 4 cm in diameter. Although mainly circular, an occasional lesion may show central clearing. There is no epidermal change; no alopecia; and no scarring.

Cylindroma (Turban Tumors)

These are pea-sized to grape-sized multiple tumors occurring mainly on the scalp, but also on the face, back, and chest. The nodules are from red to normal skin color. There is often alopecia in the covering over the tumors. They may be few or numerous, and rarely, they cover the scalp as a wig. They are ovoid or partially polypoid in shape. Cylindromas on the scalp may coexist with trichoepitheliomas on the forehead.

Nevoxanthoendothelioma (Juvenile Xanthogranuloma)

Nevoxanthoendothelioma presents in patients as a cluster of rather deep-seated (mid or lower dermis or hypoderm) papulonodules, usually occurring on the extremities or face. There are usually several large (1 to 2 cm) lesions, about which there may be smaller (2 to 5 mm) lesions. Rarely, they are solitary. Very occasionally there are hundreds of lesions associated with café au lait spots. They have a yellowish brown, almost apple-jelly color, and the lesion does not completely disappear on diascopy. At times, a reddish hue may be present. Sometimes a linear arrangement of lesions can be seen. Sometimes, the surface becomes eroded with rapid growth.

These lesions start in the first few weeks of life, grow rather rapidly until 1 year of age, and then remain stationary and eventually disappear spontaneously.

DIFFERENTIAL DIAGNOSIS

They are to be distinguished from spindle and epithelioid cell nevi (Spitz nevi), which is more red, solitary, less deeply situated, and often with lanugo hairs; from urticaria pigmentosa, which is more brown, urticates on rubbing, and which, in the solitary form, becomes bulbous after rubbing; and, more rarely, from pyogenic granuloma and sarcoidosis.

Dermatofibrosarcoma Protuberans

The basic lesion is a hard, reddish, blue, or skin-colored nodule. These nodules are usually numerous, and increase in size and number to form varying-sized, flat, freely moveable plaques resembling morphea or keloid. On the plaques, varying-sized, round, hard tumors develop and protrude like a large nipple or mushroom. Occasionally, these tumors ulcerate. The torso, thighs, and inguinal areas are favorite locations.

Nodular Deposits

Papulonodular and Nodal Calcific Deposits

I have included the calcific deposits and the osteomata under the same heading, as there are not too many of them and it is easier to consider them together.

Post-traumatic inclusion cysts and wens may become calcified. Rarely, pigmented nevi on the face may contain calcium deposits. Phleboliths may occur in varicose veins on the legs. In aged persons, calcified fat lobules the size of a grain of wheat may be seen on the inner aspect of the tibia. Some milia may be calcified. Calcification and ossification may occur in scars and in deep cystic lesions of acne vulgaris. In the latter, they may present as 1 to 2mm, dermal, blue (due to deposition of tetracycline), firm papules, scattered randomly on each cheek in patients with scarring acne vulgaris. Rheumatic nodules or nodes may calcify, become ulcerative, and discharge a chalky white material. When very extensive, scleromalacia may also be present.

Osteoma cutis is the name given to dermal and subcutaneous, calcified nodules, nodes, and plaques, sharply marginated, from 1 to 5 cm in diameter, usually occurring on the torso. The skin over them may be slightly blue and puckered, but it shows no anatomical change. They may be congenital, idiopathic, or develop as a manifestation of an abnormal calcium metabolism.

There is, of course, no way one can tell by looking and feeling (living gross pathology) whether or not a calcific deposit has or has not been ossified. In addition, some very hard fibrous tumors may raise suspicions of calcification or ossification, but only a histological examination can give a definite answer.

Scleroderma in its various forms (acrosclerosis, CRST syndrome, and localized or linear morphea) may show varying degrees of calcific plaques, usually in the dermis or subdermis. In the systemic forms, the hands are a favorite site.

Dermatomyositis, especially in its nonacute childhood and adult types, frequently shows dermal and subdermal calcific deposits. Some of these deposits may discharge. Large knobby calcium deposits may occur around the joints.

Calcifying epithelioma of Malherbe (pilomatricoma) is a firm papulonodule located in the dermis. The overlying epidermis may be skin-colored or slightly brownish. The lesion is more rubbery hard than solid hard and is only moderately well delineated from the surrounding tissue. It has an irregular or triangular border as compared to the more round or oval shape of a cyst. They are located in the shoulder area, on the outer arms, and forearms. Single lesions are the rule. On incision, they show a gritty yellowish-white calcified material.

With metastatic calcification, numerous subepidermal infiltrates are present, forming irregularly shaped plaques, papules, and streaks about the mouth, axillae, groins, popliteal fossae, nape of neck, and antecubital fossae. Farther from these flexural areas about the big joints, these infiltrates are less extensive. On pressure some are gritty, and other plaques can be felt to crack. The eruption is symmetrical. The skin over these lesions is a dusky brown. In severe cases, ulceration and necrosis may occur over some of the plaques with discharge of pieces of calcified tissue.

Calcification may occur in the pinna of the elderly particularly after repeated trauma.

References

1. Siemens HW. General diagnosis and therapy of skin diseases. Weiner K, trans. Chicago:University of Chicago Press, 1958.
2. Pinkus H, Mehregan AH. A guide to dermatohistopathology. New York:Appleton-Century-Crofts, 1969:217–219.
3. Jackson R. The many faces of basal cell carcinoma. Can Med Assoc J 1982; 126:1157–1159.
4. Jackson R, Adams RH. Horrifying basal cell carcinoma: a study of 33 cases and a comparison with 455 non-horror cases and a report on four metastatic cases. J Surg Oncol 1973; 5:431–463
5. Baston OV. The vertebral vein system. Caldwell lecture 1956. Am J Roent Radio and Nucl Med 1957; 78:195–212.
6. Enjolras O, Mulliken JB. The current management of vascular birthmarks. Pediatric Dermatol 1993; 10:311–333.

Albert Hippolyte Malherbe, 1845–1915, French Surgeon

CHAPTER 13
Nodes or Subcutaneous Nodules

A *large (over 2.0 cm) solid lesion mainly or entirely subcutaneous.*

Overview

In contrast to the raised varieties of solid lesions (papules, nodules), nodes are mainly or entirely subcutaneous and may even involve muscle or bone.[1,2] The hypoderm is closely related to the corium by the continuity of the connective tissue and elastic fibers passing from one to the other, as well as by blood and lymph vessels; furthermore, the bulbs of the largest hairs and the glomeruli of the large sweat glands are embedded in the hypoderm, especially on the scalp. On account of this inter-relationship of tissues and vascular supply, pathological processes are very apt to invade the two layers together or successively, so that many pathological processes are dermo-hypodermic. Because of their deep situation, such masses have a very flat dome if they rise above skin level. While I have considered only location as the basic definition of a node (in fact, the term subcutaneous nodule could be used instead of node), it is unusual for nodes to be as small as a pea; usually they are egg-sized or larger. It may be necessary to put tension on the skin and use side lighting to see them. Of course, palpation is very important. Be sure to distinguish between node and lymph node.

The anatomic bases of node formations may be extensive inflammatory cellular infiltrates (syphilis, erythema nodosum), cellular neoplasms, tissue hypertrophies, or an enlarged lymph gland. They frequently have a destructive character and break down with suppuration. Nodes may form ulcerative processes or, still more commonly, abscesses and sinuses.

Based on their natural course, three forms can be distinguished.

Acute nodal dermatoses, of sudden onset, are of ephemeral or not very prolonged duration (up to 3 months) and always terminate by resolution without suppuration.

In this acute form, the size varies from that of a pea to that of a hen's egg; the consistency is resistant or edematous; the boundaries are indistinct, in the sense of occupying simultaneously the subcutis and the cutis, with somewhat diffuse outlines; the skin is usually congested on the surface above the node, and they are painful to touch. The abrupt appearance, in certain regions of predilection, the distinctly inflammatory character, and the tendency to resolution are suggestive of their resulting from hematogenously spread "toxic" factors.

Subacute nodes or nodal granulomas develop insidiously and last from several months to years. Volume usually varies from that of a hazelnut to that of an almond; consistency and the appearance of the skin are modified according to the course of development; these nodes are only slightly painful. Their pathological anatomy shows them to be derived from a subacute inflammatory process, frequently having a blood vessel as the point of origin. The most common nodal granuloma today is nodular vasculitis or nontuberculous erythema induratum. Other possible causes of nodal granulomas are the standard granulomatous diseases such as deep mycosis, leprosy, tuberculosis, and sarcoidosis. Some of these nodal granulomas have a well-marked tendency to softening, ulceration, sinus formation, and scarring, e.g. erythema

Portions of the Overview have been taken and modified from Darier[1] (pp. 263, 264) and Siemens[2] (pp. 53, 55).

induratum. Others, while still classed as granulomas, have less tendency to do so, e.g. nodal sarcoidosis. Another group of subacute nodes are the panniculitides not due to the granulomatous diseases. Even though histologically these lesions may have giant cells and other histological features of a granuloma, they do not fit the clinical description of a granuloma. Unfortunately, the distinction between the nodal granulomas and the panniculitides is not always clearcut, either clinically or histologically.

It should be emphasized that the nodal granulomatous diseases, because of their deep location, do not always show all the clinical characteristics as discussed in the overview on granulomas in Chapter 12.

A group of chronic nodes persisting indefinitely are the hypodermic tumors, which present in a wide variety of sizes, shapes, and consistencies.

Lymph node enlargement is not a frequent finding in skin diseases, but should be checked during examination.

Abscesses

The general term abscess is used to describe a relatively large accumulation of pus in tissues and, with regard to the skin in particular, to such an accumulation in the cutis, subcutis, or both. In order for a lesion to be an abscess, the pus should be located so deeply that it does not show on the surface except when it "points" just before discharging onto the surface of the skin. Because of its location, an abscess is scarcely raised above skin level, and its borders are more easily palpated than seen. On the surface, the horny layer over an abscess may exfoliate forming a collarette, as the inflammatory edema subsides. Most abscesses develop from an inflammatory infiltrate followed by necrosis of cells and connective tissue. The abscess wall is formed by the adjacent compressed tissues. The transformation of a nodule into an abscess manifests itself by central softening and fluctuation of the originally firm tissue. Sometimes it may be difficult or impossible to detect fluctuation if the abscess is very small or tightly filled. As the abscess cavity enlarges, perforation and drainage of pus finally takes place. Superficial abscesses open to the surface and form ulcers, while those that are deep give rise to discharging sinuses. An abscess arising from a tertiary nodal syphilitic infiltrate is called a gumma. Colliquative abscess is the term used to describe necrotic tuberculous abscesses. Other nodal infectious granulomas that break down and discharge are also abscesses.

I include scarring, nodal, primarily nonpyogenic lesions that break down and discharge (liquifying panniculitis, deep foreign body granulomas) in my definition of abscesses.

It could be argued that the previous definition of node as a solid cellular lesion in the hypoderm does not agree with inclusion of abscesses as nodes. With abscesses, the main criterion for including them with nodes is the location—not the solidness. It should be pointed out that many subcutaneous abscesses are so firm that they might be considered to be solid.

Nodal Dermatoses

Erythema Nodosum

The lesions in erythema nodosum present as large, rounded, tender, warm erythemas, the central portions of which are very gradually elevated and form hard and painful protuberances (Fig. 13.1). Later, they soften and subside, the red color changes to bluish or livid, and the affected limb appears as if it had been severely bruised (hence the former name erythema contusiforme). Finally, the cuticle becomes scurfy. Erythema nodosum affects the fore-part of the legs and thighs in young female adults, and there may be a total of 12 lesions. Rarely, the lesions occur on the forearms, arms, buttocks, and lower abdomen. When the lesions do not show bruising, they can be called nodal or nodular erythemas.

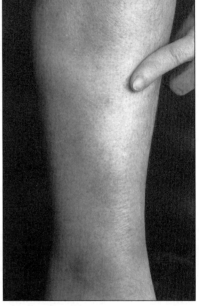

Figure 13.1 Dome-shaped subcutaneous nodules (nodes) of erythema nodosum.

DIFFERENTIAL DIAGNOSIS

The differential diagnosis consists of thrombophlebitis, in which a firm thickened vein may be felt, or deep calf tenderness and Homans' sign may be present; erysipelas, in which the tumid red plaque is usually solitary, which can occur anywhere on the leg, and which is associated with fever and regional lymphadenopathy; and acute contact dermatitis, in which there is some epidermal change, the border is diffuse the lesion, does not have a regular shape, and itching is usually present. Some drug nodular erythemas present as atypical erythema nodosum (see also "Erythema Multiforme" in Chapter 1).

Nodes of Rheumatic Fever

These present as a few to multiple small subcutaneous nodes, especially over the elbows and knees. Rarely, there are as many as 40 nodes. They occur in patients with acute rheumatic fever.

Nodal Granulomas

For foreign body granuloma, see Chapter 12.

John Homans, 1877–1955, U.S. Surgeon, Tufts Medical School

Syphilis

There are two types of syphilitic nodal lesions.

Sometimes in the course of the secondary manifestations of severe syphilis, associated in most cases with a profuse eruption of lenticular papules, nodal lesions may be found. They are hard, distinctly outlined, moveable under the skin and on the underlying tissues, round, spindle-shaped or flattened, and from the size of a large pea to that of an almond. There may be up to 20 nodal lesions, usually located on the extremities. Around the joints, these lesions are called juxta-articular nodes. As they do not break down, they are not really, from a clinical point of view, granulomas. They disappear with treatment.

The gumma is a subcutaneous, firm, rubbery, well-defined, painless indolent node. The node slowly increases in size and assumes a livid hue. Then, the skin becomes thin at one or more points, the gumma bursts, and a gummy purulent material exudes. This leads to the development of fistulous ulcers, circular or oval in shape with clearcut edges and a purulent floor often extending to tendons, cartilage, and bone. When the ulcers heal, scarring results with a brown border. They can occur anywhere but are prone to occur on the forehead, scalp, lips, and genitals. They are often multiple and may develop in crops. Gummas can also occur in the tongue, where they present as nodes with ulcerations that heal with scarring. Gummas of the soft palate usually present with regurgitation of liquids through the nose or by nasal speech.

Tuberculosis

Scrofuloderma is the name given to tuberculous ulcers or sinuses in fistulae that develop on the skin from foci of tuberculosis in structures located in the hypoderm. Thus, it is common over lymph nodes (neck, axillae, groin, presternal area) and in the skin about joints and over bones. Scrofuloderma presents as firm, well-defined subcutaneous nodes, which gradually enlarge, become attached to the skin, and subsequently degenerate, forming ulcers and then scars. The ulcers are often linear and occasionally elongated or oval, but rarely circular. The floor is uneven, with pale granulations. A watery pus can be expressed. The edges are undermined and may be thinned by stretching over fistular pockets, and may be reddish or purplish in color. The ulcer bases are attached to the subcutaneous tissue and are not deeply indurated. The crusts are not remarkable, but take the shape of the underlying ulcer. The resulting scars are corded, depressed, and irregular lines or bands that often alternate with equally irregular nodules.

Rarely, huge fungating tumors may be formed (tuberculosis fungosa cutis). Also rarely, lymphangitic scrofuloderma tuberculosis may occur similar to that seen in lymphangitic sporotrichosis.

Erythema induratum of Bazin is caused by hematogenous deposition of a small number of tubercle bacilli in the hypoderm of the calves of young women. The

Pierre Antoine Ernest Bazin, 1807–1878, French Dermatologist, Paris tuberculous process then increases in size and causes one or several, usually bilateral, deep-seated, soft, purplish nodes. These nodes are painless, show no bruising, and are not tender, which excludes a diagnosis of erythema nodosum. These soft purplish nodes extend up to the surface, undergo necrosis, and heal leaving scars and atrophy. Rarely, the lesions occur on the upper extremities.

Nodular Vasculitis (Nontuberculous Erythema Induratum)

Nodular vasculitis is a tender nodal formation, usually about the ankle, with many of the features of erythema induratum except that no evidence of tuberculosis can be found. Hence the former name nontuberculous erythema induratum. Periarteritis nodosa should also be mentioned here, as should superficial migratory thrombophlebitis as part of the differential diagnosis.

Crohn's Disease

Crohn's disease (regional ileitis) is a nodal granulomatous lesion that can produce fistulae and sinuses, ulcers associated with tremendous scarring, and inflammation. These specific lesions are usually located in direct continuity with the systemic disease and therefore occur in perianal, genital, or parastomal areas. However, specific lesions can occur in the umbilicus, or submammary and genital tissues, with no direct connection with the gut pathology. Other nonspecific dermatological findings are erythema nodosum, nodular vasculitis, pyoderma gangrenosum, and occasionally the skin manifestation of malabsorption. Ulcerative colitis rarely has specific genitocrural or perianal lesions; pyoderma gangrenosum, erythema nodosum, toxic erythemas, and vascular thrombotic lesions may be seen.

Leprosy

Hypodermic lepromas are circumscribed, round or oval, pea- to walnut-sized, and sometimes conglomerated. At first they are firm and elastic, then they become adherent to the skin, turning purplish red on the surface and forming a slightly raised or flat plaque. Occasionally they break down, discharging a watery pus.

Fungal Nodal Granulomas

Sporotrichosis of the disseminated gummatous form or of the lymphangitic type are also nodal granulomas. Cervicofacial actinomycosis and Madura foot and, on occasion, North American blastomycosis may be mainly hypodermal in location.

Hypodermic Sarcoid

These are deep, varying-sized nodes that are sometimes confluent and may be covered with normal-appearing or purplish-red skin. Sometimes other nodules or plaques may be present. The sites of predilection are the torso and anterior thighs.

Panniculitis

Many factors can cause the development of a nodal lesion in the subcutaneous fat.[3] The morphological results of some, such as erythema nodosum and erythema induratum have already been described in this chapter.

Foreign body reactions may occur in the fat as a result of deliberate injection of paraffin and from some medications given unintentionally into the hypodermis rather than the muscle. Insulin lipodystrophy and progressive lipodystrophy are basically atrophies and are not known to start as a panniculitis.

Trauma to fatty tissues such as the female breast or the buttocks can cause the development of a subcutaneous lump, which can be called a traumatic panniculitis.

Cold panniculitis can be produced by the application of a piece of ice or the wind on a cold winter day to the exposed areas on the face and legs. In children on the cheeks it is called popsicle panniculitis. It lasts as a nontender subcutaneous swelling for up to 10 days.

Relapsing febrile nodular nonsuppurative panniculitis (Weber-Christian disease) is manifest, as the name implies, by crops of tender subcutaneous nodules, usually on the thighs or buttocks, but other areas may be involved. The nodes are of varying size and present as inflammatory masses with an overlying erythematous normal-appearing skin. They do not break down or ulcerate. Fever is present at the onset. Each attack lasts about 1 month. After the inflammatory aspect is gone, the affected skin becomes permanently depressed and brown-colored. The disease is most common in middle-aged women.

A sub-variety is liquifying panniculitis, where the lesions regularly break down and discharge a greasy fatty material with resultant scarring. Other variants of Weber-Christian disease are lipogranulomatosis subcutanea of Rothman and Makai, and migratory subacute nodular hypodermatitis (Vilanova).

DIFFERENTIAL DIAGNOSIS

The differential diagnosis for panniculitis includes erythema nodosum, erythema induratum, and nodular vasculitis, which can usually be quickly eliminated by their rather specific clinical patterns, (i.e. location, acuity, sharp demarcation, ulceration). Thrombophlebitis and nodular vasculitis must also be considered, as well as traumatic fat necrosis and subcutaneous rheumatic nodes.

In pancreatic subcutaneous fat necrosis, many areas show multiple subcutaneous nodes. The patient is obviously sick, and a diagnosis of acute pancreatitis can usually be made with ease. Rarely, these nodes will be found in asymptomatic pancreatic carcinoma.

Subcutaneous fat necrosis of the newborn appears at birth or in early infancy as indurated plaques, which are sharply demarcated, symmetrical, and yellowish white.

Endre Makai, 20th Cent, Hungarian Surgeon
Max Rothman, 1868–1915, German Pathologist
Xavier Vilanova, 1902–1965, Spanish Dermatologist

The neonate is usually well. The condition is common in premature infants and heals with scarring. Cheeks, shoulders, buttocks, and calves are common sites. The skin is cold, indurated, and at times the lesion presents like an indurated hive. There is no pitting. In contrast, sclerema neonatorum does show pitting, the neonate is sick, and the lesion disappears with no scar.

Lupus profundus presents as a panniculitis. It may coexist with discoid or systemic lupus erythematosus. Discoid lesions may be present in the scar of a healed lupus profundus ulcer.

Miscellaneous Nodal Abscesses

Hidradenitis suppurativa (see "Acne Conglobata" Chapter 20) is manifest by numerous intradermal or subdermal abscesses from the size of an almond to that of a large nut. These abscesses develop slowly and are perceptible by palpation. Gradually they form a demonstrable, hemispherical, red, nonacuminate prominence. They may undergo absorption, but more often, they soften and open through the thinned and reddened skin, emptying a bloody purulent material. Each abscess lasts about 2 weeks. Scarring may be marked; it tends to be linear. They are located on the areas with apocrine glands, in the axillae, the groin, the buttocks, and the submammary areas.

Other acne lesions of the deep granulomatous and furunculoid type, as well as large and double comedones, are often present in the nonapocrine areas such as the chest, back, and face or in the scars of old acne; the skin may be coarse, pitted, and oily. Sometimes deep cystic nodules and nodes with sinus formation may be present on the scalp.

Acneform granulomas present as nodal, well-defined, skin-colored swellings, usually located on the cheeks or jawline. They are usually single, and the usual stigmata of polymorphous acne may be present. On incision, these granulomas show a grayish, semigelatinous translucent material. They are not true cysts.

Myiasis may be deep enough to be considered as nodal, but side pressure will cause the fly larvae to appear and make the diagnosis obvious.

In pyococcal septicemic states, as part of the overall clinical picture, nodal lesions may appear, and they are hot and tender. On puncture, creamy pus may be obtained.

Nodal Tumors

There are innumerable nodal tumors, and since many have similar morphology and require biopsy to establish a definite diagnosis, this portion of the text will not list them all. Also, many nodal tumors are not in the realm of dermatology.

I have classified nodal tumors into two types, as follows.

The first type consists of nodal tumors that are part of a disease with other obvious abnormal findings. Metastatic carcinoma, for example, usually shows other evidence of disease before extensive frank nodal tumors are present. The same applies to nodal tumor deposits of the leukemias, lymphomas, and mycosis fungoides. Rarely, nodal pulsating fist-sized lesions may be seen in metastatic deposits from renal cell carcinoma. The varying-sized nodal plexiform neuromas of neurofibromatosis are associated with café au lait spots, the pedunculated skin papules, and nodules. Deep, erosive, recurrent basal and squamous cell carcinomas may have a large nodal component.

The second type consists of tumors in which the nodal tumor is primary and unassociated with other obvious clinical disease. Lipomas, deep cavernous angiomas, cystic hygromas (often on the face or neck of children), epidermal inclusion cysts (especially on the scalp and back) are examples. Malignant rare nodal tumors are reticulum-cell sarcoma, fibrosarcoma and other adnexal tumors.

A subcutaneous soft bulging of the skin in the scaphoid and triangular fossa of the pinna is a seroma (pseudocyst). It is to be distinguished from a hematoma, which follows trauma, is very painful and leaves a permanent deformity. Seromas are common in Asiatics.

For calcific deposits, see "Papulonodular and Nodal Calcific Deposits" in Chapter 12.

On the thighs and buttocks, particularly in women, deposition of excessive subcutaneous fat is uneven because the fibrous septae joining the skin to the deep fascia limit swelling of the subcutaneous tissue. This results in an irregular, dimpled surface called cellulite.

Pezogenic pedal painful papules are herniations of fat into the dermis which develop on the medial side of the arch and heel of the foot on standing.

References

1. Darier J. Textbook of dermatology. Pollitzer S, trans. Philadelphia:Lea & Febiger, 1920.
2. Siemens HW. General diagnosis and therapy of skin diseases. Weiner K, trans. Chicago:University of Chicago Press, 1958.
3. Michelson HE. A consideration of some diseases of the subcutaneous fat. Arch Dermatol 1957; 75:633–641.

CHAPTER 14
Ulcers and Erosions

> Ulcer: Loss of the covering epidermis or epithelium and underlying tissue so that scars are left after healing. If externally caused, they are called wounds.

> Erosion: Defect from loss of a portion of the epidermis, commonly following vesicles or bullae; usually nonscarring.

Overview: Ulcers and Crusts

Ulcerations of the skin are losses of substance resulting in scarring.

In general, ulcers have a marked tendency to persist for a long time or indefinitely.[1,2]

The concept of indolency is a good part of the concept of many ulcers. As an example, a traumatic leg ulcer on the lower shin area of those over 65 years of age will take as many months to heal as it is centimeters wide in its largest diameter. If there are aggravating factors such as edema or the sequelae of stasis, the time for healing will be much longer.

Cutaneous gangrene is death of an extensive area of tissue. It may be accompanied by death of the underlying tissue.

General Features

The variable depth of the loss of substance of the skin permits a distinction between (1) excoriations and erosions, which are superficial, involving only the epidermis and often resulting from a blister or a superficial pustule, and which heal without a scar, leaving a simple brown macule; and (2) true or dermic ulcerations, which encroach upon or destroy the dermis and are necessarily followed by scar formation.

The majority of skin ulcers do not start on the surface, but rather from below. The deeper the starting point of the destructive pathological process, the deeper will be the ulcer and the steeper its edges. If the pathological process is so deeply situated that it is invisible and connected with the surface merely by a duct, the lesion is called a sinus even though there may be a small ulcer at its orifice. A sinus originates from an abscess that perforates to the surface (e.g. dental sinus, tuberculous sinus).

It is important to be able to state, after examining an ulcer, whether the ulcer occurred in normal skin or resulted from some pathological process in the skin itself. The ulcer itself often causes some reactive change in the surrounding skin so one should discount some surrounding local inflammation and swelling in making this determination. Examples of pre-existing lesions causing ulcers are the presence in the edges of knobby and protuberant basal cell or squamous cell tumor, the sclerotic bound-down depressed lesion of necrobiosis lipoidica diabeticorum, the board-like sclerotic brown of stasis sequelae, or the telangiectatic lardaceous sclerosis of chronic radiation sequelae.

As implied in the preceding paragraph, the clues as to whether or not an ulcer is occurring in normal skin are best found in the surrounding or peripheral tissue on examination for pre-existing abnormalities such as sclerosis, induration, and in the base of the ulcer, which must be inspected for infiltrates and so on (Fig. 14.1). Having looked for these findings in the periphery and in the base, one can consider other aspects of the ulcer in search of diagnostic clues. These include location, size, border, discharge, floor, lymph node involvement, pain, and course of disease.

Location may be helpful in assembling tables of differential diagnoses. The conditions causing ulcers on the face, genitals, and lower legs are quite different.

Portions of the Overview have been taken and modified from Darier[1] (pp. 277–279) and Siemens[2] (pp. 114–119).

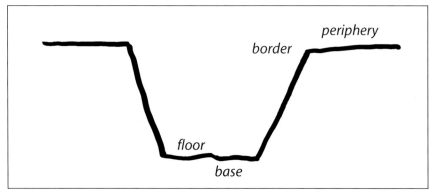

Figure 14.1 The important areas to study when examining ulcers for pre-existing local disease are the periphery and the base.

The configuration or shape of the ulcer borders can be helpful. Is it sharp and linear? Is it round, oval, polycyclic, or reniform? Some ulcers are made up of many small separate foci of disease and when each of these foci ulcerates they make a retiform or colandar-like pattern. The scar of an ulcer may take several patterns. If it heals evenly from the periphery, the scar will be circular in shape at the periphery. If it heals on one side, but progresses on the other, serpiginous, clover-leaf or kidney-shaped ulcers may occur. The colour of the border is occasionally useful, e.g. the deep purplish red of rapidly growing acute pyoderma gangrenosum. The border itself should be examined. The verrucous small pus pocketed dark brown border of blastomycosis is characteristic; the peripheral undermining of a Fournier's gangrene may be seen.

The discharge may be of varying sorts, from bloody to serous to purulent. If crusts are present, they should be removed. At times it may be necessary to soak them off with compresses. The various sorts of crusts and their significance is covered later in this chapter.

The floor may be level or uneven, granular, papillomatous, "worm-eaten", crateriform, raised, or otherwise. In exceptional cases, the floor of an ulcer may vegetate to such a degree that it rises above the level of the surrounding skin, giving the impression that there is no defect, but rather an increase in tissue substance, in spite of the absence of the upper layers of the skin (e.g. proud flesh, or tomato tumors of mycosis fungoides).

The lymph nodes, especially the regional ones, should always be examined.

Pain is a feature of some ulcers, particularly those occurring in areas of sclerous radiation sequelae, the neuroanesthetic ulcers are relatively pain-free.

The course of the ulcer can often be suggested by the clinical findings. The rapidity of development of the ulcers is usually of more value in determining the acuity of the process than in making a diagnosis of the cause of the ulcer.

Jean Alfred Fournier, 1832–1914, French Venereologist

Papules

As a rule, the lesions of secondary papular syphilis undergo resolution without ulceration. Malignant syphilis presents with papulocrusted lesions, which ulcerate under their brownish or grayish crust. These lesions are disseminated and progressively increase in size and depth. Mucosal ulceration also occurs. Ulcerative secondary syphilis consists of irregularly scattered eruption of ulcerations, which develop and enlarge rapidly; they have a round or more often oval form; perpendicular purplish borders, a cupola-shaped floor; bloody pus filling; and a soft base. A bomb-explosion arrangement may be seen. The peripheral extension and the desiccation of the pus that they secrete sometimes give rise to ostraceous crusts, which are thicker in the center, like the shell of an oyster (rupial syphilis).

Papular Tumors and Ulcers

Almost all of the papular tumors that show ulceration are malignant (Fig. 14.5). Of the black or brown papulonodular tumors, the pigmented basal cell carcinoma, malignant melanoma, and ulcerated pigmented dermatofibroma should be considered. Of the malignant papular tumors, basal cell carcinoma of the superficial multicentric or grass fire type and their differential diagnosis are also to be considered. The varying forms of histiocytosis X may present as ulcerating papules.

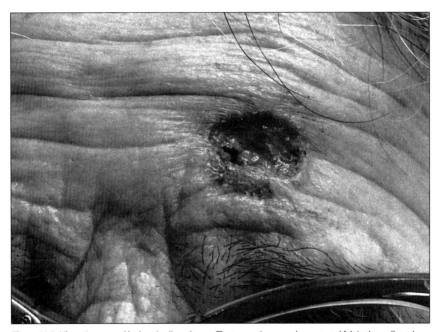

Figure 14.5 Ulceration caused by basal cell carcinoma. The tumor tissue can be seen and felt in the walls and floor of the ulcer, but there is no rolled border.

Nodes and Nodules

Realizing that the nodal and nodular ulcerative forms of syphilis and tuberculosis are now rare in well-developed countries, I have left them in here for completeness.

Granulomatous Syphilitic Ulcers

Noduloulcerative tertiary syphilis develops ulcers with polycylic borders, usually solitary with extensive degrees of honey-combed scarring. Frequently, one side shows rows of punched out polycylic ulcers discharging pus or covered with thick, hard, adherent, sometimes ostraceous crusts of a greenish-black color. Sometimes the nodular element is not obvious and only a polycylic, sharply demarcated, rather shallow, scarring ulcer is present.

Nodal ulcerative tertiary syphilis (or gummas) may present as solitary, rounded or kidney-shaped ulcers with loose, soft, or edematous borders. It results from the disintegration and evacuation of a nodal lesion arising from deep tissues such as lymph nodes or bone. Sometimes massive destruction of tissue occurs with bones, tendons, and vessels being exposed. On the tongue and legs, a sclerous nodal ulceration may occur. They arise in scarred tertiary syphilis and are characterized by their woody or sclerotic character.

Tertiary syphilic ulcerations may arise from mixed nodal and nodular lesions.

DIFFERENTIAL DIAGNOSIS

The differential diagnosis mainly includes large basal or squamous cell carcinoma, the deep mycoses, and tuberculous ulcers.

Granulomatous Orificial Tuberculous Ulcers

These occur on the lips, tongue, or elsewhere in the mouth or pharynx or about the anus. These ulcers are ovoid, polycylic, or irregular in shape and are of varying size, up to 2 cm in diameter. They have ragged contours, perpendicular or detached borders, a reddish or purplish color, and an uneven roughened granular floor that is dotted with hemorrhagic points, and often covered with gray debris. The ulcers are superficial and shallow. On the floor or at the periphery, numerous small yellow colored granules of a pinhead size may be seen. There is a small amount of bloody discharge. The regional lymph nodes are frequently enlarged. The ulcers are tender and basically nonhealing. Rarely, the ulcer has a linear component especially at the commissures of the lips or on the tip of the tongue. Occasionally they may be verrucous.

DIFFERENTIAL DIAGNOSIS

The differential diagnosis includes traumatic ulcers, which heal rapidly; chancroid, which is exceptional outside the genitoanal region, has an abundant suppuration, has a rapid course, and is autoinoculable; syphilitic ulcers, which have a more regular form and an indurated base; ulcerated squamous cell carcinomas, which usually have a firm rubbery feel. For diagnostic purposes, a deep biopsy including muscle and tissue scrapings, or material from the floor of the ulcer or margins should be sent for bacterial and fungal studies. Crohn's disease should also be considered.

Lupus Vulgaris Ulcers (Nodular Tuberculous Ulcers)

The borders are slanting, the adjoining tissue is purplish or brownish-yellow, tense, infiltrated, and more or less transparent. The shape of the ulcer is round or oval. The floor is slightly depressed, friable and of spongy consistency. The ulcer bleeds easily, is of a spongy consistency, and is readily lacerated. The base is the site of a soft infiltration, and it is usually nonadherent to the underlying tissue. The secretion is turbid, bloody, and dries in a thin adherent grayish yellow crust that may be deeply imbedded in the lesion.

Ulcerative Tuberculides (Nodal Tuberculous Ulcers)

The ulcers of erythema induratum have rather deep depressions, a grayish, reddened floor with an extensively infiltrated base, and the area about the lesion has a purplish hue.

The ulcers formed in scrofuloderma have a shaggy, nonindurated border. There frequently are one or two sinus openings from which a small amount of material can be expressed.

The ulcers of leprosy have a variable appearance. Severe loss of tissue is a feature of these ulcers. Lepers may also develop neurotrophic ulcers due to nerve damage. Ulcers may also follow the bullous lesions of leprosy.

The ulcerations of the deep mycoses, e.g. sporotrichosis, blastomycosis, and actinomycosis, should be considered in the differential diagnosis.

Other granulomata (sarcoidosis, foreign body, cutaneous leishmaniasis, necrobiosis lipoidica diabeticorum, bromoderma, and iododerma) may and often do have an ulcerative component. However, only rarely do they present basically as ulcers. The draining sinuses of some of the forms of panniculitis may also have an ulcerative component.

Nodal and Nodular Ulcerative Tumors

Of the nodal and nodular tumors, only a few present with a large ulcerative component. These are squamous and basal cell carcinoma, malignant melanoma, mycosis fungoides and metastatic deposits. Of these, only the deeply invasive often recurrent basal cell carcinoma occasionally present a problem in differential diagnosis. Rapidly growing malignant cutaneous lymphomas may show surprisingly great ulceration.

Verrucosities

Only the verrucous granulomas and verrucous cancers regularly show ulcers, but in all cases, the verrucous element gives away the basic underlying lesion.

Scleroses

Many sclerosing conditions can develop ulceration. Stasis sequelae on the leg (see later), late radiation sequelae, necrobiosis lipoidica diabeticorum, systemic scleroderma, morphea-like basal cell carcinoma, and sclerosing breast cancer are some examples that come to mind. Ulcer formation is secondary.

Folliculoses

A few bacterial and fungal folliculoses produce ulcers that scar.

Onychoses

Ulcerative conditions of the nail and periungual tissues are usually due to squamous cell carcinoma and malignant melanoma (sometimes amelanotic). Occasionally, traumatic ulcers may be seen.

Stasis Leg Ulcers (Gravitational)

The most common site of leg stasis ulcers is on the inner aspect of the leg just above the ankle in the spat or gaiter area (Fig. 14.6). Anywhere in the lower half of the leg or about the ankles may be involved, except that the anterior aspect of the ankle and the dorsum of the foot are almost never involved. In these leg ulcers, the obvious lesion is the ulcer, although other underlying changes are present.

The ulcers may be single or multiple. If multiple, there is a tendency to coalescence. The shape is basically oval, but many have rather irregularly shaped borders. The size may go up to 15 cm, and rarely, they may encircle the leg. The floor is bright red or purplish, proliferating, oozing, or covered with a thick crust with drainage of a bloody purulent material. The borders are adherent and gently sloping or perpendicular. The periphery of the ulcer is erythematous and sclerotic. The other changes of stasis are also present, namely atrophy,

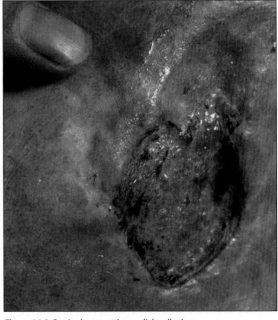

Figure 14.6 Stasis ulcer over the medial malleolus.

brown and black pigmented areas, purpuric spots, edema, atrophie blanche and noire, and eczematous dermatitis. Scars from previously healed ulcers may be present. Rarely, a full blown pyogenic infection such as cellulitis or erysipelas is in progress. The overall picture is that of an ulcer occurring in thickened, smooth, tense, unfoldable skin with a mottled white, brown, or purplish color. Above and below this, large deep varicose veins may be seen. Rarely, an elephantiasis-like picture may occur (see Chapter 19).

Over the years, I have been impressed at the frequency of arterial ischemia factors in aggravating and causing a continuation of stasis ulcers. It stands to reason that any deep stasis ulcer damages the small arterial blood supply. As these ulcers are more common in the elderly, the circulation is already decreased by arteriosclerosis. Once an ischemic element is introduced the ulcers will, of course, be deeper, slower to heal, and more painful, especially on raising the foot — a procedure which makes the plain stasis ulcer less painful. Occasionally, painful ulcers in the stasis or spat area of the ankle may be due to large vessel arteriosclerosis.

I am also impressed by the degree of dermatosclerosis that can precede the ulceration, almost as if the sclerosis were the main underlying lesion predisposing to ulcer formation (see Chapter 18).

DIFFERENTIAL DIAGNOSIS

The main differential diagnosis includes the nodular and nodal lesions of syphilis and tuberculosis, which are now very rare. The underlying changes are usually obvious if sought on examination.

Ulcers: No Basic Skin Lesion

Vascular Ulcers

Hypertensive: Ischemic

These ulcers occur on essentially normal skin. They occur on the skin of the lateral ankle or on the shin. They are painful, punched out, oval lesions about the size of a quarter (2.3 cm diameter). The floor is red, and the sides are perpendicular. The ulcers are indolent. There is no inflammatory reaction and other signs of stasis are not present.

Other ischemic ulcers occur on pressure points in individuals whose circulation is impaired permanently by such ailments as arteriosclerosis (especially in diabetics and smokers) or thromboangiitis obliterans. In these patients, the feet and lower legs are common sites of ischemic ulcers. The ulcer may start rather acutely with a bulla, often hemorrhagic, under which a deep ulcer develops as the result of tissue death.

When the pressure is temporary, a bulla may be formed. This is the case in patients comatose from an overdose of drugs where the bullae develop at sites of pressure (often in bizarre placcs) due to pressure ischemia. These bullae usually do not produce ulcers. When the pressure is prolonged, ischemic decubitus ulcers result. They can also occur on amputation stumps.

Ulcers with Rheumatoid Arthritis

On the legs (especially the shins), varying-sized indolent ulcers may be present. They tend to be oval in shape, with a regular unimpressive border. The floor is poorly vascularized, and so looks pale, and may have a seropurulent exudate. Healed lesions show scarring. There are often other findings of vasculitis, such as ulcers, urticarial lesions, purpura, and bullae.

On the palms and palmar surfaces of the fingers, usually three to four punched out ulcers are present. They are tender and may have a purpuric element and scar on healing.

Ulcers may occur over nodal or nodular calcium deposits. Calcific material may be discharged. The CREST syndrome and the calcification of the dermatosclerosis of stasis are examples.

Livedo with Ulceration on the Soles

Livedo with ulceration is the name given to rather deep scarring fissures on the plantar skin on the heel or on the forefoot portion of the sole. The cracks measure up to 3 cm in length and up to 5 mm in width. Black (the remains of hemorrhage) color is often present in these cracks. They follow the lines of cleavage of the plantar skin. Sometimes they are directly on weight-bearing areas, other times they are not. One, two, or even more lesions may be present. Semilinear white atrophic scars may be present at the site of prior lesions.

Other factors assisting with diagnosis are the presence of livido reticularis involving the whole foot and sometimes the rest of the extremity, other ischemic ulcers on the malleoli or lower leg, and a cool, hairless, pale, foot.

DIFFERENTIAL DIAGNOSIS

The differential diagnosis includes the frequent cracks and fissures from miscellaneous tylotic conditions of the palms and soles. Scarring and livido reticularis are not present in these latter conditions.

Vasculitis

Drug-induced erythemas may have a vasculitis component, which may produce ischemic vasculitis as manifest by ulceration. These ulcers are of varying size and location, although the legs and feet are common sites. Other vasculitis ulcers can be seen in connection with the collagenoses such as systemic lupus erythematous periarteritis nodosa and rheumatoid arthritis. Systemic scleroderma may produce ischemic ulcers on the pinna of the ear, the elbows, knees, and on the knuckles, as well as at the tips of the fingers and toes.

Neuroanesthetic Ulcers

Mal Perforans Plantaris

Mal perforans plantaris begins as a corn or callous, usually under the head of the first metatarsal or on other pressure points (Fig. 14.7). The corn then becomes

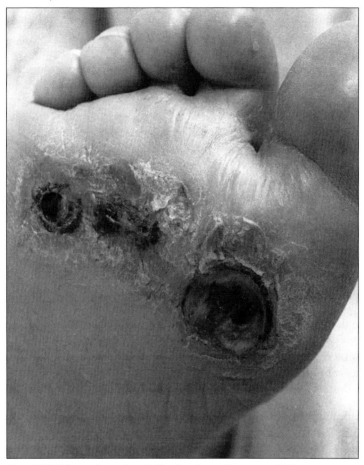

Figure 14.7 Malum perforans plantaris. Note flexed toes of the neuropathic foot.

hemorrhagic or crusted. With paring of the horn or removal of the crust, a rounded ulcer is found, with a gray dead-looking floor, perpendicular walls, surrounded by hyperkeratosis. It may burrow deeply. In fact, the shape of some of these ulcers is like that of an iceberg, i.e. the deep portion is larger than the surface portion. Early, the lesion may appear just as a hemorrhagic corn or callous. It is impossible to make a diagnosis unless the crust or covering horn is removed by paring. Excessive horn formation is seen around any neuroanesthetic ulcer on the sole. It presumably represents nature's attempt to protect the ulcer from further trauma. At times this may be extensive and verrucous, suggesting an HPV infection or verrucous squamous cell carcinoma (epithelioma cuniculatum) (see also under verrucous carcinomas, Chapter 16).

Trigeminal Trophic Syndrome

Ulcers in Neurotrophic Skin

A typical case might be as follows:

Mrs. M.D., estimated age 75, was first seen in July, 1963, having been referred with a clinical diagnosis of basal cell carcinoma on the left upper lip and left external naris. In 1941 she had had a section of the posterior root of the left fifth cranial nerve for "major" tic douloureux.

On examination, the patient showed almost complete anesthesia on the left side of her face, including her upper lip and the side of her nose. There was more flacidity in the muscles of expression on the same side; a dimple was present in the center of the left cheek; the left naris was considerably larger than the right. There was a sharply demarcated crescentic ulcer about 2.5 by 1.0 cm involving the upper portion of the left upper lip (skin surface) and extending onto the lower portion of the left side of the nasal septum. The base of the ulcer was clean; the border was smooth and not rolled. The patient was a mentally confused recluse; she stated the lesion had been present for about 6 months. She denied ever touching the lesion, even though she was seen to pick and rub at the ulcer while waiting to be examined.

The clinical differential diagnosis was self-induced ulcer in neurotrophic skin or rodent ulcer. Histological examination of two punch biopsies, one from the ulcer and one from the adjacent skin on the left upper lip, showed no evidence of tumor. When the area was permanently occluded, the ulcer healed completely.

This brief case report illustrates a common cause of the so-called neurotrophic ulcer. The basic cause for the patient's scratching and picking is a parasthesia.

Phagedena

Phagedenic ulcers have the following characteristics.[3]

Death of Tissue: While considerable necrosis occurs in many phagedenic ulcers, true gangrene is rare. Remember that gangrene means a severe and irreversible type of massive destruction, ending in complete devitalization. Admittedly, there are transitional zones between simple necrosis and true gangrene.

Burrowing, Eating Away of Tissue with an Undermined and Sometimes Verrucous Border: The ulcer involves the total thickness of the skin and so, after healing, there will be extensive scarring. Frequently, too, deeper structures such as muscles, tendons, nerves, and blood vessels may be exposed at the base of the ulcer. The borders are commonly surrounded by a red and indurated zone from 1 to 2 cm wide. Rarely, the death of the epidermis presents a picture of a circular flaccid superficial bulla at the periphery of the ulcer. The border is commonly undermined. It also may be elevated, verrucous, and eaten away and pocketed by small, pea-sized collections of pus. The floor contains thick maloderous pus, which when cleared away may show a yellowish, difficult to remove, adherent dead tissue. More commonly, the floor is red, granular, sometimes with reepithelialization on one side or scattered throughout the base. The border may show some crusting, but this is not a major feature.

Arcuate or Serpiginous Borders: The configuration of the ulcer is sometimes irregular, often polycylic. When two ulcers meet, a figure-8 appearance may be found. Other variations of circle formation may be present. Geometric phagedena is a term used for these peculiar-shaped lesions.

Palm-Sized or Larger Ulcers: Most phagedenic ulcers are large, and usually there are two or three of them. At times there is one huge (up to 20 cm) ulcer. Nonhealing progressive chickenpox or smallpox can produce a crop of 4 to 5 cm phagedenic ulcers.

Chronicity with Periods of Rapid Growth: Most phagedenic ulcers are chronic, i.e. they last longer than three months. At the onset, particularly, there may be a period of very rapid necrosis and spread of the ulcer. Ulcers 10 cm across may develop in a period of two to three weeks. Thereafter, progress may be slow and unremitting or the ulcers may grow in fits and starts. New ulcers may continue to appear. Frequently, one side progresses while the other side heals.

Some Underlying Weakened Systemic State Is Often Present: Alcoholism, diabetes, postoperative states, ulcerative colitis, or regional ileitis are examples. However, this is not always the case, and in some patients, the search for underlying abnormalities will be fruitless.

I have never seen phagedenic ulcers on the palms or the soles.

Severe scarring is common with strand-like epidermal bridges, skin tags, and a generally disorganized scar. Cribriform is an often-used adjective, but colander-like is probably more accurate.

Phagedenic ulceration is a morphological concept, not an etiological one. Large burrowing ulcers of known cause, e.g. malignant secondary syphilis, tertiary syphilitic ulcers, tuberculous ulcers, and cancerous ulcers, are by tradition not identified as phagedenic ulcers. Phagedenic ulcers now seem to be less common. Presumably, potent antibiotics and systemic corticosteroids have arrested or controlled these ulcers. This is particularly true in ulcers that start as banal bacterial infections.

Specific Types and Names

Pyoderma gangrenosum and geometric phagedena are the names used by dermatologists to describe phagedenic ulcers in patients who often have ulcerative colitis or regional ileitis, myeloproliferative conditions, and rheumatoid arthritis. The ulcers are multiple, are common on the ankles, knees, and buttocks, and have most of the features of regular phagedenic ulcers. These patients also have small furunculoid lesions that develop at sites of injury. Sometimes these lesions turn into ulcers.

The early lesions may include juicy red papules and plaques, papulopustules, or pustules with a marked erythematous halo. Sometimes, a small central necrotic area is present. Some, but not all, of the lesions rapidly enlarge to produce the typical deep necrotic ulcer with heaped up edges.

Meleney's (chronic undermining) ulcer and postoperative progressive serpiginous ulcer are names used by surgeons to describe phagedenic ulcers that develop in surgical patients. They seem again to start from some injury, incision, draining sinus, abscess, or ruptured lymph node. Operations involving the large bowel or anal area have been the starting point for most of these ulcers that I have seen.

Progressive synergistic bacterial gangrene is similar to the above listed types, but has more death of tissue. Fournier's gangrene (of the scrotum) is another variant following again on lower bowel surgery (see also under "Gangrenous Infections" later in this chapter).

Circumscribed phagedenic ulcers (infectious multiple gangrene of the skin, dermatitis gangrenosa infantum, gangrenous impetigo) are multiple phagedenic ulcers arising from pyogenic bacterial or viral skin infections that have spread embolically.

Tropical phagedenic ulcers are varied, usually occurring on the feet and legs of patients who go barefoot and have a low general standard of hygiene and nutrition.

Coumarin necrosis is most frequently seen in obese middle-aged women in such fatty areas as the thighs, buttocks, abdomen, and breasts, usually after 3 to 10 days of receiving the drug. The first presentation is that of a tender red plaque up to 15 cm across. Purple ecchymoses, blistering, and necrosis follow. The border is red, elevated, and indurated.

Miscellaneous

Chancroid (soft chancre) has a round or oval, relatively deep ulceration up to the size of a silver dollar (2.7 cm diameter); the borders are perpendicular, undermined, or slightly detached; often they are cracked or fissured. The floor is of a creamy yellow or yellowish-gray color, irregular, and appears worm eaten. The surrounding tissue is red and swollen, but induration is not marked. There is an abundant purulent discharge. As a rule, several ulcers are present. The regional lymph nodes are usually swollen and painful, one of which is much larger than the rest. These lymph nodes suppurate and discharge forming a sinus, ulcer, or bubo, usually unilateral. The genitals and the genital regions are the usual sites; in men on the penis, in women on the vulva. Occasionally, "kissing ulcers" are present. Rarely, extragenital soft chancres are found.

Patients with glanders (due to Pseudomonas mallei) have ulcers. The ulcers have irregular shaped, livid purplish, ragged margins, an irregular floor, with a soft base, and fluctuating nodosities and small abscesses at the periphery. Mutilating glanders is usually in the center of the face and causes severe disfigurement. Syphilitic chancre is usually an erosion, but in the immunologically exhausted patient, a deep painful infiltrating burrowing ulcer may occur. Ankle or lower leg ulcers may be found in blacks with sickle cell anemia.

Frank Lamont Meleney, 1889–1963, U.S. Surgeon

Overview: Cutaneous Erosions and Excoriations

There are different levels of skin loss.[2] Figure 14.8 illustrates levels of skin loss produced by scratching.

Lightly scratching the skin surface, removes only the horny layer, i.e. the scales. The result is a dry streak surrounded by horny-layer debris. If the scratching fingernail penetrates to the malpighian layer, the track of the scratch will be moist, with clear serum oozing forth. If the injury reaches still deeper, the papillae are torn off. Thus a punctate or, if a larger area is involved, sieve-like hemorrhage results. These superficial lesions are called erosions. If the injury penetrates into the connective tissue proper, the bleeding is more uniform and copious, and the lesion is called a wound. If connective tissue is disrupted, scarring results. This scarring is the hallmark of wounds and ulcers.

Erosions are not caused only by trauma, but may develop by detachment of the uppermost epidermal layers usually aggravated by maceration (eczemas between the toes and under the breasts, erosive balanitis, and the primary lesion of syphilis). Most frequently, erosions originate in the epidermis or between the epidermis and the dermis from a vesicle or bulla that has lost its top. The vesicular or bullous genesis of an erosion can be diagnosed by its outline and the remnant of the blister top (collarette) remains at the edge. However, such an epithelial collar around erosions does not necessarily tell the tale of its development from a blister, as the example of erosio interdigitalis blastomycetica show. In these conditions, the epithelial collar is caused by undermining of the periphery. Erosions following vesicles of mucosal surfaces (aphthae) retain the round or oval outline.

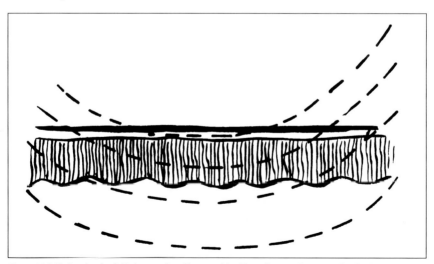

Figure 14.8 Various levels of skin loss produced by scratching. Top to bottom: Desquamation; Erosion; Excoration; and Wound.

Marcello Malpighi, 1628–1694, Italian Anatomist
Portions of the Overview have been taken and modified from Siemens[2] (pp. 76, 81, 84, 85, 86).

Some postbullous erosions characteristically form vegetations instead of healing smoothly (pemphigus vegetans). In other instances, healing of the blister floor is accompanied by the formation of tiny epithelial inclusion cysts called milia (in, for example, epidermolysis bullosa, porphyria cutanea tarda, or traumatic scars).

Although scratching, tearing, or abrasions may cause excoriations in normal skin, damage may be done much more readily when the papillae of the cutis are elongated so that their tips can be easily torn off. Such a situation is most pronounced in psoriasis. Therefore, punctate sieve-like bleeding on vigorous scratching is regarded as a diagnostic sign of psoriasis, and is called psoriasiform bleeding (Auspitz's sign).

After healing, erosions and excoriations frequently leave brown hyperpigmentation or hypopigmentations (melanodermas or leukodermas), which may persist for some time (see "Dyschromias", Chapter 17, for definition). These should not be confused with the depigmentation occurring in scars.

Erosions and excoriations appear most frequently and in the largest numbers as the result of scratching (scratch marks). Itching, however, does not always lead to scratch marks. There exist two different types of itching: (1) rub itching or pressing or kneading; and (2) scratch itching. Rub itching occurs in urticaria and some lichenifications, while scratch itching occurs in scabies, body lice, papular urticaria, and atopic dermatitis.

The shape of the scratch marks may give a clue to the cause of the itching and are therefore of diagnostic significance. On morphologically normal skin, scratch streaks form and, if they go deep enough, bleed and become crusted. Rubbing tends to abrade the hair follicles, leaving small, round crusts arranged at strikingly equal distances from one another. If papules and vesicles are destroyed by scratching, as, for instance, in papular urticaria or atopic dermatitis, punctate and small circular scratch marks appear. These marks are not as regularly arranged as the follicular ones. Linear scratch marks are frequently oblong with pointed ends and are wider in the middle, where the scratching nail can penetrate most deeply into the edematous or inflamed tissue. If the scratching is very violent, one sees long, parallel, or sometimes crossing groups of scratch marks, frequently with linear purpura. Some of the lesions may be only scaly, whereas others may be covered with thin bloody scabs. The parallel arrangement indicates simultaneous scratching with several fingers.

Just as excoriations can be viewed to determine the type of itch producing the excoriations, the pattern of the excoriations can also be examined.

In general, excoriations fall into three types: (1) long linear scratches; (2) erythema and lichenification with eventual browning from rubbing; and (3) small circular crusted erosions or circular excoriations from picking. Although, of course, the three varieties may coexist, the type and pattern of the excoriation is often the same.

The linear scratch mark is best seen on the torso of patients with body lice. Pubic lice also may cause the patient to produce scratch marks on the thighs and abdomen. Maculae ceruleae (blue spots) on the sides of the torso can be seen. Linear scratch marks can also be seen in jaundice and uremia.

Rubbing and picking to produce an erythematous brown lichenified eruption with a circular excoriated area is common in atopic dermatitis, in lower leg xerotic winter eczema, and in lichen simplex chronicus.

Circular excoriated areas can be produced by scratching some weakened structure of the skin, so that the scratching removes the skin, blister tops, or crusts, producing a circular excoriated lesion, for example, in the excoriated papulovesicles on the elbows and knees in dermatitis herpetiformis, the excoriated turgid papulovesicles of nummular eczema, and the numerous round scalp excoriations in an infestation of head lice (frequently with secondary pyoderma). Picking can also produce circular excoriated areas as in acné excoriée des jeunes filles. In such cases, though, there is also an element of squeezing, which can be recognized by the presence of a perilesional brown color and also by lichenified and acneform enlargement in some areas, particularly the ear lobes and retroauricular crease.

The excoriations of Hodgkin's disease tend to begin as the circular excoriated type, but rapidly become papular and develop into prurigo nodularis. The excoriations of insect bites tend to be of the small circular type.

It is worthwhile to mention that in some reportedly itching dermatoses there may be no morphological excoriated lesion. This is often the case with urticaria. Neurotic excoriations are dealt with separately. Frequent, prolonged and severe scratching produces nail changes. Briefly, these consist of buffing of the distal one-third, an open V-shaped defect in the center of the free edge of the nail, and a general wearing away of the nail tip (see "Traumatic", Chapter 22).

All itching skin eruptions, which lead to scratching, can be complicated by various types of cutaneous pyodermas (impetigo, ecthyma, furuncle, erysipelas). If pyogenic infection has set in, small wounds previously covered with little, thin, dark red, bloody scabs become covered with thick, moist, turbid, brown to greenish purulent crusts surrounded by inflammatory red halos. Pyogenic ulceration of the skin may also be present. The continued scratching spreads the pyogenic infection, giving rise to primary impetigo blisters and crusts, folliculitides, and abscesses far away from the underlying initial pruritic lesion. The presence of secondary pyoderma from scratching plus possible secondary irritation or contact reaction from topically applied preparations can indeed produce a confusing picture, making the diagnosis of the underlying condition difficult, if not impossible. In longer-lasting diseases with constantly repeated rubbing and excoriation, the cumulative effect of the irritation causes thickening, brown hyperpigmentation, and hyperplasia of epidermis and cutis. The skin of the involved areas takes on a dirty brown color interspersed with numerous light, small scars. This skin is rough, desquamates easily, and becomes thickened. Longterm infestation with body lice can produce the morphological changes just described. It has been called Vagabond's disease. In this case, some of the color change is also due to associated nutritional deficiencies.

Self-Inflicted Lesions

There are, of course, innumerable ways that self-induced injuries (including excoriations) can be produced on the skin or mucosa.[4] Butterworth and Strean have described these in some detail.[5] As they are not part of the usual dermatological practice, a mere listing of the means by which skin can be excoriated (or injured) is sufficient here to suggest the possible wide spectrum of morphological changes produced. The list includes biting, bumping, clenching, cutting, excoriating, grinding, injury by chemical, thermal, or other means, licking, picking, pressure, pulling, rubbing, striking, and sucking.

One condition seen on the extremities of young girls is the flaccid collapsed superficial friction bulla produced by pushing hard on the skin with a finger for a long period of time. The lesions are multiple, on the dorsa of the hands, forearms, arms, and thighs. Sometimes an associated bruise may be seen. There is usually some surrounding erythema. Compare this with the autoerythrocyte sensitization phenomenon in Chapter 3, "Purpura".

Stokes and Garner in an early article classified self-inflicted lesions into two types: neurotic excoriations and dermatitis artefacta.[6]

The morphological criteria for making the diagnosis of dermatitis artefacta are three. First, they are almost always destructive, varying from a physical or chemical burn to an ulcer to gangrene. Second, they all have bizarre shapes, for example, squares, lines, tails, or other odd non-natural shapes may be assumed. Third, the lesions are all on accessible sites. The characteristic psychological features of these patients are impossible to confine in writing. One almost needs a sixth sense to make a diagnosis of self-inflicted lesions in certain cases. An important finding is that a particular eruption is not just typical of any known eruption or lesion; a bizarre lesion in a bizarre patient. This of course, implies a considerable degree of experience on behalf of the observer. Dermatitis artefacta as a differential diagnostic possibility in a patient with a chronic ulcer should always be considered — then it will not be missed.

Occasionally, the type of sclerosis or scarring may be highly suggestive of the diagnosis. On the faces of patients who dig deeply to remove "ingrowing hairs", a deep irregular and at times linear scar formation develops — often at times mixed with deep shaped edged, irregular, varying sized ulcerations.

Another area to be considered are lesions inflicted by occupations.[7]

Traumatic lichenifications are covered in Chapter 11 "Papules".

Mutilations are loss of tissue such as bone, cartilage, tendons, and so on, along with destruction of skin. Some are self-inflicted. Many are due to disease, e.g. lupus vulgaris or leprosy.

Neurotic Excoriations

Neurotic excoriations is the term given to superficial self-inflicted lesions consisting of circular or ovoid whitish, slightly atrophic areas from 2 to 8 mm in diameter.

Interspersed among the atrophic areas are varying stages of small wound formation: some are eroded with oozing; some show a fresh bloody crust; some show a dry loosely attached crust; and some show an atrophic red area. The lesions may or may not scar; most do not. The scars may accentuate the follicular orifices. The borders of each lesion are sharply demarcated. The eruption is symmetrical, located primarily on the outer aspect of the arms, the upper back and shoulders, and the head and neck, i.e. the readily accessible areas. However, the lesions may be more widely disseminated to such areas as the outer aspect of the forearms and the clavicular areas. Some of the skin between whitish areas appears darker brown than the skin in other areas. I am impressed that a minor degree of acne vulgaris is often present and that the eruption is common in the areas usually afflicted by acne (acné excoriée des jeunes filles). Neurotic excoriations are less common in men. Rarely are neurotic excoriations, dermatitis artefacta, and prurigo nodularis seen in the same patient.

DIFFERENTIAL DIAGNOSIS

The differential diagnosis between excoriated papular urticaria, dermatitis herpetiformis, and neurotic excoriations is discussed under "Papular Urticaria" in Chapter 2.

Inflammatory Erosions: Syphilitic Chancre

A syphilitic chancre has the following characteristics.
1. It is a slight erosion (not an ulcer) generally of the size of a dime (1.8 cm diameter).
2. It has a round regular form.
3. It has no marked borders, being on the same level as the surrounding tissue.
4. The color varies from red fleshy color with smooth, moist, glazed, or finely granular surface to a grayish color with diphtheroid surface scattered with ecchymotic points and sometimes covered with a thin brownish crust.
5. There is an indurated base which is recognized by grasping the chancre between the thumb and the index finger across its diameter and slightly raising it.
6. The chancre is accompanied by a satellite bubo. This bubo has its seat in the glands corresponding to the lymphatic territory of the chancre. It consists of a group of hard, ovoid, movable, painless, noninflammatory glands; one or two of these glands are apt to be larger than the rest and may present a very evident protuberance. The bubo appears from 6 to 10 days after the chancre and survives it for a number of months.

The chancre heals in a fortnight to 6 weeks; the induration may persist for several months. A cicatrix is seen in only about one-half the cases.

The varieties of syphilitic chancre are innumerable, but the typical form is by far the most common. There occur dwarf chancres, or giant chancres; papular hypertrophic or ulcerative chancres; or ecthymatous chancres covered with a fairly thick crust. Although the chancre is, as a rule solitary, multiple chancres (two or three

---

Portions of this section have been taken and modified from Darier[1](pp. 614–616).

or more) are encountered in some patients. The chancres are simultaneous or successive, which may be due to a variable inoculation, successive contaminations, autoinoculations, or to a chancrous lymphangitis that has given rise to local erosion.

Localization

Genital chancre in men is frequently located on the balanopreputial groove and the sides of the frenulum, but may occur on any other point of the penis, the scrotum, or the pubis. Intraurethral chancre of the meatus is rare. In women, the labia majora and minora, the fourchette, the clitoris, and more rarely the meatus are the seat of the chancre, hardly ever the vagina. Chancre of the uterine cervix is rare, but should be looked for during the examination.

Extragenital chancre is localized on the head in most cases. A common location is the mouth, especially the lower lip. When it straddles the free borders of the lip, it is crusted in its cutaneous portion, erosive in its mucous portion. Chancres also occur on the tongue and tonsils. The latter is unilateral, erosive or ulcerative, of woody hardness, relatively painless, lasts for a number of weeks, and is associated with rather prominent regional lymphadenopathy. This adenopathy is a striking feature of chancres of the face, scalp, and mouth.

A badly healing or proliferating wound on the fingers, about the nails, or over the joints should raise the possibility of an extragenital chancre. Chancres can also occur on the breasts and in the perianal area. Darier in 1920 claimed that most extragenital chancres were "innocently acquired" by tattooing and family contacts. In 1994, I doubt that this is still true. The nonsexual innocently acquired origin of extragenital syphilis in adults must now be very rare. The same is not true of treponematoses such as yaws and bejel.

Complications

The indurated chancre can become inflamed after traumatism, improper treatment, or secondary infection; it then becomes painful, bleeds, and suppurates. Sometimes the bubo itself breaks down and discharges. Superficial gangrene and phagedena are rare complications. Simultaneous chancres from the *Treponema* pallidum and from Ducrey's bacillus are rare, but may occur. Gonorrhea may coexist with a syphilitic chancre.

Recidives

Most recidives (French meaning relapse) or relapsing lesions on the body are the grouped secondary papular lesions. On the genitalia and mucous membranes, these are moist eroded papules, condylomata lata, and mucous patches predominate. Relapse of the primary chancre, usually in secondary syphilis, is spoken of as a monorecidive chancre or chancre redux. This is not the same as pseudochancre redux; the latter is a tertiary gummatous lesion at the site of the original chancre.

Augosto Ducrey, 1860–1940, Italian Dermatologist

Malignant Erosions: Paget's Disease of the Nipple

This is a superficial, sharply demarcated, oozing, erosive, sometimes crusted lesion. Some epidermal papulation may be present. Polycyclic borders and superficial or deep loss of nipple and areolar tissue may occur. The periphery may be scaly. The lesion is unilateral. A node of tumor deep in the underlying breast tissue may occasionally be felt. Another unilateral, oozing, often warty, nipple lesion is erosive adenomatosis.

Scabetic and postpartum eczema are bilateral, have a poorly demarcated border, and do not show any loss of nipple or areolar tissue.

For the differential diagnosis of all malignant erosive lesions see "Malignant Papular Tumors", in Chapter 11.

Mucosal Erosions and Ulcerations

The lips consist of a superior and inferior fleshy fold surrounding the mouth orifice that are covered by mucosa internally (the mucosal lip), by semimucosal on their appositional surfaces (the red or vermilion lip), and by cutaneous integument externally (the white lip). When the jaws are in physiologic rest position, the lips are in natural apposition, and the area exposed externally is referred to as the prolabium or vermilion area. Occasionally, the terms such as the red zone, transitional zone, semimucosa, or dry region of the lips are used to define this area. The frequently used term vermilion border, usually refers to the junction of the outer border of vermilion area (red lip) and the skin surface (white lip). This is of some importance surgically. It should be remembered that there is also an inner border of the vermilion area which is at the junction of the red and mucosal lip surfaces. In black patients, the preferred terms are the skin surface of the lip, the semimucosa of the lip and the mucosal surface.

Not all of the mucosae are covered in this text. Specifically, the conjunctivae, nasal mucosae, and the pharynx are not discussed separately. In general, I stress the mucosae that are easily visible without mechanical aids.

For convenience, other nonulcerative lesions reasonably specifically localized to the oral[*][8] and genital mucosa are discussed in this chapter under the heading "Miscellaneous Nonulcerative Mucosal Lesions".

In making a diagnosis of mucosal erosions and ulcerations, a complete examination of the patient including all of the skin and all of the mucosae should be undertaken, especially in bizarre presenting conditions.

All vesicles and bullae of the mucous membranes are rapidly transformed through maceration and trauma to erosions by a loss of the detached epidermal layer. They may have a pseudomembrane. Crusts and scales do not appear in the mouth.

Portions of this section have been taken and modified from Darier[1] (pp. 614–616).

*Readers interested in studying the oral living gross pathology in more detail should consult Reference 8. In Eversole's text the diseases discussed are cataloged according to their most common presenting features in a manner similar to that used in this text.

In general, the mucosae do not show as specific diagnostic morphological patterns as does the skin. Factors responsible for this probably are the continuous moist environment, the continuous trauma, and the generally unspecialized nature of the covering epithelium.

The areas in the mouth to be examined by sight and feel are the buccal mucosae, the alveolar ridges, the floor of the mouth, the hard palate, the soft palate, and the tongue.

Full descriptions of diseases are not given here except where the mucosal lesions are the only lesions and there is some specificity to the lesions. Full descriptions will be found under the appropriate basic cutaneous lesion.

Mucosal Erosions

A canker (aphthous erosion) is a 2 to 5 mm, round or oval discontinuity in the oral mucosa, which presents as an erosion. The base is yellowish, and the periphery, indurated with surrounding erythema. At times the erosions may be up to 2 cm in diameter.

Early, there is a small localized oval area of redness. Then a superficial yellow to grayish membrane surrounded by a 1 mm zone of erythema develops. A superficial slough occurs 2 to 3 days later, leaving an erosion, the base of which soon becomes covered with grayish granulation tissue. Peripheral induration is variable. After 1 to 6 weeks, the lesions heal without scarring. These can be classified as minor <1.0 cm, major >1.0 cm, or herpetiform. Major lesions may scar.

Aphthae are located on all parts of the oral mucosa and in the inner and red portion of the lip.

Other small erosive mucosal lesions are primary herpes simplex (which at times can form multiple red ∩-shaped erosions on the gum line—one above each tooth; occasionally with skin lesions), zoster (usually with skin lesions), varicella, hand-foot-and-mouth disease, herpangina, and other viral diseases. Rarely, recurrent herpes simplex occurs on the hard palate.

Various bullous diseases may produce large erosive areas, sometimes becoming confluent and forming extensive erosive areas. Pemphigus vulgaris commonly involves the oral mucosa and there may be no other skin lesion; more unusually, vesiculobullous lesions of dermatitis herpetiformis or linear IgA bullous dermatosis are present. Of patients with bullous pemphigoid, 30% may have oral lesions.

The bullae of erythema multiforme are commonly present in the mouth. They cover rather large round areas and are quite superficial. Drug reactions of the erythema multiforme type, of the fixed drug type, or just erosive areas (as with methotrexate) should be considered in the differential diagnosis. Some of these have been called Stevens-Johnson Syndrome or toxic epidermal necrolysis.

Both lichen planus and systemic lupus erythematosus may present with erosive lesions. Usually these are located on the buccal mucosae with other nonerosive lesions of lichen planus and lupus erythematosus. Other cutaneous or systemic findings may help make the diagnosis.

The scaly whitish fissured pattern of solar cheilitis may be seen on the adjacent exposed lower red lip. Many of these patients have a protuberant lower lip, allowing greater exposure to sunlight.

Behçet's disease, when fully developed, consists of recurrent, rather deep, large, painful, nonscarring erosions located anywhere on the conjunctiva, oral mucosa and lips, and vulvar or penile mucosae. The erosions have a small red inflammatory halo and are covered by a yellowish exudate. A considerable amount of edema may also be present. The erosions come in crops with periods of partial or complete remission. Other findings include erythema nodosum–like lesions on the shins, furunculoid lesions on the arms and upper torso, and a wide spectrum of neurological abnormalities. In minor cases where only one mucosal surface is involved, it may be difficult to distinguish from aphthae.

Infectious mononucleosis, cyclic neutropenia and leukemic states can produce erosive lesions on the mucosae. Reiter's disease can show mucosal erosions.

Rare now are syphilitic mucous patches and chancre, and diphtheritic angina and stomatitis.

Nonscarring oral erosions can also occur from bites, trauma from ragged or jagged teeth, and by direct irritation by contact with caustics, e.g. aspirin. Contact stomatitis may become erosive, although usually the reaction is more marked on the vermilion area of the lips and perioral tissues.

Patients who have some type of tardive dyskinesia also can produce and prolong ulcers and erosions on the side of the tongue. Some of these can look quite frightening.

DIFFERENTIAL DIAGNOSIS

In the differential diagnosis of oral mucosal erosions, thrush (oral candidiasis) should be mentioned. It presents as a white or creamy adherent layer on an erythematous base, which when detached results in bleeding of the underlying mucosa. It occurs on the tongue, cheeks and isthmus. Factitial cheilitis of varying degrees of severity must always be considered.

I have not included Vincent's stomatitis or angina because it is rare in dermatological practice.

Mucosal Ulcerations

The scarring true mucosal ulcers are not now common.

Syphilitic chancre of the mouth, in contradistinction to tonsillar chancre, is rarely ulcerative. Ulcerative secondary syphilis and malignant syphilis develop rapidly, are deep, and have a sharp circular outline. Ulcerative gumma and sclerogummatous ulcerations also occur.

Henri Vincent, 1862–1950, French Physician

Tuberculosis tongue ulcers, neurotrophic ulcers, and noma (buccal gangrene) may also cause ulceration. Noma in children begins with a red swelling of the cheeks, becomes blistery, and then develops a grayish slough. The loss of this slough leaves an ulceration which rapidly spreads and burrows. It has a ragged border and a bloody irregular floor, sometimes perforating the cheek. The teeth fall out and the bone becomes necrotic. Death was the usual outcome. This could be classified as a type of phagedenic ulcer.

The deep fungi, especially sporotrichosis and actinomycosis, may produce ulcerative mucosal lesions.

On very debilitated patients, dermal oral ulcerations may occur. This is particularly so in patients on potent anticancer chemotherapy. Radiotherapy may cause extensive localized erosions and ulceration, frequently with later dryness and telangiectasis and scarring. Cicatricial pemphigoid may cause scars in the conjunctiva and mouth. The same is true of dystrophic epidermolysis bullosa. Crohn's disease may show specific ulcerative, fissured, scarring, discharging sinuses and crevices in the genital and perianal area. Discoid lupus erythematosus scars the oral mucosa.

Ulcerative Tumors

Squamous cell carcinoma is by far the most common ulceration in the mouth. These nodular ulcers may occur on the tongue (especially laterally and inferiorly), soft palate (especially on the tonsillar pillars), floor of mouth, and occasionally elsewhere. The ulcers can measure up to 2 cm in diameter or larger. The base consists of friable red granulating tissue which bleeds easily. The border is hard and elevated. It is sharply demarcated. Loss of mucosal and bony tissue may be obvious. Adjacent areas may show a slightly infiltrated, speckled, white plaque (leukoplakia) sometimes with fissuring or erythroplakia. Caries, neglected, tobacco-stained teeth, and an alcoholic breath may also be present. The disease is more common in males. Early lesions may present as small sharply marginated velvety red plaques. Oral florid papillomatosis, verrucous carcinoma, and hyperplastic Bowen's disease of the oral mucosa are probably all variations of well-differentiated squamous cell carcinoma.

Basal cell carcinoma occurs as a firm, pearly, ulcerative papulonodule, occasionally occurring on the semimucosa of the perianal area, the semimucosa of the lips, and the nasal vestibule, probably also arising on the adjacent glabrous skin.

Miscellaneous Nonulcerative Mucosal Lesions

Author's Note: As explained on page 285, this portion, up to *Genital Erosions and Ulcerations* on page 291, is included here, not as an example of ulcers and erosions, but for convenience only.

Granular-cell myoblastoma is a single, small, slowly growing, clinically indistinctive nodule. About one-third of these lesions occur in the tongue. Mucosal polyps are pedunculated, fibrous, mucosa covered, rubbery soft tumors up to about 1 cm in diameter. They occur mostly in the buccal mucosa along the bite line and on the inner aspect of the lips. Perianally, mucosal tags and soft protuberant polyps may be seen.

Epulis is a hypertrophy of the gum tissue in the inner dental regions. Cheilitis glandularis is a disease of the lower lip, which becomes swollen, tumid and tense, and is studded with pinpoint to hemp seed-sized elevations representing mucin-secreting glands with dilated orifices. These orifices can be probed, causing a thin mucoid material to be exuded. Cheilitis exfoliativa is a scaly and crusting affliction on the semimucosa of the lips. Removal of crusts causes bleeding. Associated seborrhea is often present. Granulomatous cheilitis (Melkersson-Rosenthal syndrome) consists of gross lip edema, recurrent facial palsy, and scrotal tongue.

Granuloma fissuratum (irritation hyperplasia) occurs in a labioalveolar sulcus of the mouth as a solitary papulonodule and arises from the mucous membrane at the junction of the upper (or lower) lip and gum. The tumor is raised 2 to 3 mm and is conspicuously indented by a fissure in the coronal plane which divides the tumor in half and continues at either extremity into the normal mucosa. The fissure is usually eroded and sometimes the eroded area involves most or all of the inner aspect of the indentation. The lesions are smooth and paler pink than the surrounding mucosa, though the fissure is bright red. The lesions are firm, but not as firm as a squamous cell carcinoma, with no induration of the base, and can be freely moved over the underlying bone. The borders are sharply raised and smoothly rounded. Granuloma fissuratum arise from trauma from ill-fitting dentures. A similar lesion may be seen in the posterior aspect of the pinna just anterior to the retroauricular crease, presumably from rubbing by the frame of a spectacle. The name is, of course, incorrect: in no way is this a granuloma.

Black hairy tongue is produced by an overgrowth of the epidermis of the filiform papillae, which gives the clinical appearance of hairs. The epithelial filaments may measure from 0.5 to 1.5 cm in length. The color is black or dark brown. The black area occurs most frequently in the middle of the dorsum of the tongue in front of the circumvallate papillae. The lesion is darkest in the center and fades and becomes browner and less prominent at the periphery. The lesion may occur with or without prior administration of broad spectrum antibiotics.

Glossodynia (painful or burning tongue) is most commonly seen in the elderly female. The sensations are reported from the anterior portion of the tongue. No visible abnormality is seen apart from occasional traumatic erythema from rubbing of the painful tongue on the teeth. Other orolingual paresthesias without visible organic disease are also occasionally seen in elderly patients. An analogous condition is present in the vulva (vulvodynia), on the scrotum (the red scrotum syndrome)[9] and on the lips.

Scrotal tongue is a congenital, usually familial, condition in which the tongue is lobulated and furrowed almost like giant lichenification on the skin. The villous surface is studded with prominent fungiform papillae. There is a soft consistency. Rarely, the folds and crypts may become inflamed. Geographic tongue may occur on scrotal tongue.

Median rhomboid glossitis is a benign permanent abnormality occurring only in adults. The lesion is located on the dorsal aspect of the tongue in front of the circumvallate papillae. It is sharply defined, pointed anteriorly and broadened into a wedge shape posteriorly where it fuses with the papillae. From front to back it might

Ernst Gustaf Melkersson, 1898–1932, Swedish Physician
Curt Rosenthal, 20th Cent, German Psychiatrist

be 3 cm in length. The lesion itself is reddish and mammillated, being composed of papular lobes separated by folds. The lesion has the firm sclerotic consistency of rubber, but is freely moveable over the underlying tongue.

Oral submucous fibrosis shows sclerotic fibrous bands especially in buccal, labial, and palatal mucosa. Atrophy of the overlying epithelium as well as hypopigmentation or irregularly mottled pigmentation are also present. Supposedly from highly spiced foods and betel nut sucking, it is common in South-east Asia. Eventually the mouth becomes smaller.

Torus palatinus is a 2 by 1 cm or larger regular hard bony excrescence on the midline posterior portion of the hard palate. The mucosal tissues over this knot are normal. The lesion is longer than it is wide. The central portion slopes down gradually like the keel on a rounded boat. The lesion is permanent. Torus mandibulae is the same type of bony excrescence on the lingual surfaces of the mandible in the biscuspid area.

Stomatitis nicotina consists of numerous, 1 to 2 mm or larger, dome-shaped papules of normal mucosal color with a small central depression. The lesions are confluent in the central portion of the posterior hard palate and become more scattered laterally and anteriorly. The lesions are firm to the touch. Evidence of tobacco staining on the teeth, particularly on the inner aspect of the lower incisors, is always present.

Denture sore mouth is the accumulation of numerous small polypoid hyperplasias on the part of the oral mucosa covered by the denture. At times it can be finely verrucous.

Other tumors may be found in the oral cavity. These include mucocele (see Chapter 24), hemangioma, pyogenic granuloma, neurofibroma, pigmented and blue nevi, mixed tumors, and verrucae, which are described elsewhere. Multiple mucosal neurofibromas located mainly on the tongue, but also on the lips, conjunctiva, and larynx are seen in multiple endocrine adenomatosis in association with thyroid carcinoma, pheochromocytoma, and hyperparathyroidism.

Other surgical dental conditions in the mouth may be seen. Ranula is a cyst of the sublingual or submaxillary salivary glands. Abscesses, Dilantin hyperplasia, and reactions to topical medicaments, dentures, and periodontal disease (gingivitis, pyorrhea, periodontal abscess) occur.

Scarlet fever and measles also have mucosal lesions. Severe nutritional deficiencies can cause a red smooth tongue and perlèche. These are now rare.

The pigmentary changes are described under dyschromias. Fordyce's disease are misplaced sebaceous glands on the vermilion area of the lips and anterior portions of buccal mucosae.

Hemorrhoids are thickened varicosities occurring about the anus. They present as dilated, compressible, reddish purple, cystic structures up to about 1.5 cm in diameter. They may be multiple and contiguous, forming a circle or parts of a circle about the anus. Divisions between the various enlarged venous sacs form a ridged pattern. Occasionally, thrombosis occurs in the hemorrhoid producing a tender, purplish red, firm, polypoidal structure. They are to be distinguished from mucosal tags and verrucae.

Other conditions to be considered are prolapse of the rectum. This presents as a red ring of mucosal tissue about the anus with the orifice in the center. Fissure in ano is a superficial tender break in the semimucosa and mucosa about the anus. The lesions run radially. Fistula in ano shows an external opening sometimes with the appearance of a pyogenic granuloma, which on examination may have connection with the rectum.

Ischiorectal abscess presents as a redness and swelling between the anal verge and the tuber ischiale. All of these conditions must be distinguished from perianal intertrigo and its superadded variants.

Genital Erosions and Ulcerations

Most of the erosive or ulcerative affections occurring in the mouth may also be encountered on the genital mucosae or semimucosae of both sexes. Herples simplex is common; syphilis, aphthae, and diphtheria are rare. Eczema, psoriasis, and scabies occur on the genital semimucosae, but not in the mouth.

Traumatic erosions due to coitus, scratching, and rape may be seen. Chancroid also is present. Gonorrhea may cause a diffuse inflammation or a few punched out erosions.

Bruises, burns, bites, and traumatic hair loss are seen in some cases of child abuse.

Candidal balanitis is not uncommon, especially in those with a long redundant foreskin. Granuloma inguinale also occurs on the genital mucosae. It is manifested by ulcero-verrucous nodules with granulation tissue, scarring, and eventually elephantiasis. It is basically a tropical disease.

Fissures

Fissures or rhagades (plural; Greek, meaning chink or rent), caused by excessive tension or diminished elasticity in the skin are classified with the erosions and excoriations. These linear cracks are found mostly where the elasticity of the skin suffers the greatest strain, i.e. in the natural folds of movement over the joints, and on the transitional areas between skin and mucous membranes, i.e. the semimucosae of the angle of the mouth and anus. The fissures always run crosswise to the direction in which the skin is stretched and are very superficial.

Fissures represent only a loss of continuity, a crack of the skin, as a rule, without any loss of substances. Often they are located on an infiltrated plaque (psoriasis, eczema, or syphilitic papules in the angles of the mouth). An inflammatory infiltrate is the most frequent cause of the loss of elasticity that favors the tearing of the skin. In other cases, the cause may be found in excessive tension in the less elastic horny layer, e.g. over acutely inflamed red and swollen skin or on shrunken scars. The stratum corneum is the least extensible layer of the skin and is able to extend its surface only by straightening the skin relief furrows. If these furrows are absent, as is often the case on scars, the horny layer is bound to tear if it is stretched to any extent. In the depths of fissures, the malpighian rete or the uppermost part of the cutis lies

Portions of this section have been taken and modified from Siemens[1] (pp. 81, 83).

bare, with oozing or bleeding. Rarely, the cracks become deep enough to leave thin linear and furrowed scars. This type of scarring around the mouth is often sufficiently characteristic to make a diagnosis possible (congenital syphilis and late sequelae of excessive radiation therapy). Of course, fissures may become secondarily infected and ulcerated. Fissures can be the portals of entry for serious infections with, for example, recurring attacks of erysipelas and lymphangitis.

They occur on the extremities including the palms and soles as complications of hyperkeratosis, or at the circumference of the natural orifices, at the lips, the nipples, very frequently the anus, and the prepuce. Under the influence of movements of extension, the keratotic, macerated, or eczematized epidermis cracks and the lesion reaches down to the cutis. The borders of the crevices are perpendicular, the floor is bright red, sometimes bleeding; pain is often very severe; healing may take place without scars.

A common condition of this type is angular cheilitis. It should be again stressed that in affluent countries angular cheilitis is almost always from ill-fitting dentures and not from a vitamin deficiency.

Around the anus, persistent fissuring should make the clinician suspicious of an underlying regional ileitis. Fissuring is very common on eczemas of the palmar or plantar skin.

Cutaneous Gangrene

Full thickness death of a large portion of the integument means cutaneous gangrene. It may be accompanied by death in the underlying tissue. When it is abrupt, complete, and localized it is called necrosis; when slow and incomplete it is called necrobiosis. The dead portion is called a slough.

Gangrene manifests itself first as a change in the color of the skin, which at the same time becomes cold and anesthetic to touch or pricking, and becomes tender. With dry gangrene, the skin becomes yellow, then brownish, and promptly hardens through desiccation, becoming depressed below the normal level. Moist gangrene begins with bloody purulent bullae, the floor of which become necrotic. In a few days, the slough in both types becomes surrounded by a congestive halo, sometimes bullous at its periphery.

On the line of demarcation between the dead and living tissue, a deep groove is formed. Suppuration at this area may occur. The slough becomes dark brown or black, retracts, and finally falls off, leaving an ulcer covered with debris, or sometimes pink and verrucous tissue.

The distinction between gangrene and gangrenous ulcerations is discussed later.

Direct Local Gangrene

This results from an external injury directly affecting the skin and the subcutaneous and deeper tissues.

Traumatic gangrene may occur from severe crushing, contusions, and war wounds. Prolonged compression as from a plaster cast may cause a slough. Decubitus ulcers are a form of local gangrene due to pressure over bony prominences (sacral, trochanteric, scapular, and heel regions). The decubitus ulcers occur in immobilized patients, often where the general nutrition is low and the vascular tone and sensation is poor. Physical causes such as trauma, frostbite, cutaneous flow diathermy, spark gap apparatus, or excessive x-ray exposure may cause gangrenous patches. Chemical agents, such as strong acids or alkalis, or zinc chloride, may also cause gangrene.

Most direct local gangrene is caused by stasis or thrombosis or destruction of the cutaneous blood supply.

Vascular Gangrene

Ergot of rye used to cause ergotism, a painful mutilating gangrene of the extremities.

Diabetic gangrene, usually of the lower extremities, is mainly due to an increased and more severe atherosclerosis of the muscular arteries of the lower extremities. In this type, an initial bulla with subsequent necrosis is often present, and if the lesion progresses, there may be a peripheral bulla. Diabetics are more prone to gangrenous infections. This lack of resistance may be due to either a reduced blood supply or a decreased resistance to infection.

The up to palm-sized smelly black thick-walled bullous gangrenous ulcers on and about the heels of severe diabetics are quite characteristic. Trauma is presumably an irritating factor. They are to be distinguished from the mummifying ischemic gangrene involving the acral portions of the toes.

Blood vessel rupture, ligation, compression, embolism, or thrombosis produce a dry gangrene especially on the feet. It begins with one or several toes, attacking the skin and deep tissues including the bone. Arteriosclerosis and thromboangiitis obliterans are examples of causes of dry gangrene.

Rarely, gangrene is seen with systemic scleroderma and more rarely Raynaud's disease.

Gangrenous Infections

Gangrenous infections can be classified into two groups. The first group is directly infected gangrene, such as gangrenous zoster, gangrenous varicella, syphilitic chancre, and so on. These are due to excessive virulence of the causative agent, diminished resistance of the host, or the secondary introduction of necrotizing agents.

Another example of this type is necrotizing streptococcal gangrene (streptococcal fasciitis). This is basically a very virulent erysipelas often associated with a debilitating disease or immunosuppressive therapy. Commonly located on the legs, ankle, and foot is a pustular bullous hemorrhage with large (up to 10 cm) areas of tissue necrosis or gangrene. The underlying tendons may be exposed. The whole area is grossly edematous and shows a bright red, inflammatory erythema.

Another example of the first type is Fournier's scrotal gangrene. Scrotal gangrenous ulceration presents as a foul-smelling, palm-sized or larger area of ulceration on top of which there is a black eschar-crust consisting of dead necrotic tissue, blood, serum, and dried pus. When this crust is removed, there is a raw denuded area extending deeply into the tissues. Laudable pus and a bloody exudate are seen. The ulcer is relatively anemic. The border is sharply marginated with, at most, 1 cm of inflammation. There is no heaping up the border and no undermining. There is at the onset no fever, no lymphadenitis, and surprisingly little systemic reaction. It can follow operations on the bowel or inguinal areas.

The second type of gangrenous infections develop from bacterial emboli to the skin. There is first an extensive eruption of erythematous, urticarial, or purpuric spots, then bullae or pustules may appear and multiply. The center turns black, the slough spreads, then becomes surrounded by a suppurative groove and loosens, leaving a perpendicular or dome- shaped ulcer with a bloody floor. Several lesions may coalesce. Sloughing may destroy a portion of the nose, lips, ear lobe, external genitalia, or fingers and toes. Nodose lesions and abscesses may also be present. The eruptions may occur anywhere. Sometimes the purpuric element may be marked, and initially, before the necrosis develops, one may justifiably classify these as basically a severe purpuric eruption. These embolic gangrenes were once more common in children than in adults.

Most of the gangrenous infections are now seen in patients who have had their immune systems depressed by long term, high dose adrenal corticosteroid therapy, by high dose anticancer chemotherapy, or in patients with AIDS. The derelict alcoholic of large cities, or the malnourished country recluse or hermit may also be prone to these infections. Occasionally, an abdominal operation may be the initiating factor.

Briefly, the characteristics of a phagedenic ulcer are repeated here in order to distinguish them as much as possible from the infectious causes of gangrene. Phagadenic ulcers usually show death of tissue, a burrowing eating away of tissue with an undermined and sometimes verrucous border, a border that is arcuate or serpiginous, palm-sized or larger in size, chronicity with periods of rapid growth, and association with some underlying weakened systemic state.

References

1. Darier, J. Textbook of dermatology. Pollitzer S, trans. Philadelphia:Lea & Febiger, 1920.
2. Siemens HW. General diagnosis and therapy of skin diseases. Weiner K, trans. Chicago:University of Chicago Press, 1958.
3. Jackson R, Bell M. Phagendena: gangrenous and necrotic ulcerations of skin and subcutaneous tissue. Can Med Assoc J 1982; 126:363–368.
4. Lyell A. Cutaneous artefactual disease. J Am Acad Dermatol 1979; 1:391–407.
5. Butterworth T, Strean LP. Behavioural disorders of interest to dermatologists. Arch Dermatol 1963; 88:859–867.
6. Stokes JH, Garner VC. The diagnosis of self-inflected lesions of the skin. JAMA 1929; 93:438–443.
7. Ronchese F. Occupational marks. New York:Grune & Stratton, 1948.
8. Eversole LR. Clinical outline of oral pathology. Philadelphia:Lea & Febiger, 1978.
9. Fisher BK. The red scrotum syndrome. Cutis 1977; 60:139–141.

CHAPTER 15

Keratoses

A localized moderate thickening of the horny layer.

Overview

The name keratosis is applied to a localized dermatological lesion that consists of a moderate thickening of the horny layer.[1,2] Under normal conditions, the horny layer is formed by layers of lamellar cells, which are composed of keratin and some fat, but have neither cytoplasm nor nuclei. These corneal cells represent the last stage in the process of epidermal development. Beginning with multiplication of the cells of the basal cell layer, the malpighian cells are gradually pushed up by the newly generated cells and reach the granular layer. There, they show keratohyalin granules. Then they become keratinized. The corneal cells adhere to each other and persist for a certain time on the epidermal surface, where they make a resistant, supple, and selectively permeable protective covering. Being no longer alive, the stratum corneum cannot react biologically to irritants of any kind. The corneal cells are finally shed. The stratum corneum is thicker in the black race. Thickness of the stratum corneum varies greatly in different areas of the body.

In the skin diseases with a thickening of the horny layer, the degree of hyperplasia is variable. In some, there is slight thickening accompanied by a powdery scurfy desquamation; in others, it is considerable, and produces a carapace that is hard and liable to crack. In ichthyosis, all degrees are met with, from a simple dry skin to the most pronounced sauriasis (lizard skin). In general, keratoses are scaly.

When the horny layer is very hyperplastic, the granular and malpighian layers are often also abnormally thick. The dermis is usually congested and there is a tendency to produce papillary elevations or verrucosities. Circumscribed hypertrophy of the horny layer, forming a tumor, can produce a cutaneous horn. With the callous scale formations and the cutaneous horns, may be grouped the keratotic verrucosities occurring either in circumscribed areas or spread widely over the body surface. If the individual protrusions tend to be round, one may speak of granular papular keratoses (Darier's disease). If these keratoses are larger, their sides become compressed and they present mosaic or cobblestone-like arrangements. If the prominences are long and pointed, one may call them porcupine scales. See also "Overview" in Chapter 16.

For keratoses that are clearly or mainly follicular, see Chapter 20.

The keratoses can be classified by their distribution into two groups: (1) diffuse or disseminated keratoses spreading over almost the entire body, or at least over large surfaces, although with evident predilections, and (2) circumscribed keratoses, composed of distinctly limited keratotic surfaces. Some are scattered without apparent order; others assume a regional or symmetrical arrangement. The distinction between disseminated and localized is, at times, not clear cut.

Many skin diseases can show keratotic lesions to a more or less extensive degree. Flat warts and common warts have been described elsewhere (see Chapters 11 and 16). Ostraceous psoriasis, hypertrophic lichen planus, hypertrophic lupus erythematosus, verrucous tuberculosis, angiokeratomas and lymphangiomas are some examples in which the thickening of the horny layer is secondary to a definite

Portions of the Overview have been taken and modified from Darier1 (pp. 194–196) and Siemens[2] (p. 110).

process of a different character. They are mentioned here to provide examples of secondary keratosis formation.

Palmar and plantar keratoses are called keratodermas. Although the epithelium of the mucous membranes, especially of the mouth, does not under normal conditions become keratinized like the epidermis, local pathological lesions are seen which I call keratoses of the mucosae.

Disseminated
Xerosis (Asteatosis)

In xerosis, the skin is abnormally dry to the touch and is prone to desquamation, fissuring, and chapping. The legs are a common location for xerosis; the flexural areas are usually spared.

Many diseases have a xerotic component, e.g. ichthyosis, nummular eczema, and atopic dermatitis.

In the elderly, dry skin is common on the back and legs. It is aggravated and becomes itchy and frankly eczematous in the winter when there is a marked lack of humidity in heated rooms. This results in "winter itch". This, of course, is worsened when excessive daily washing and bathing remove what little sebum there is in the elderly and by the wearing of woolen clothing.

Local xerosis is seen on the hands of people who repeatedly use strong soaps, detergent, and other cleaning agents.

Ichthyoses

Table 34 provides a comparison of the different ichthyoses.

Table 34: **Differential Diagnoses of Ichthyoses**				
	Age of Onset	Type of Scale	Localization	Associated Findings
Ichthyosis vulgaris	Childhood	Shield-shaped	Extensors	Keratosis pilaris Atopic dermatitis
Lamellar ichthyosis	Newborn	Collodion then large coarse shield-shaped	Worse in flexures, palms and soles	Ectropion
Bullous congenital ichthyosiform erythroderma (epidermolytichyperkeratosis)	Newborn	Brown verruciform scales	Flexures and intertriginous areas	Some normal skin
X-linked ichthyosis	First year of life	Shield-shaped	Extensors, trunk, and neck	Corneal deposits deposits

Ichthyosis Vulgaris

Ichthyotic skin is dry and scaly (Fig. 15.1).[3,4] In cases of moderate severity, the integument is roughened, parchment-like, and covered with dry scales, which have been compared with fish scales or the shingles on a roof (see "Overview" in Chapter 6). The scales are of variable size, being largest and most prominent on the legs. They are thin, white, brown, or gray, more or less detached, and constantly renewed. The scaliness is arranged in parallel rows or in diamond pattern, and consists of polygonal

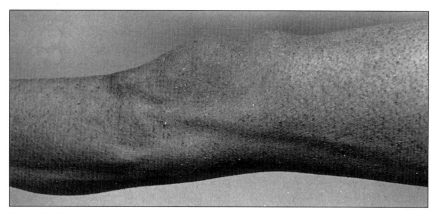

Figure 15.1 Ichthyosis vulgaris.

or shield-shaped areas of scaling intersected by white furrows. The peripheral portion of each scale is less well attached than the center. Some of the scales on the back have a pasted-on appearance. Varying degrees of a dirty gray-brown-black pigmentation may be present. The eruption is symmetrical and is most pronounced on the extensor surfaces of the limbs, especially on the elbows, knees, lower legs, and to a lesser degree on the trunk. The scalp has a diffuse dry scaliness. The palms and soles are very often dry and wrinkled with accentuation of the palmar and plantar markings. The articular folds and genital areas are almost always reasonably free, as is the face. Many degrees of ichthyosis can be seen. In xeroderma, the skin is merely dry, and the desquamation is powdery and almost imperceptible. Ichthyosis nitida (shiny) or nacreous (iridescent) ichthyosis, with thin and silvery lamellae, is the most common form. In black ichthyosis, the scales are black. In serpentine ichthyosis, the scales are long and polygonal. Large and thick scales occur in sauriasis (lizard's skin), whereas in ichthyosis hystrix, prominent warty or pointed hair excrescences are seen, suggestive of porcupine skin.

Ichthyosis vulgaris is not present at birth. It develops in the first years of life. Ichthyosis persists throughout life, although it may decrease in severity. It is worse in the winter, and occasionally in old age. The hair may be normal or less than normal; the downy hairs on the extensor surfaces are fine, resembling lanugo hair. Keratosis pilaris is invariably present. The nails are usually normal; rarely, dry and brittle. Sweat secretion is greatly reduced.

Although normally associated with dry skin, normally worse on the lower extremities, and normally present or noticeable at an early age, occasionally rather marked ichthyosis on the torso (sparing the creases and extremities) may develop in young adulthood.

Atopic dermatitis may be present and when it is, lichenification and excoriations are seen.

Ichthyosis hystrix is really not an ichthyosis. It is a disseminated epidermal nevus following the lines of Blaschko (see later). Associated ichthyosis may be present. Several drugs (triparanol, butyrophenones, nicotinic acid) may cause diffuse scaling of the skin. Essential fatty acid deficiency may also cause scaling. Acquired ichthyosis may develop in middle or late life as a result of some underlying disseminated cancer or lymphoma or in hyperthyroidism.

Ichthyosiform sarcoidosis has been reported in blacks; biopsy of an acquired ichthyosis revealed a sarcoidal reaction in the dermis.

Lamellar Ichthyosis

A very rare form of ichthyosis, lamellar ichthyosis (nonbullous congenital ichthyosiform erythroderma) starts with the newborn infant being encased in a tight, shiny envelope, which cracks in some areas. Eversion of the eyelids and lips may occur. After the first few days of life, the collodion-like membrane is replaced by a coat of coarse scales, which persists through life. The scales are large (0.5 to 1.5 cm in diameter), gray-brown in color, and frequently adherent at the centers with detached, slightly raised edges. These scales follow the wrinkle lines of the skin, but do not overlap. Follicular orifices may have a crateriform appearance. Ectropion can persist and sometimes causes corneal damage. The skin on the palms and soles shows moderate hyperkeratosis. The eruption is generalized, worse in the flexures.

Epidermolytic Hyperkeratosis

In epidermolytic hyperkeratosis (bullous congenital ichthyosiform erythroderma), at birth the skin is red, moist, and tender, with some remains of the thick scaly mantle being present. Then the skin becomes dry and scaly. The condition is lifelong. Thick gray brown, often verruciform, scales are noted over most of the body, but are most prominent in the flexural areas and other intertriginous areas. These verruciform lesions occur in the wrinkle lines of the skin. Small or large bullae appear during childhood and persist until adulthood. These bullae occur year round and develop in smooth and ichthyotic areas. No scarring occurs from these bullae. There is often an overall patchiness to the eruption, caused by the intermingling of areas of normal-colored smooth skin and brown, more or less verrucous areas. Rarely, the disease is unilateral, associated with other congenital defects.

X-linked Ichthyosis

This rare condition is not present at birth, but develops during the first year of life. The mild scaling in males increases during childhood and is most prominent on the trunk, extremities, and neck. The flexural creases tend to be less involved. The palms and soles are supple. In adult females, scaling of the legs may be present. Corneal deposits are often present.

Miscellaneous Ichthyotic States

There are other very rare, congenitally determined scaling disorders associated with abnormalities of the nervous system and other organs. The harlequin fetus is very rare. Death usually occurs shortly after birth. They have generalized plaque-like scales.

Ichthyosis linearis circumflexa is a rare, generalized, erythematous, scaly eruption present at birth. The lesions are annular and serpiginous, with areas of diffuse erythema and scaling. The serpiginous lesions show a band 4 to 6 mm wide with a "double edge" scale. Diffuse scaling is present on the scalp. Mental retardation and trichorrhexis invaginata are often present as is atopic dermatitis and the atopic state. This is probably the same disease as Netherton's syndrome. These children are usually blond and of the female sex.

Collodion baby is not a disease entity but may represent a stage of ichthyosiform erythroderma, X-linked ichthyosis, or Sjögren-Larsson syndrome. One must be careful in assigning the term collodion baby to one pigeonhole or another until some time has passed and other ancillary investigations are performed. Harlequin fetus is, of course, a different matter and should not be confused with collodion baby.

Erythrokeratodermia

Erythrokeratodermia denotes the association of hyperkeratosis and erythema in persistent circumscribed areas.

Erythrokeratodermia variabilis has two types of lesions: (1) symmetrical, thick, comma-shaped, polycyclic, persistent, circinate, sharply marginated, scaly plaques; and (2) patches of transient erythema. The sites of predilection are on the trunk, buttocks, thighs, face (mouth and eyes), and genitalia. The condition occurs mainly in females. It is considered to be a variant of congenital ichthyosiform erythroderma.

Erythrokeratodermia symmetrical progressive shows sharply marginated plaques of erythema with hyperkeratosis, scaling, and hyperpigmented border on the feet, front of shins, knees, and the backs of hands and fingers. The palms and soles are not involved.

Pachyonychia Congenita

This is a rare congenital anomaly characterized by dystrophic changes in the nails, palmar and plantar hyperkeratosis, anomalies of the hair, leukoplakia, follicular keratoses of the acneform type particularly about the knees and elbows, and dyskeratoses of the cornea. Verrucous lesions are described as occurring on the knees, elbows, popliteal regions, buttocks, legs, and ankles. Bullae are common and occur chiefly on the plantar surfaces of the feet. All, or only a few of the above, may be found in each case.

The keratotic stage of incontinentia pigmenti shows linear keratotic lesions, mainly on the areas exposed to trauma on the extremities. The linear streaks and whorls of gray pigmentation usually make the diagnosis obvious.

Dyskeratosis congenita is a very rare disease characterized by bluish gray pigmentation and hypopigmented atrophic areas on the trunk, neck, and face. Leukoplakia is present on the tongue and mucous membrane. The skin of the hands and feet is atrophic, and the nails are dystrophic or absent. It is not easy to know

Larsson
Henrik Samuel Conrad Sjögren, 1899–   Swedish Ophthalmologist

where to put this disease. It could be classed with the dyschromias, under the poikilodermas, or with the keratoses of the mucosae.

Hyperkeratosis Lenticularis Perstans

In hyperkeratosis lenticularis perstans, which is also called Flegel's disease, (dyskeratotic psoriasiform dermatosis) we find keratotic papules and small psoriasiform plaques varying in color from light brown to pink to red and in sizes from 2 to 5 mm. On light scratching of the keratotic surface of the larger lesions, a silvery white color results. Force is necessary to remove the keratotic covering, and it comes away in one block. The underlying surface is often elevated over the surrounding skin, and it is uneven with some deep pits showing some capillary bleeding points.

The lesions are most profuse on the distal portions of the limbs, but may occur anywhere. They are increased in number over the knees, elbows, buttocks, and dorsa hands and feet. On the palms and soles there are numerous punctate keratoses.

DIFFERENTIAL DIAGNOSIS

The differential diagnosis includes Darier's disease (including the lesions of acrokeratosis verruciformis on the dorsa of the hands), tar keratosis, early seborrheic keratosis, stucco keratosis and Kyrle's disease, which is follicular (see Chapter 20 - Tables 45,46).

Darier's Disease

Darier's disease (follicular dyskeratosis, keratosis follicularis) is a papulocrusted eruption, often but not always follicular. The scale-crust is grayish-brown or black, and moderately adherent. On removal, there is a funnel-shaped depression with raised margins. The small base may have a glistening or moist appearance. In severe cases, vegetations may occur in the moist areas, the crusted areas become confluent and verrucous, and the patient's skin assumes a dirty appearance.

Sites of predilection in Darier's disease are temples, nasolabial folds, scalp, presternal and interscapular grooves, the belt line, the perigenital region, and the large articular folds.

On the backs of the hands, elevations identical with flat warts are often seen; the palms and soles may show a punctate keratosis composed of yellowish translucent points; the nails are striated and brittle, wedge shaped at the distal end of the nail plate with subungual keratoses; and the tongue may have villous white plaques.

Occasionally Darier's disease may disappear entirely and recur at intervals.

Acrokeratosis verruciformis is probably Darier's disease of the dorsa of the hands and feet.

For a fuller description of Darier's disease, see Chapter 20.

Acanthomata Following Eczema

In acanthomata following eczema, a large number of small, slightly raised, verrucous, epidermal, gently sloping, white or faint yellow keratoses, measuring a few millimeters to 1 cm in diameter, are diffusely scattered over the back and front of the chest or arms.[5,6] More often, the acanthomata are located among the already existing seborrheic keratoses. These appear after the generalized or widespread eczema starts to subside. As the eczema disappears, the acanthomata fall off without leaving sequelae.

Disseminated Superficial Actinic Porokeratosis

This porokeratosis has, as its early or primary lesion, a tiny conically shaped papule, 1 to 2 mm in diameter, usually follicular in its location, and topped with a small keratotic plug. It usually is brown or brownish-red. The plug sometimes falls out, leaving a minute central depression. The papule then enlarges centrifugally, usually leaving a somewhat depressed or atrophic area surrounded by a fine slightly raised, hyperkeratotic, sharply defined ridge. Sometimes the central area remains pigmented, erythematous, or both, and it often is separated from the border by a hypopigmented zone; some show keratotic papules with delling. The center is usually devoid of hairs. The lesion gradually enlarges, making a round or oval shape with a peripheral ridging of brownish-gray. Disseminated superficial actinic porokeratosis occurs only on sun-exposed areas, especially on the anterior portion of the legs in women.

Disseminated Porokeratosis with Palmar and Plantar Lesions

This porokeratotic condition is nonactinic and has the following characteristics. The initial lesion is a red or brown, tiny (1 to 3 mm), keratotic papule. These papules enlarge, leaving a depressed, sometimes atrophic central area which is skin colored or slightly red-brown. The lesions are annular or gyrate and vary from 5 to 15 mm in diameter; they are superficial, with a slightly elevated, nonfurrowed, hyperkeratotic margin, which is less than 1 mm in height. The eruption is symmetrical, with most of the lesions being on the extremities. The lesions occur everywhere, even on non-sun-exposed areas such as the breast and intergluteal fold. The face and mucosae are spared, although the palms and soles may have as many as fifty keratoses, which tend to be more numerous on the pressure areas of the heel and metatarsal regions. These lesions are round or oval, 3 to 5 mm in diameter, and most of them have a fine elevated border.

Disseminated Spiked Hyperkeratosis

Non-follicular thin (0.5 mm) whitish gray, hard, spiked keratoses, 2 to 4 mm in length, are present over the upper extremities and torso, particularly the flanks.[7,8]

Localized

Epidermal Nevi

One of the most distinguishing features about epidermal or epithelial nevi is the linear arrangement along the lines of Blaschko[9] (Fig. 15.2). The features of these lines are the v-shape over the vertebral column, the open s-shape on the sides of the torso and lower abdomen, the inverted U-shape on the anterior arm and adjacent chest wall, and the linear (nondermatome) pattern on the extremities. Another feature of epidermal nevi is that almost any single or combination of skin structures may be included in these congenitally determined abnormalities. Some examples are linear epidermal nevus, linear sebaceous nevus, comedo nevus, pigmented hairy epidermal nevus (Becker's nevus), unilateral nevoid telangiectasia, systematized achromic nevus, and "zosteriform" lentiginous nevus. It is also interesting, that many inflammatory skin diseases, e.g. linear scleroderma, lichen planus, and lichen striatus, may also occur along these lines.

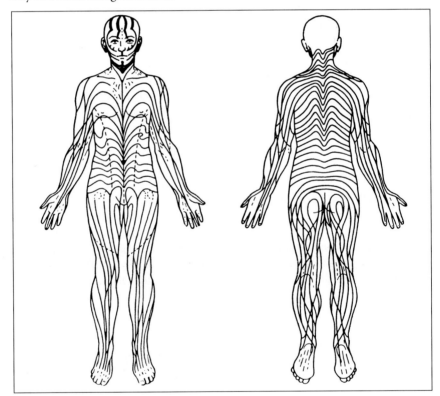

Figure 15.2 The lines of Blaschko.

Samuel William Becker, 1894–1964, U.S. Dermatologist

If epidermal nevi are regarded in this manner, many of the long descriptive names appear inane and lack a unifying concept, which is obviously intrinsic. The morphological approach to a linear lesion following Blaschko's lines (as distinct from other linear lesions related to nerves, e.g. zoster, or to lymphatics, like sporotrichosis) is to decide which normal skin structure is involved. This usually is not difficult to do.

As previously indicated, not all epidermal nevi will be strictly epidermal and keratotic, so in this book they are found in several chapters, depending on the most prominent basic lesion. Remember, though, that their arrangement must be determined by the same factors.

The keratotic epidermal nevi (including ichthyosis hystrix) show warty keratoses, vary in size from that of a millet seed to that of a pea or larger, and are brownish, yellow-brown, or black in color. The lesions are hard, and when confluent they are frequently furrowed. Streaks and curves of black-brown pigmentation are often present. In some cases, most of the lesion may consist of this type of pigmentation. On the buccal mucosa, a linear whitish plaque may be seen in cases in which linear epidermal nevi are present on the cheeks. Although a few may be present at birth, most become apparent in early childhood, slowly increase in size and extent, deepen in color until young adulthood, and then remain constant. A few show no change with time.

Very extensive lesions are rare. Most occur in limited areas, e.g. one arm, upper torso, and most are unilateral. In some cases, the lesion may be so limited that it is not possible to see immediately the linear pattern of Blaschko's lines.

Epidermal nevi may be histologically indistinguishable from seborrheic keratosis. Occasionally, a brisk inflammatory response may be seen throughout the linear lesion with scaling, lichenification, and excoriations present. This is inflammatory linear epidermal nevus (ILEN). It can be very psoriasiform.

A very rare form is the bilateral brown warty keratosis on the areola and adjacent skin of each breast. This has only been reported in women.

The epidermal nevus syndrome shows, in addition to the already described cutaneous changes, involvement of other body systems, e.g. skeletal, neurological, and ophthalmological.

Rarely, basal cell carcinoma, and more rarely, squamous cell carcinoma may develop on epidermal nevi.

Cutaneous Horn

A cutaneous horn is just that—a horn growing out of the skin (Fig. 15.3). The horn is composed of hard, yellowish-brown keratin of varying length and thickness, which tends to taper to a point. There is usually some curving and twisting of the horn, like a ram's horn. They may be 2 cm wide at the base and up to 5 cm in length, although they are usually about 2 cm long. Some horns appear to arise on normal skin, and some arise like a neck from a circular shoulder of epidermis at the base. Most arise

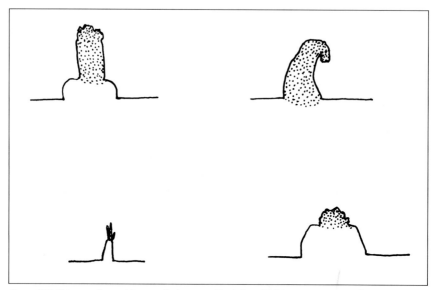

Figure 15.3 Cutaneous horn arising on solar keratoses *(Top, Left and Right)*; a verruca *(Lower Left)*; and a keratoacanthoma *(Lower Right)*.

on solar keratoses, and so occur on sun-damaged skin. Many other conditions can give rise to cutaneous horns, e.g. seborrheic keratoses, squamous cell carcinoma, and keratoacanthoma. In a way, a filiform verruca is a thin tapered horn; where about half of the total length is the underlying verruca. The central keratin core of a keratoacanthoma may extend above the large shoulders. It, however, is not tapered, and the protruding core obviously forms only a minor portion of the total lesion. Sometimes cutaneous horns may develop on amputation stumps.

Solar (Actinic) Keratosis

These lesions are sharply demarcated localized thickenings of the horny layer occurring on the sun-exposed skin (Fig. 15.4). The mustache area is a frequent location particularly in women and particularly at the junction of the red and white lip. Also the temples, forehead, nose, upper cheeks, and bald pates are favorite sites. They are more common and extensive in fair-skinned, blue-eyed, light-haired individuals, especially those with outdoor occupations and/or the findings of dermatoheliosis. They are a dirty grayish, yellowish, or whitish color. The keratotic layer is more elevated in the center and is extremely adherent. Removal of the keratosis gives rise to small hemorrhages. The amount of thickening may vary from a thick scale to a horn; sometimes the scale or horn falls off by itself and a new one regrows. Occasionally, these lesions have an irregular, atrophic, red, telangiectatic, rough surface with a sharply marginated, irregular, map-like border (Fig. 15.5). In all cases, the lesions are much more easily felt than seen; they are hard and spiky in

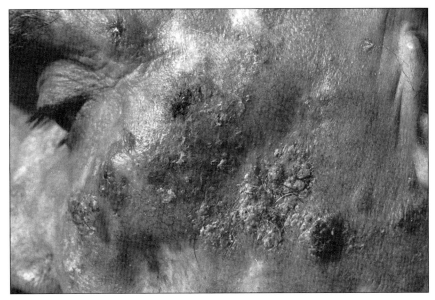

Figure 15.4 Solar keratoses.

texture, and often, quite tender. Some-times large areas of sun-exposed skin may be involved in this process. In some, there may be dotted black and/or brown pigment quite clearly evident below and in the scaly keratosis. These dots are often clustered and are more common at the periphery, or they may be asymmetrically clustered at one side or another.[10]

On the dorsa and sides of the hands and fingers, the keratotic

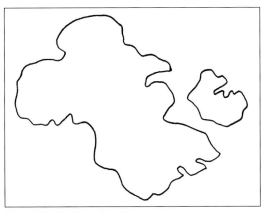

Figure 15.5 Map-like outline of solar keratoses.

element may not be striking, and the lesion may be basically an erythematosquame. The border is sharply demarcated. There are varying amounts of white scale, which in places is firmly adherent. With trauma, some areas may become eroded. The lesions are often multiple and may be up to several centimeters in diameter. The usual changes of skin damage from habitual exposure to sun are present (epidermal atrophy, telangiectasia, and leather-like yellowing and browning) on and about the affected parts and also on other sun-exposed areas.

DIFFERENTIAL DIAGNOSIS

On the face, discoid lupus erythematosus and multiple superficial basal cell carcinoma should be considered. In xeroderma pigmentosum, chronic sequelae of excessive radiotherapy (radiation keratosis) and arsenical keratosis, the individual isolated lesion may be indistinguishable from solar keratosis. Keratoses from tar are also very similar to solar keratosis, except they occur almost entirely on the dorsa of the fingers, hands, and forearms in individuals who have for years been exposed to crude coal tar products. There are frequently also hypo- and hypermelanotic spots. Small solar keratosis lesions may be difficult to distinguish from small seborrheic keratosis. Lichen planus-like keratoses are lichenoid, scaly, sometimes brown, papules on the upper torso or forearm. They are rarely diagnosed before biopsy.[11] Actinic granuloma has a scaly border with a central, slightly atrophic area. Chrondo-dermatitis nodularis chronica helicis is a firm, 5 mm round, red papule with a flattish surface, often covered by an adherent tough scale, occasionally with a central crust. It is located on the areas of the helix and antehelix that are exposed to pressure. This lesion is very tender.

The other erythematosquamous disorders should be considered in the differential diagnosis of actinic or solar keratosis, especially discoid lupus erythematosus, psoriasis, and parapsoriasis en plaque, as well as Bowen's disease.

Seborrheic Keratosis

These are numerous circular or ovoid, elevated papulonodular lesions varying from 0.5 to 2 cm in diameter. These papulonodules are firm, raised, light tan to pitch black, and have a verrucous, greasy, and furrowed or pitted surface. The brown pigment often has an ill-defined muddy hue. On the surface, the 1 mm circular areas, representing the opening of horn cysts, are often more evenly blackly pigmented than the intervening network.[12] The border is well defined. The lesions have a "stuck-on" appearance, i.e. they are mostly above the level of the epidermis. Large lesions may be polypoidal in shape. The face and back are common locations and the temple is a favorite site. On the back, the long axis of the ovoid lesions appears to follow lines of cleavage of the skin (Christmas-tree effect). In the intramammary crease and on the adjacent underside of the breasts and upper abdominal skin, there may be clusters of seborrheic keratoses. These may be arranged in lines running horizontally. In patients with widespread eczema or psoriasis, perilesional eczema or psoriasis may be present. Dermatosis papulosa nigra has the same histological picture as seborrheic keratosis. It has been proposed that eruptive seborrheic keratosis can come from an underlying malignancy — the sign of Leser-Trélat. This myth has finally been exposed.[13]

Edmund Leser, 1852–1916, German Surgeon
Ulysse Trélat Jr., 1828–1890, French Surgeon, Bordeaux

Variations

Two-toned lesions are not unusual. The central portion is usually a darker brown and the periphery a lighter brown. In these lesions, the muddy opaque brown color is often quite apparent in the periphery. This is in marked contrast to the Hutchinson freckle (which also commonly occurs on the face as does the two-toned seborrheic keratosis), which has sharply demarcated drops, nets, or networks of dark-brown pigment. Occasionally, seborrheic keratoses are whitish (keratosis alba) or dark red. Lesions on the pale skin of the torso may have an orange red color, especially those which present as slightly elevated plaques.

Some lesions are up to 10 cm in diameter. Some have a donut-shaped appearance with the keratosis forming the halo with normal skin in the center. Others are two levelled lesions with the central portion thicker and surrounded by an almost flat large periphery and are common on the face.

Most of the liver spots or solar lentigos on the backs of the hands of the elderly are just palpable seborrheic keratoses. The scalp frequently has many seborrheic keratoses, at times they may be as diffuse on the scalp as on the back. Seborrheic keratoses can occur in the external auditory canals.

Small 2 to 3 mm skin-colored papules sometimes covering large areas such as the forearms are an unusual pattern of seborrheic keratosis. A herpetic arrangement is sometimes seen with a cluster of small islands of keratoses with normal skin in between.

Psoriasis and eczema can occur throughout and about seborrheic keratoses. Solar keratoses and verrucae can occur on seborrheic keratoses—usually on the face. I have seen a keratoacanthoma and a seborrheic keratosis occur side by side (a so-called collision tumor). Although quite rare, there is no question that red fungating and bulky bowenoid squamous cell carcinomas can arise in seborrheic keratoses.

Lifelong linear seborrheic keratoses are probably linear epidermal nevi.

DIFFERENTIAL DIAGNOSIS

The differential diagnosis of seborrheic keratosis includes the localized keratoses listed in this portion of the text. As well, one should review the black or brown papulonodules, especially dermatosis papulosa nigra (see Chapter 11). In the supra-pubic area and on the shaft of the penis, they may resemble viral verrucae and actually have DNA virons. They also can resemble bowenoid papulosis. Some papilloepitheliomata, on the neck especially, may show the histological picture of seborrheic keratosis and have been called papillomatous seborrheic keratoses.

There is some argument about into which morphological category seborrheic keratosis fits. In addition to being keratoses, they are also epidermal papules or nodules, and they also are often verrucous. I suppose their complete description could be verrucous, epidermal, papulonodular keratoses.

Keratosis Alba

These lesions are 0.2 to 0.5 cm, hypochromatic, slightly elevated epidermal papules. The surface is irregular, forming numerous small, slightly divided lobules. They occur only in blacks and are located on the torso. They are probably variants of seborrheic keratosis.

DIFFERENTIAL DIAGNOSIS

The differential diagnosis includes verruca plana, which are not hypopigmented, are more of a papule than a keratosis, and consist of small 1 to 2 mm lesions.

Stucco Keratosis

These are grayish, white, brownish-gray, or dirty gray in color and are usually found about the ankles, on the dorsal and lateral aspects of the feet, on the outer aspects of the arms and forearms, and on the dorsa of the hands. The individual lesion is a discrete keratotic papule with a flat or convex surface, the long axis of the oval lesion usually parallel to the skin lines. These lesions are from 2 to 5 mm in diameter, oval or round, with a hard, rough, dry surface. If the keratotic portion is scratched off, there is no bleeding, but a fine scaly collarette is left. As with other keratotic lesions, some are more easily felt than seen. The skin in the area is usually dry and wrinkled. Seborrheic keratoses are often present.

DIFFERENTIAL DIAGNOSIS

The differential diagnosis includes seborrheic keratosis, acrokeratosis verruciformis, verrucae planae, epidermodysplasia verruciformis, solar and arsenical keratosis, and Flegel's keratosis (see Chapter 20).

Acrokeratosis Verruciformis

These are hyperkeratotic and verrucous lesions on the dorsa of the hands and feet. They may precede or occur with Darier's disease. They are probably part of the picture of Darier's disease (see Chapter 20).

Epidermodysplasia Verruciformis

Morphologically, this is a variety of verrucae planae. Other findings may be reddish, almost flat, verrucous keratoses, reddish plaques on the trunk, and scaling brownish or achromic lesions resembling tinea versicolor. On the backs of the hands, the warty lesions are larger than those seen in Darier's disease. The lesions are accentuated in sun-exposed areas.

Porokeratosis of Mibelli

This is a progressive keratoatrophoderma. Fully developed, it consists of an atrophic, whitish center with hairs, surrounded by an arcuate elevated border 1 mm in height. In cross-section, the border is triangular in shape. In the top of this triangular wall is a slender furrow or groove. There is sometimes some scale on the inner aspect of the encircling ridge. The lesion slowly extends peripherally. The lesions appear most commonly on the hands and extremities, the face, and the genitals. Occasionally, they are linear, extensive, and follow Blaschko's lines.

Precancerous Dermatosis of Bowen

Bowen's disease (dyskeratosis lenticularis et discoides) shows sharply demarcated nummular discs, usually solitary, often with arcuate nonserrated borders, covered with thick scaly crusts. Occasionally, atrophic areas are present. The disease is common on the extremities and is very slow growing. Occasionally, a frank squamous cell carcinoma tumor develops in one corner. Rarely, the lesions have a black brown pigmentation. Bowen's disease of the face and dorsa of the hands probably should be classified as Bowenoid solar keratosis. Bowen's disease does not occur on the palms, soles, or mucosae.

The border of this disease is arcuate, composed of large smooth arcs. This should be distinguished from superficial multicentric basal cell carcinoma, which is arciform, but also finely serrated.

Miscellaneous

Some of the basically verrucous lesions may have a keratotic aspect to them. These may include verrucae, acanthosis nigricans, verrucous tuberculosis, and diffusely verrucous or keratotic hypertrophic discoid lupus erythematosus. These are described under the verrucosities.

Localized traumatic lesions such as corns, calluses, and verrucae which consist mainly of hyperkeratosis, can be classified as localized keratoses. As most occur on the palms and soles, they have been described under the keratodermas in Chapter 15. Knuckle pads are fibrous thickenings on top of which marked hyperkeratoses may occur. Some are familial, but most are from trauma ("gnaw warts"). The familial type arises in young adulthood, are more numerous, and in areas not easily traumatized. Gonococcal keratodermas are discussed under the keratodermas.

Acrokeratosis paraneoplastica has a constellation of findings including browning or purpling, erythema, scaling, and fissuring of the palms and soles. The ears and sun-exposed areas of the face are also involved.

Perforating dermatoses are often quite keratotic (see Chapter 20, and "Papules", Chapter 11).

Localized: Mucosal

On mucosae and semimucosae, the macerated horny thickenings that appear white are called leukoplakia. By definition, leukoplakia does not occur on hairy skin. Leukoplakia should not be confused with macerated epithelium or with pseudomembranes. Sharply localized thickenings of the mucosal horny layer are called leukokeratoses.

Admittedly, many leukoplakias are not plaques in the correct sense (plaque = slab), but really are patches. However, the term leukoplakia is so well entrenched that I cannot see it being replaced by "leukopatchia".

As indicated above, most mucosal keratotic lesions appear as white areas of varying degrees of thickness of the epithelium. Lesions of both the mucosae and semimucosae will be considered in this portion.

Leukoplakia

Favorite locations for leukoplakia are the mouth, lips and vulva. It is rare on the prepuce, glans penis, and in the perianal area. In the mouth, the anterior half of the tongue, especially on the top and sides, the inner aspects of the cheeks, and the lower alveolar troughs are common sites. The inner aspect of the lower lip and the vermilion border of the lower lip may be involved. On the vulva, leukoplakia is most common on both labia and the clitoris. Leukoplakia does not occur on the skin; this can be an important point in the differential diagnosis.

Leukoplakia is composed of spots or patches of extremely variable dimensions. Usually there is more than one patch, sometimes clustered together, sometimes widely spread apart. The border is usually sharply demarcated, although occasionally there is a gradual tapering off into normal mucosa. The white or gray-white keratotic layer is firmly adherent and can only be removed by very strong pulling, which causes bleeding. The degree of thickening varies. Sometimes it is very thick and may have fissures or irregular knobby surface projections. At times, pieces of this keratotic material fall off, but new ones appear. Occasionally a verrucous surface is present. Some cases show a firm, hard, ulcerative nodule, which represents a squamous cell carcinoma. However, this tumor formation is by no means inevitable; leukoplakia may exist for many years without significant change. It is, in general, persistent, although there may be some waxing and waning of its extent and thickness. Sclerosis is not a feature.

It should be stressed that poorly cared for, diseased, carious, rough-edged, and tobacco-stained teeth are commonly found in patients with leukoplakia. Alcoholic breath may also be present. It should also be stressed that leukoplakia is a diffuse change and can exist histologically in areas that may show surprisingly little visible gross morphologic change.

It is now quite clear that most leukoplakias do not develop into carcinoma. The early cancer or precancerous lesion in the oral mucosa is a friable red irregular patch or plaque, not a well demarcated white patch. At times, like erythroplasia of Queyrat in the glans penis, the mucosal erythroplasia may be present for years before a histologically proven carcinoma can develop. Speckled leukoplakia has an intermediate malignant potential.

Pseudoepitheliomatous, keratotic, and micaeous balanitis is probably a variety of hyperplastic mucosal leukoplakia.[14]

Lichen planus presents as a confluent or lace-like, purplish- white film on the red and inner mucosal portions of both lips. The same may also be seen on the buccal mucosa. Occasionally, eroded areas are present. Lesions are also seen on the genitalia. Characteristic skin lesions should be looked for on examination. Very rarely, a nodular squamous cell carcinoma may develop on chronic, erosive, buccal lichen planus, almost always in smokers.

Discoid lupus erythematous involves the hard palate, buccal mucosa, or lips as a sharply demarcated, atrophying, telangiectatic plaque with a purplish-white color and an elevated, slightly indurated edge. Erosions or ulcers are rare. On the lips, the adjacent skin is often involved. Quite severe scarring may occur.

Thrush (candidiasis) presents as a white filamentous film widely distributed in the oral mucosae. As it can be rubbed off, it is not leukoplakia.

Geographic tongue is manifest by circinate patches, rings, or other designs on the top and sides of the tongue. The spots have a white border 1 to 2 mm wide, within which lies a desquamated bright red surface. The lesions start as white spots that enlarge and become confluent. The change in size, extent, and shape from week to week can be quite dramatic. Fissured or scrotal tongue is often present.

Secondary syphilitic lesions such as smooth patches, opaline mucous patches, and papillomatous papules may occur. Tertiary syphilis, such as the tuberculoulcerative types, gummas, and sclerotic glossitis, should be considered, although all of these forms are now rare.

Psoriasis has been reported to occur on lips and tongue.

Cheilitis exfoliativa is a scaly and crusted eruption, often associated with seborrhea.

For a differential diagnosis of the white lesions of the vulva, see "Lichen Sclerosus et Atrophicus" in Chapter 11.

Solar Leukokeratosis of the Red Lip

Although this condition may be regarded as a type of leukoplakia, I think it has more in common with epidermal solar keratosis and so prefer the term leukokeratosis. (Solar cheilitis is not a good term because it includes the acute photosensitivity eruptions.)

Solar leukokeratoses occur in blue- or green-eyed, blond, fair-skinned individuals who have had habitual exposure to sun, either as an occupation or as leisure. Other changes from habitual exposure to sun, e.g. brown leather-like skin, solar keratosis, erythromelanosis colli, and telangiectasia, are usually present in those with solar leukokeratoses.

The changes are located on the vermilion area of the lower lip, which often is more protuberant in patients with these leukokeratoses. Marked leukokeratosis is rare in women, presumably because of the protection from the sun's rays afforded by lipstick.

The epithelium of the lower red lip is somewhat thickened, whitish or grayish white, and smooth with vertical lines. This change is more pronounced in the central portion. Fissuring may occur. The lesion gradually blends into the mucosal lip surface and onto the adjacent skin with the loss of the usual sharp demarcation. The skin just below is often slightly puffy. In some areas, clear-cut keratoses can be found; in others, the keratosis formation has a reddish, eroded surface. At times there may be some exfoliation.

Erythroplasia of Queyrat

Erythroplasia of Queyrat (carcinoma in situ on the glans penis), is a well-defined keratotic plaque with a brilliant red velvety surface. The border may be just palpable as slightly elevated and firm. Lesions up to 3 cm in diameter may be seen. Papules or nodules of squamous cell carcinoma may develop on large lesions. Frequently, only one portion of the plaque shows this carcinomatous change. There is no sclerosis. Although occurring mainly on the semimucosae of the glans penis and prepuce, a similar lesion may be seen on the vulva or buccal mucosa and tongue.

DIFFERENTIAL DIAGNOSIS

The differential diagnosis includes candidal balanitis and psoriasis, both of which are rarely persistent. They are not velvety. Balanitis xerotica obliterans shows also sclerosis, telangiectatic blood vessels, and eventually meatal stenosis.

Traumatic White Lesions

While trauma may play a role in the development and localization of leukoplakia, there are many white thickenings of the epithelium of the mouth that are caused by chronic chewing, rubbing, or irritation alone. These lesions are less white, less thick, and less well defined than leukoplakia. There is usually a specific source of obvious irritation, and removal of the trauma results in the disappearance of the lesion. In my experience, these lesions are usually located on the buccal surfaces. They can also occur under dentures.

White Sponge Nevus of Cannon

The white spongy nevus of Cannon (epidermal nevus of oral mucosa) is a white, soft, folded keratosis involving various parts of the oral mucosae. The lesion may have a linear component; there is no extensive thickening, fissuring, or induration; it may be unilateral; and it is present from an early age and does not change. Occasional patients with extensive linear epidermal nevi may have epithelial nevi on the buccal mucosa.

Other multiepithelial congenital abnormalities such as pachyonychia congenita, parakeratosis variegata, dyskeratosis congenita, hereditary benign intraepithelial dyskeratoses, and others may have white plaques in the mouth, usually on the buccal mucosa.

Localized: Keratodermas

On the palms and soles, accumulated, hard, firmly adherent masses of keratin are called keratodermas.* They may be punctate, circumscribed or diffuse (Table 35). These tylotic or callus scale formations may be in the form of pinhead-sized papules located in the major crease lines. After a time these lesions often lose their keratotic centers (keratosis palmoplantaris papulosa). They may also result in lentil-sized to silver dollar-sized (up to 2.7 cm diameter) horny pads (calluses) on palms and soles or may tend to cover the skin in a more diffuse manner (tylotic eczemas, keratosis palmoplantaris diffusa), giving the affected areas a yellow wax-like color and blurring the normal skin surface relief. Callus horn formations have the color of horny materials, namely yellow to yellowish-brown, often greenish-black if of long duration, and milky white if macerated by sweat. Surfaces of these lesions may be smooth without visible exfoliation, pitted, covered with more or less loose scales, or verrucous. They may also show cracks or pits surrounded by collarettes. If there are no cracks, the surface relief may be coarsened and may exhibit deep furrows, so that one is reminded of lichenification. However, in lichenification, the thickening of the skin, which is the cause of the coarse relief, is situated in the rete pegs (histologically acanthosis) and in the cutis (histologically an infiltrate), whereas in keratosis, the thickening is in the horny layer. The two phenomena should not be confused with each other or with the insignificant accentuation of skin relief found in macerated sweaty hands. The lack of elasticity in calloused skin areas may cause superficially squamous or sometimes deeper cracks or fissures that penetrate into the papillary body, eventually causing severe pain and offering a portal of entry for infections. The location of calluses is frequently very typical, because they form in places exposed to constantly repeated pressure and rubbing. Knowledge of their exact location and shape frequently permits conclusions as to the activity or vocation of the patient (rowers, cleaning women, cobbler, milker, sculptor) or, in some countries, the type of clothing worn (wooden shoes).

It is interesting to note how many diverse conditions involving the plantar and palmar skin are confluent only on the palms and soles. When the lesions extend

Table 35: Examples of Keratodermas

Punctate
- Psoriasis
- Arsenical
- Verrucae
- Hereditary
- Idiopathic

Circumscribed
- Psoriasis
- Traumatic (burns of all sorts)
- Porokeratosis
- Lichen simplex chronicus
- Linear
- Lichen planus
- Striate
- Peridigital dermatitis *ENTA*
- Gonococcal
- Syphilis

Diffuse
- Hereditary
- Psoriasis
- Pityriasis rubra pilaris
- Tylotic eczema
- Moccasin type tinea
- Parapsoriasis en plaques

*Keratoderma is the generic term for keratoses of the plantar and palmar surfaces. Some would restrict this term to conditions that involve all or almost all of the palmar and plantar surfaces. Conditions not involving the total surfaces, they would call keratoses. The problem with this is that there are several conditions where both total and partial involvement may occur, e.g. psoriasis and arsenical keratoses.

beyond this skin they become scattered and not confluent (e.g. moccasin type tinea, psoriasis, pityriasis rubra pilaris). There must, therefore, be something different in the palmar and plantar skin.

All solitary keratotic lesions of the soles and palms should be pared before a final diagnosis is made. Moistening the skin with mineral oil or glycerin may make the easier identification of papillary skin lines and capillaries.

Verrucae

On the soles and palms, verrucae (Fig. 15.6) present as circular, dirty brown keratotic lesions that spread apart the print lines. On paring, the sides of the lesion are straight and numerous small capillary vessels perpendicular to the surface can be seen. Some of the vessels are clotted. On deep paring, these centrally located capillaries bleed. The border is usually elevated. Callus usually is present over the wart, especially over areas of pressure. A wart tends to be most painful when side pressure is applied, a corn when direct pressure is applied. When it is resolving, the lesion sometimes suddenly becomes a gray black color, and on removal of the callus a friable desiccated tissue is seen. This tissue is easily picked out, leaving a depression.

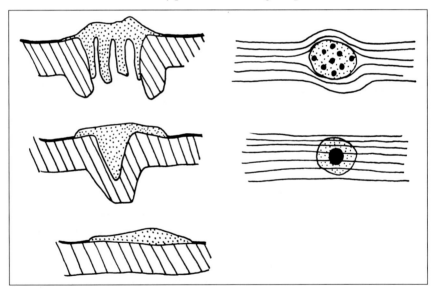

Figure 15.6 *Top:* Verruca, cross-section and plane view. *Middle:* Corn, cross section and plane view. *Bottom:* Callus, cross section.

The size, number, and arrangement in plantar verrucae are variable (see "Verrucae" in Chapter 16). Sometimes only a solitary lesion is present; sometimes multiple lesions are present; and sometimes a mother-daughter or bomb-explosion type pattern is present. Occasionally, a wart may occur in a corn. Verrucae occur commonly, but not exclusively over pressure points. An average wart size would be from 0.5 to 1 cm. Occasionally, in patients with sweaty feet, verrucae with a vegetative or papillomatous and proliferating nature are seen, especially on the sides and plantar surfaces of the toes. These look similar to moist or venereal warts. Also, multiple plantar warts seem to be more common in those with marked hyperhidrosis.

Myrmecia as defined by Lyell and Myles are solitary, painful, red, swollen, and deeply set plantar, palmar, or periungual verrucae.[15]

A mosaic wart, almost always on the soles, occasionally the palms, is made of many 2 to 3 mm, superficial, keratotic, nontender lesions, each one showing the characteristics of small plantar warts. The individual satellite lesions at the periphery are circular, but in the center they appear to have angular borders because they are so closely packed. Mosaic verrucae have arcuate borders. This type of verruca may cover large areas of the plantar surface. The most striking feature is their lack of tenderness on walking or on lateral or direct pressure.

Keratotic Verrucae

These lesions are 2 to 4 mm sharply marginated, round keratoses present singly or aggregately on the palms or soles. Paring reveals the bleeding capillaries of the cut papillae. The print lines of palms or soles go around the lesions. Some are amazingly scaly and keratotic, and even seem to have an arcuate border. The lesions have a yellowish cast, with a tendency to small central keratotic core formation. They may be more common and extensive on the traumatic areas of the first and second digits of the palmar surface of the hands. On the nonpalmar skin, vulgar or flat viral warts may be seen. In areas of confluence, especially over the flexural areas, fissuring may occur.

DIFFERENTIAL DIAGNOSIS

Keratotic verrucae of palms and soles must be distinguished from arsenical keratoses and from the lesions of isolated keratotic palmar and plantar psoriasis.

Callus

A callus or callosity (see Fig. 15.2) is a hard keratosis of variable extent, round or oval, with a gently sloping border, thick and solid on palpation, of a yellowish-white color, and occurring at sites of repeated trauma, especially on the soles and palms. Occasionally, linear callosities are present as a result of pressure over a linear bony surface; sometimes there are even numerous small corns in these linear lesions, e.g. on medial side of each big toe. The exact shape and extent of callosities and corns depends on the nature of the trauma and the shape or arrangement of the underlying bony prominence or resistance. Occasionally, emotionally upset individuals relieve their tensions by intensive pacing for hours on end. This may produce very extensive plantar callous and corn formation.

In orthopedic circles, there is a slight difference in terminology for the localized trauma-produced lesions on the feet. The term corn refers to those lesions occurring over the interphalangeal joints; the term clavus (Latin for nail) is used to describe those lesions occurring over the repeatedly traumatized areas on the sole of the foot. I have not made this distinction and have used corn and clavus interchangeably.

Corns

A corn (clavus) (see Fig. 15.6) is a keratotic lesion which, in contradistinction to verrucae, does not spread apart the print lines. Sometimes these print lines are thicker in the corn than in the adjacent noninvolved skin. It is funnel-shaped with sloping sides, and is composed of a yellowish, translucent, horny keratin material, often with a 1 to 2 mm white central core, and contains no capillaries. On deep paring, bleeding occurs peripherally. Corns occur only on pressure areas. Callus is present at the periphery. A corn tends to be most painful on direct pressure. Hemorrhage into corns is not unusual.

On the weight-bearing sole, particularly in the center of the anterior arch, pressure calluses and corns may take the form of 1 to 3 mm corns, arranged, along with considerable callus, in basically an anterior-posterior line. Paring reveals these small corns to have all the features of larger ones. I have seen similar lesions in the calloused creases of the palms and fingers of men who do heavy manual labor.

Porokeratosis plantaris discreta is a single or a group of sharply marginated hyperkeratotic plugs that press into the sole skin to a depth of 4 to 5 mm. The plugs are opaque, rubbery, and devoid of blood vessels.

A moist or soft corn (the eye of a partridge) is most painful on pressure on the external side of the fifth toe. A moist corn must be distinguished from epidermophytosis, which has an arcuate undermined border, frequently with small vesicles, which shows only maceration and not keratosis formation, and also frequently extends onto the non-weight-bearing areas of the under surface of the toe. Also, in epidermophytosis, involvement of only one interdigital web area is most unusual.

Moist interdigital psoriasis is not basically a keratotic lesion. The lesion is more widespread, and frequently away from the web space basic psoriasis lesions may be seen. Again, involvement of interdigital psoriasis in one web space would be most unusual.

Chinese Foot-Binding Syndrome

The so-called "Chinese foot-binding syndrome" occurs mainly in women, and consists of varying degrees of one or more of the following symptoms.[16,17]

1. Hard corns or callosities on the tips of the toes, some subungual, on the dorsa of the phalangeal joints, on the dorsolateral aspect of the fifth toe, on the medial aspect of the big toe, over the medial aspect of the first metatarsal-phalangeal joint, over the lateral and medial and central portion of the anterior arch of the

sole, and in the central portion of the sole, anterior to the central portion of the anterior arch. Rarely, calluses may be present over bony prominences on the dorsa of the foot.

2. Soft corns at the sides or base of the third or fourth interdigital toe space.

3. Compression of the toes, especially the four lateral ones, with loss of the interdigital spaces and squaring of the tips.

4. Lateral deviation of the first and second toes, and medial deviation of the fourth and fifth toes, to such an extent that the fifth toe may be pushed under the fourth and the second under the third.

5. Elevation of interphalangeal joints to form an inverted V, usually on the second and third toes (claw toes).

6. Presence of an enlarged, medially extending first metatarsal-phalangeal joint over which a large callus is present, and associated with at least some lateral deviation of the big toe (bunion).

7. Compression and deformity of the toenails in association with compression of toes. Sometimes, longitudinal horny hypertrophy of the toenails occurs. The sides of the toenail may be buried in the lateral nail fold, and hence cause ingrowing toenails. The nails may also show subungual keratosis, forming the nail plate to an inverted U shape. The keratosis is made up of very firm, whitish, keratin material. The plate is lifted up towards its distal end and may show whitish areas. In effect, this is a callus of the nail.

8. A feature of most of these changes is their symmetry.

If all the above listed findings are present, there need be no question of the diagnosis. Confusing or complicating findings may be as follows.

1. Presence of definite verrucae vulgares (of the solitary, mother-daughter, or mosaic type) about the corns and callosities. Occasionally a solitary wart may exist in a corn.

2. The presence of a congenitally shortened first metatarsal (Morton's toe) may cause some of the changes listed above.

3. Occasionally, congenital (lateral deviation of the big toe) or acquired (post-poliomyelitis, postinfantile hemangioma radiation damage to metatarsals) factors may produce a few of the changes listed.

4. Other keratotic lesions have been dealt with elsewhere.

5. Although the Chinese foot-binding syndrome is seen more often and with more extensive involvement in women, it may also occur in men.

6. As has been implied, this syndrome is from ill-fitting shoes. When these shoes are also occlusive, the effects of hyperhidrosis will be exaggerated (more maceration, more odor), and blistering tinea will be found more often and be more active.

Thomas George Morton, 1835–1903, U.S. Surgeon, Philadelphia

Late Radiation Sequelae

On the sole, chronic radiodermatitis presents similar features to those found on other areas of the body, viz. atrophy of epidermis; sclerosis and atrophy of dermis, hypoderm, and appendages; telangiectatic blood vessels; usual circular or square area; and occasional ulceration. On the sole, keratosis formation is not unusual and this must be pared off to make the diagnosis. This hyperkeratotic lesion contains in part the varying-sized telangiectatic capillaries that run in all ways—both perpendicular and longitudinal to the level of the sole skin. Some of these capillaries contain only clotted blood and present the finding of telangiectatic purpura in that the blood cannot be compressed out of these capillaries. The overall structure of the lesion after paring is irregular, and the normal papillary lines of the skin are interrupted. The amount of loss of tissue apparently depends on the source, dose, and fractionation of the original ionizing radiation. In severe cases, after paring off the keratotic surface, a malodorous discharge will come from a shaggy-based, lifeless, dirty gray ulcer. These ulcers occupy the central portion of the radiodermatitis. Some lesions are quite rigid and firm and are attached to underlying structures. Spontaneous pain is often a feature. In very severe cases, actual deformity of the bony structure of the foot occurs, especially if excessive radiation was given before the bones had stopped growing.

Surgical or Electrosurgical Scars

These present as small linear or stellate lesions often covered with a hyperkeratotic mass. Occasionally, one or two small corns are present in the scar. Also, at the periphery, small verrucae may be seen, especially of the mosaic type. The border is reasonably well demarcated; telangiectasis is not a feature, but the skin lines are disturbed. Recent surgical scars may be hypertrophic. Pain with direct pressure or with walking is a feature on weight-bearing areas. This pain is not as severe as the pain in radiodermatitis.

Foreign Bodies

Foreign bodies, especially hair, may present as a localized tender keratotic plantar lesion. Paring reveals the foreign body, making the diagnosis. In some cases, some erythema, sinus formation, and pyoderma may occur.

Peridigital Dermatitis in Children of Enta

Peridigital dermatitis in children (juvenile plantar dermatosis, glazed foot, sneaker dermatitis), is a reasonably well-demarcated, usually symmetrical, erythematous scaly eruption on the plantar and palmar skin of prepubertal children (see also Chapter 5, "Hands and Feet"). The lesion is really a scaly plaque involving, most frequently, the tips of the fingers and toes and often the adjacent palmar and plantar skin. The involvement of the palms and soles is never complete. The instep area and center palm areas are often spared, as are the heels. The eruption has an irregular (and not arcuate) border, and there may be some undermining, with no vesiculation, at some of the borders. The scale is nondescript and adherent. There is marked fissuring.

In psoriasis, the border is arcuate, the lesion more purplish-red in color, and the scale more mica-like and thicker. Also, other psoriatic lesions, particularly on the nails, are usually present.

The dyshidrotic pattern seen in atopics shows vesiculation on the sides of the fingers and toes, the palms or instep area.

Nonblistering tinea pedis (as from *Trichophyton rubrum*) shows a duller red eruption, a moccasin-type arrangement, and almost always involvement of the toenails or intertoe-web spaces with the features of tinea pedis. Unilateral palmar skin involvement is not unusual.

Some contact eczemas may present with a subsiding scaly phase, but the eruption is usually symmetrical, often on pressure areas only, and may show some vesiculation.

The congenitally determined keratodermas are usually thicker, more extensive, do not clear in summer, and are familial.

Atopic dermatitis with lichenification, postinflammatory browning or whitening, and excoriations may be present on the palmar or plantar skin. Usually, though, it is present more on the dorsal surfaces, from where it extends onto the thicker skin.

Traumatic keratoderma may at times present a rather diffuse process, but its occurrence on areas of pressure and the presence of callus should clearly separate this condition.

Striate Keratoderma

Linear unilateral keratoderma presents with striate keratotic bands about 1 cm in width. Characteristically, the flexor surfaces of the fingers, with extension onto the palm, are involved. This condition is presumably a variety of linear epidermal nevus.

A similar condition is symmetrically striate keratoderma, which shows thick, linear, keratotic, dirty gray-yellow bands on the flexor aspects of the fingers that extend onto the palms, where the linear arrangement is not as obvious and there are more and larger lesions at sites of trauma. There is a purplish 2 mm erythema at the border. The soles show extensive, yellow, horny, hyperkeratotic areas on sites of pressure, some on the anterior portion over the whole foot. The instep is clear. Hyperhidrosis of the palms and soles is often present, as is ichthyosis vulgaris of a moderate to severe degree.

The lesions start in infancy. They are persistent.

Collagenous Plaques on the Hands

Collagenous plaques on the hands, at sites of trauma, occur in outdoor workers in sunny climates. They consist of small warty papules, yellowish or flesh-colored, extending in a narrow band, sometimes telangiectatic, at the junction of palmar and dorsal skin from the tip of the thumb around the web to the radial side of the index finger. The ulnar portions of the hand may also be involved.

Arsenical Keratoses

Arsenical keratoses, due to ingestion of As_2O_3, occur especially on the palms and soles, but may be found anywhere on the cutaneous surface. In its most characteristic form, there are punctate keratoses of the palms and soles. The condition is marked by numerous, small, horny, corn-like elevations, usually 2 to 5 mm in diameter. They occur frequently as epidermal pegs, which can be picked out of their keratotic beds. They are frequently situated on the thenar and hypothenar eminences of the hand, on the palmar and side surfaces of the fingers, sometimes also on the back of the phalangeal joints. On the soles, the sites of predilection are the heels and the anterior portion of the soles. There may be a confluence of a group of these corns, forming wart-like excrescences, but differing from true warts by having no papillary structure and by not pushing apart the skin print lines. Sometimes the palms only or the soles only are affected. Rarely, there is a more diffuse keratosis of the palms and soles, giving the skin a leathery appearance (diffuse keratoderma). The punctate horny thickenings may be situated on an erythematous base, or a horny patch may be surrounded by an erythematous halo. Rarely, the punctate keratoses are combined with the keratoderma. The keratoses of palms and soles are usually symmetrically distributed. Fissures may occur on the keratoses. If cancer develops on these keratoses, it has the characteristics of squamous cell carcinoma, especially of the verrucous type. Multiple superficial basal cell carcinoma may be present on the torso. It has been claimed, but not proven, that systemic cancer of the gut, respiratory tract, genitourinary tract, and liver occur as a result of long-term ingestion of inorganic trivalent arsenic.

DIFFERENTIAL DIAGNOSIS

The differential diagnosis of these punctate keratoses may include keratotic verrucae, multiple keratotic corns, keratotic psoriasis, and unusual types of keratosis punctata. A very rare combination of keratoses closely resembling those due to arsenic is seen in combination with a peculiar neuropathy characterized by painful legs and an athetosis of the toes.

Psoriasis

Psoriasis occurs in three forms on the palms and soles: regular, pustular or vesiculopustular, and keratotic. The keratotic form will be considered here. In this condition, there are 1 to 2 mm keratoses with a hard yellow scale. On pressure areas, the lesions may be confluent. An arcuate border is often present.

Pityriasis Rubra Pilaris

In pityriasis rubra pilaris, the palms and soles are seen to be diffusely dry, hyperkeratotic, and thickened, with a peculiar yellowish tinge. In the creases, there may be some dark lines. There is almost no desquamation.

Lichen Planus

Lichen planus shows scattered flattish papules; more or less confluent keratotic spots, each with a central depression; finely scaly plaques; totally nonspecific-looking keratoderma; or, rarely, destructive bullous lesions. Lichen planus lesions are usually present on other sites of the skin or mucosae other than palms and soles.

Blistering Tinea

Blistering tinea may superficially resemble a keratoderma, but basically it is a vesiculobullous eruption with peripheral undermining and is often located in the intertoe-web spaces as well as on the soles and insteps. It does not occur on the palms, but a "dyshidrotic" id may be seen in association with an acute blistering tinea.

Nonblistering Tinea

Nonblistering tinea is an erythematosquamous eruption covering almost all of the plantar skin. The toenails are commonly involved. Unilateral palmar involvement may be present; the so-called two-foot-one-hand tinea.

Gonococcal Keratoderma

This is probably a form of pustular psoriasis or Reiter's disease and presents as thick, juicy, hyperkeratotic or crusted, acuminate papulonodules surrounded by a dark red halo. The palms and soles are affected, but so also are the elbows, knees, and ankles.

Pitted Keratolysis

In pitted keratolysis (basketball feet), a peculiar change occurs in individuals with very sweaty feet who indulge in heavy and frequent physical activity while wearing nonpermeable footwear (see Chapter 23). The change seen is a whitish or purplish maceration containing easily felt clusters of small circular depressions. These depressions are isolated at the periphery, but in the center they are confluent and present themselves as a very superficial defect. They are really not keratoses, but depressions.

Pitting of Palms and Soles

These are pits not keratoses. Many normal people have them, especially blacks. They are also seen in Darier's disease and the nevoid basal cell carcinoma syndrome.

Parapsoriasis en Plaque

This is an erosive, arcuate, scaly plaque on the palms and soles (Fig. 15.7). Fissuring, crusting, and bleeding are quite common. The diagnosis is made on the basis of findings elsewhere.

Occupational Keratodermas

These lesions occur in individuals who do heavy manual work.

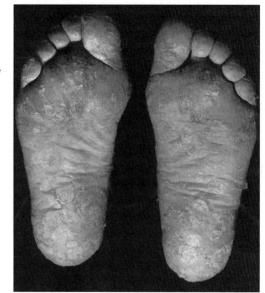

Figure 15.7 Parapsoriasis en plaques. Note also the square-shaped toes from foot binding (from shoes).

Keratotic (Tylotic) Eczema

Keratotic eczema may extend over the entire palmar and plantar skin or only small areas. It is often symmetrical in both degree and extent. Only rarely are both palms and soles involved. It has poorly defined borders, spreading along the large creases. The thickened horny layer splits, and some exfoliation occurs. Vesicles are rarely seen. They are small, deep-seated, and do not break readily as do eczema blisters elsewhere. Other areas of eczema are often present on the sides of the fingers and toes and on the dorsa of the hands and feet.

For further discussion of eczemas of the hands and feet, see Chapter 5, "Localized Varieties".

Lichen Simplex Chronicus

This type of rather poorly demarcated, nonarcuate keratoderma more often affects the palms than the soles. It may be bilateral but is more often unilateral. Evidence of excoriation or traumatization is usually present. There are no blisters. Middle-aged women frequently have this disease, hence the term keratoderma climactericum. It is freely admitted that the distinction between this condition and keratotic eczema or psoriasis is at times very difficult or impossible.

Psoriasiform Palmar And Plantar Syphilides

Secondary syphilis consists of multiple lesions consisting either of flat lenticular papules of a dusky red or cooked ham color, slightly keratotic and scaly, or of depressed nummular spots, surrounded by a keratotic ridge. Occasionally the lesions may be frankly horn-like.

In the tertiary stage there are round or polycyclic spots of a dark or coppery red, may be markedly hyperkeratotic or wrinkled or cracked, sometimes surrounded by a papular border. These lesions are often unilateral. They may be found anywhere on the plantar or palmar surfaces. Occasionally the lesions may be infiltrated, and they may encroach onto the nonpalmar and nonplantar skin. Scarring may occur.

Scarring discoid lupus erythematosus may be present on the palms.

Familial Keratoderma

Familial keratoderma (mal de Meleda) is an ordinarily congenital, sometimes acquired disease that frequently attacks several children of the same family and has a marked tendency to hereditary transmission.[*18]

The palmar and plantar skin are the sites of a horny thickening. The borders are marked by a purplish or bluish pink edge from 4 to 5 mm wide. The hyperplastic horny layer may be smooth, soft, of a waxy or brownish yellow color, and made up of large adherent lamellae. Local hyperhidrosis is frequently present. In some cases, the hyperkeratosis is dry, hard, roughened, and thickened; it is fissured in the folds or divided into polygonal blocks.

The underlying skin is often red, usually tense, sclerotic, and atrophic. In severe cases, the skin is so retracted at the end phalanges that the fingers appear conical and tapering, as if enclosed in a very tight-fitting yellowish and horny case. The nails are thinned. Movements of the hands and fingers are impeded and painful; walking is difficult.

Other areas may be involved in mal de Meleda. The flexor aspect of the wrist and the achilles tendon area are often involved in continuity. Localized, thick, brownish-red, keratotic plaques may also be present on the elbows and knees.

Keratosis Punctata

Keratosis punctata is characterized by small, sometimes very hard, scattered or grouped, miliary horny masses. Pitting may also be seen. Keratosis punctata may occur independently or may occur in many other skin diseases, e.g. lichen planus, Darier's disease, palmar and plantar keratotic nevi, sequelae of arsenical ingestion, familial keratoderma, hyperkeratosis lenticularis perstans (Flegel's disease), and porokeratosis with palmar and plantar keratoses. Keratosis punctata may also show small horny plugs in small cup-like depressions in the palmar flexor creases of the fingers or palms (see corns). Spiny keratotic lesions can be seen on the palmer and plantar skin.

Miscellaneous

There is a long list of rare keratodermas that are often familial, with other rather dramatic findings.[19] From a morphological point of view, the separation of these various types is made by other findings. A partial listing is included here. The group includes such conditions as keratoderma with carcinoma of the esophagus,

Meleda (An island in Dalmatia, former Yugoslavia)
*For a listing of diffuse palmoplantar keratoderma with autosomal dominant inheritance and associated features see Reference 17.

mutilating keratoderma with ainhum-like constriction of the digits, progressive keratoderma, disseminate keratoderma with corneal dystrophy, Papillon-Lefèvre syndrome, circumscribed with mental deficiency, polykeratosis, hidrotic ectodermal dysplasia Naegeli's syndrome, pachyonychia congenita, disseminated porokeratosis with palmar and plantar lesions, and Clouston's hidrotic ectodermal dysplasia.

A diffuse dry keratoderma is seen on the palms and soles after a cast is removed or following a long period of immobility when there is no friction to remove the normally shed stratum corneum.

On occasion, after paring a localized keratotic lesion, a small (0.5 cm) intact epidermal inclusion cyst can be found.

Other ulcerative conditions such as malum perforans, ischemic ulcers, and ulcer-producing tumors (especially an amelanotic malignant melanoma) may have a covering of soggy keratotic mass, which obscures the basic nature of the lesion until it is pared off.

References

1. Darier J. Textbook of dermatology. Pollitzer S, trans. Philadelphia:Lea & Febiger, 1920.
2. Siemens HW. General diagnosis and therapy of skin diseases. Weiner K, trans. Chicago:University of Chicago Press, 1958.
3. Frost P. Ichthyosiform dermatoses. J Invest Dermatol 1973; 60:541–552.
4. Frost P, Van Scott EJ. Ichthyosiform dermatoses. Arch Dermatol 1966; 94:113–126.
5. Berman A, Winkelmann RK. Seborrheic keratoses appearance in course of exfoliative erythroderma and regression associated with histologic mononuclear cell inflammation. Arch Dermatol 1982; 118:615–618.
6. Gupta AK, Siegel MT, Noble SC, Kirby S, Rasmussen JE. Keratoses in patients with psoriasis: a prospective study in 52 patients. J Am Acad Dermatol 1990; 23:52–55.
7. Frank E, Mevorah B, Leu F. Disseminated spiked hyperkeratosis. Arch Dermatol 1981; 117:412–414.
8. Goldstein N. Multiple minute digitate hyperkeratosis. Arch Dermatol 1967; 96:692–693.
9. Jackson R. Blaschko's lines: a review and reconsideration of observations on the cause of certain unusual linear conditions of the skin. Br J Dermatol 1976; 95:349–360.
10. James MP, Wells GC, Whimster IW. Spreading pigmented actinic keratoses. Br J Dermatol 1978; 98:373.
11. Laur WE, Posey RE, Waller JD. Lichen planus-like keratoses. J Am Acad Dermatol 1981; 4:329–336.
12. Provost N, Kopf AW, Rabinovitz HS et al. Globulelike dermascopic structures in pigmented seborrheic keratosis. Arch Dermatol 1997; 113:540–541.
13. Rampen FHJ, Schwengle LEM. Letter to Editor. J Am Acad Dermatol 1990; 23:153.
14. Read SE, Abell E. Pseudoepitheliomatous, keratotic and micaceous balanitis. AMA Arch Dermatol 1981; 117:435–437.
15. Lyell A, Myles JAR. Myremcia: a study of inclusion bodies in warts. Br Med J 1951; 1:912–916.
16. Jackson R. The Chinese foot-binding syndrome. Observations on the history and sequelae of wearing ill-fitting shoes. Int J Dermatol 1990; 29:322–328.
17. Cohen PR, Scher RK. Geriatric nail disorders: diagnosis and treatment. J Am Acad Dermatol 1992; 26:521–531.
18. Nielson PG. Hereditary palmoplantar keratoderma and dermatophytes. Int J Dermatol 1988; 27:224.
19. Lucker GPH, Van de Kerkof PCM, Steijlen PM. The hereditary palmoplantar keratoses: an updated review and classification. Br J Dermatol 1994; 131:1–14.

Howard Rae Clouston,1889–1950, Canadian Physician
Paul Lefèvre, 20th Cent, French Dermatologist
Oscar Naegeli, 1885–1959, Swiss Dermatologist
M. M. Papillon, 20th Cent, French Dermatologist

CHAPTER 16
Verrucosities

Wave-like proliferations of the malpighian layer and the papillae, with or without a thickened stratum corneum.

Overview

Verrucous proliferations or verrucosities are more or less prominent multiple excrescences, which may be conical, filiform, or resembling a cauliflower growth in cross-section.[1,2] They are arranged as papules, plaques, and may be spread out over large areas. Each proliferation really corresponds to several papillae, united on the same connective tissue vascular stalk. As a general rule, the malpighian layer hyperplasia, known as acanthosis or hyperacanthosis, is the original disturbance (Fig. 16.1). It is not understood why this sometimes gives rise to a simple epidermic papule (for instance, the flat juvenile wart) or sometimes to a papillomatous elevation (for instance, the vulgar verrucous wart).

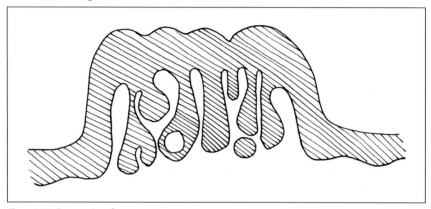

Figure 16.1 Cross section of a verrucosity.

The horny layer covering the proliferations may have normal thickness, it may be thinned as in the venereal warts, or thickened as in common warts. Hence, some have a smooth pink surface; others have the normal color of the skin; and still others are of a grayish-yellow color, firm consistency, and obviously keratotic. There may be gradations between a keratosis (a localized thickening of the horny layer) and a verrucosity (a localized thickening of the dermal papillae and malpighian layer). Occasionally both are present in the same lesion.

Verrucous changes are common in the perianal, perigenital, inguinal, and axillary regions. This is probably because adjacent parts rub together and the warm, damp conditions.

The former term for verrucosities was papillomatous and proliferating lesions, but I have not used the term papillomatous because the basic lesion is not a tumor of the papilla, but of the malpighian layer. The papillary overgrowth is secondary.

Eruptions that consist of many small, closely packed, sometimes round, sometimes pointed or thread-like projections are called vegetations. Vegetations may be of fine or coarse caliber, they may appear in small, rounded aggregations looking like

Portions of the Overview have been taken and modified from Darier[1] (p.237) and Siemens[2] (pp. 75, 76).

raspberries, or they may form beds covering areas of almost any size. Vegetations may be found below the level of the skin in wounds and ulcers, they may simply sit on the skin, or they may occur on top of other prominences such as nodules.

The vegetations in ulcers are called granulation tissue and are glossy and bright red.* They represent an early stage of scar tissue and are rich in blood vessels and cells which promote secondary healing. If vegetations become excessive, they are referred to as hypertrophic granulations or proud flesh. Vegetations sitting on non-ulcerated skin, even on papules and tumors, often appear bright red, glossy, and moist. These are naked or erosive vegetations. They may be bulging or smooth, or consist of round or pointed papules. If they have developed on the floor of a blister, the remnant of the blister top is usually still visible as a coarse collar of scales. The surface of vegetations may be ulcerated. The entire bed of vegetations may be constricted at the base or may be situated on a stem reminiscent of a raspberry or a cauliflower or, if the surface is smooth, of a pea or a marble (pyogenic granuloma). If the vegetations are covered with intact epithelium, they are, of course, dry and more or less skin-colored. These are called verrucous vegetations or verrucosities.

Essentially Verrucous Dermatoses

Verrucae

Verrucae are keratotic excrescences presenting as dirty grayish, brownish, rounded, prominent, distinctly circumscribed elevations with a mamillated surface studded with protuberances of a hard, rough consistency.

The basic shape of all verrucae (except verrucae planae and mosaic warts) is that of a small cauliflower with a narrowed base, umbrella-shaped top, and in cross-section a radial formation from a lower central point (Fig. 16.2).

All of these findings are characteristic of verrucae in many different locations and in different assortments of sizes and numbers (Fig. 16.3). In many instances, some of the above mentioned features are exaggerated, while in others they are minimized. Some examples of these will be described.

On the face and neck, on small thread-like stalks, radially arranged verrucae may be seen. In moist mucosal warts, the peripheral

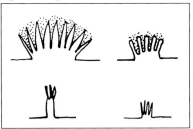

Figure 16.2 Cross-sections illustrating radiating cauliflower-like shapes of verrucae.

umbrella portion of the verrucae may be tremendously hypertrophic, and fist-sized lesions may be present. Presumably the warmth and moisture is the underlying factor in such cases, and similar lesions may be seen in warm moist areas between the toes. Periungual verrucae may cause a temporary linear indentation of the nail plate.

The arrangement of verrucae is varied (Fig. 16.4). One solitary lesion or many discrete solitary lesions may be present. At times, solitary lesions may be confluent.

*There is some question as to whether granulation tissue, proud flesh or pyogenic granulomas should be included here. I have done so, as to consider them with angiomatous papules or plaques seemed less satisfactory.

Bomb-explosion (corymbose) and mother-daughter types are not uncommon. Verrucae usually occur over sites of trauma (elbows, knees, periungual areas, fingers, on the beard area in men, on the legs of women, soles, genitals, and perianal area). Linear lesions are common, especially with verrucae planae, which are described with their differential diagnosis under papular lesions, as the radial cauliflower appearance is not present. Linear lesions also occur with so-called vulgar verrucae. Occasionally, viral verrucae may develop in healing lesions of pyoderma and in surgical or electrosurgical scars. On the palms and soles, the so-called mosaic pattern may exist (Fig. 16.5). Verrucae may have a rim pattern following cantharidin. Kissing warts between the toes are occasionally seen. Sometimes a wart will grow within a blister produced by liquid nitrogen.

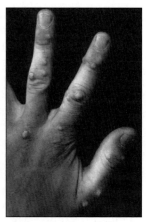

Figure 16.3 Verrucae.

Occasionally, mosaic plantar warts take on a similar arrangement to vulgar warts (mother-daughter, solitary, bomb-explosion).

Condylomata acuminata are verrucae that occur on the genital organs and the neighboring folds. They maintain the same basic radial arrangement, but presumably because of warmth and moisture they grow luxuriantly, becoming pedunculated, large, and confluent. Between the confluent verrucosities there may be a bright red oozing surface with an offensive odor. Smaller pedunculated or papular verrucae are usually present on the periphery. The hypertrophic mucous patches of secondary syphilis, condylomata lata, are basically papular, becoming hypertrophic. Oozing is a common feature. There are no small satellite lesions.

Plantar warts and their differential diagnosis are described in Chapter 15, "Localized keratoderma".

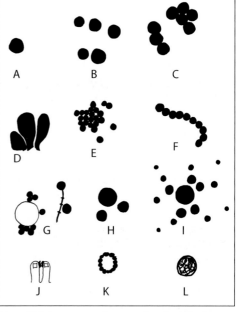

Figure 16.4 Arrangement of verrucae. *From Top Left to Bottom Right: A,* Solitary; *B,* Multiple solitary; *C,* Grouped solitary; *D,* Condylomatous (in moist areas, on soles in immunocompromised); *E,* Mosaic; *F,* Linear; *G,* Verrucae in scars; *H,* Mother-daughter; *I,* Bomb-explosion type; *J,* "Kissing"; *K,* Halo verruca following cantharidin; *L,* "Blister" verruca following liquid nitrogen.

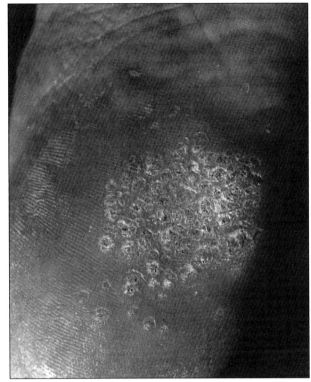

Figure 16.5 Mosaic verrucae on heel.

Verrucae can occur on many pre-existing lesions. Some of these are seborrheic keratosis, linear nevus sebaceous, linear epidermal nevus, atopic dermatitis, pigmented nevus, and superficial scratches (verrucae planae). The occurrence of these secondary verrucae seem to be more common on the face and scalp.

Verrucae may be more luxuriant and extensive in patients with disorders or who receive treatments that result in the impairment of the immune systems. Condylomatous and papillomatous and proliferating warts may be seen on the plantar surface in the severely compromised.

DIFFERENTIAL DIAGNOSIS

The differential diagnosis varies, depending on the morphological type of verrucae and location. Hypertrophic mucosal or semimucosal verrucae must be distinguished from the verrucous mucosal squamous cell carcinoma of Ackerman in the mouth and from florid oral papillomatosis. Also, condylomata lata should be considered on the mucosae and semimucosae. In the suprapubic area and on the penile shaft and foreskin, light brown seborrheic keratosis must be considered in the differential diagnosis. With newer techniques it seems that some of these lesions contain human

Lauren V. Ackerman, U. S. Pathologist, Columbus, MO

papilloma virus and so probably represent true verrucae. Early keratoacanthomas, verrucous psoriasis, verrucous lichen planus, lichen simplex chronicus, stucco keratoses, and disseminated superficial actinic porokeratosis may at times resemble verrucae, especially when they occur on the legs and ankles.

Verruciform xanthoma is a solitary warty lesion usually in the mouth. At times it can have a yellow hue.

Two other conditions to be considered are postpyodermal verrucous keratoses and the pseudorecidives that may occur following radiotherapy for cutaneous cancer, usually basal cell carcinoma. Both these lesions may be single or multiple, and it is amazing how closely they can morphologically approximate the sessile cauliflower shape of a verruca. With the postpyogenic lesions, there is usually the surrounding erythematous brown peripheral halo. These lesions do not appear while the frank pyodermatous lesions are present. In some cases these postpyodermal lesions may even be linear in arrangement. The postradiotherapy pseudorecidives (as described by Belisario[3]) are usually solitary, and of course show the erythematous browning and peeling of subsiding acute radiation sequelae in the surrounding skin.

There can be a marked verrucous appearance to the surface of the atrophic and scarred balanitis xerotica obliterans.

Nevi

Many of the so-called linear epidermal nevi may be verrucous, but these will be considered with the keratoses. The hamartomatous tissue involved may be primarily the epidermis, the sebaceous glands, the apocrine glands (nevus syringocystadenomatosus papilliferus), the melanocytic cells (as manifest by brown pigmentation or depigmentation) or nevus cells, the hair follicles, or the vascular or lymphatic system.

Many of the disseminated keratoses are also examples of verrucosities, e.g. verrucous varieties of ichthyosis hystrix.

Many of these follow Blaschko's lines (see keratoses).

Acanthosis Nigricans

Acanthosis nigricans shows two features of note. One is a dirty dark brown pigmentation. The second is a roughened condition of the skin with scattered or grouped verrucous elevations. The roughened velvety skin is due to an exaggeration of the normal folds and fissures, which do not disappear on stretching the skin. This irregular surface is studded with verrucous protuberances of a brown or black color. These protuberances are soft, sometimes scaly, and are either sessile or pedunculated. The eruption is symmetrical with somewhat diffuse borders and is located on the axillae, neck, anogenital region, inner aspect of the thighs, and rarely in other large body folds.

John C. Belisario, Australian Dermatologist

In addition to the true acanthosis nigricans (adult or juvenile type), a pseudoacanthosis nigricans eruption is frequently seen in the genitocrural areas of very obese patients.

DIFFERENTIAL DIAGNOSIS

To be considered in the differential diagnosis is the papillomatous light brown verrucous change in each axilla which occurs in the skin over the ectopic hypertrophic breast tissue (so-called axillary tail of Spence) in the last few months of pregnancy. This change is present only in the axilla, only in late pregnancy, and the ectopic hypertrophied breast tissue can be seen and felt beneath the acanthosis nigricans–like change in the axilla. Papilloepitheliomata show no change in the underlying skin.

Cutaneous Papillomatosis (Gougerot and Carteaud Syndrome)

This is manifest by numerous brown, round, flat-topped, well-defined verrucous protuberances about 4 to 5 mm in diameter. As they increase in number, they form confluent reticular plaques. The eruption is located in the intramammary and epigastric areas and extends from there down to the pubic areas and also the axilla. The back can also be involved. The neck and axillary skin is thickened, roughened, and brown. This condition is very rare; some consider it an unusual variant of tinea versicolor.

Verrucous Carcinomas

Verrucous and proliferating carcinomas (Table 36) may be seen in the oral mucosa, on the external genitalia, perianally, and rarely, verrucous carcinomas can occur on the palms and soles, sometimes arising from arsenical keratoses. Bowen's disease may be verrucous. These carcinomas must be distinguished from blastomycosis and verrucous tuberculosis.

Table 36: **Types of Verrucous Carcinoma**

Proposed Names	Involved Areas	Involved Areas
Panoral verrucous carcinoma	Oral cavity Nasal cavity Larynx Esophagus	Oral florid papillomatosis
Anogenital verrucous carcinoma	Penis Scrotum Vulva Anus Rectum Vagina Cervix Buttocks	Giant condyloma acuminata (Buschke and Lowenstein Disease)
Plantar-palmar verrucous carcinoma	Plantar surface Palmar surface	Epithelioma cuniculatum

Alexandre Carteaud, 1897–   French Dermatologist, Paris
Lowenstein
James Spence, 1812–1882, Scottish Surgeon, Edinburgh

Occasionally Verrucous Dermatoses
Syphilis

Verrucous syphilides are either secondary or tertiary forms of syphilis.

Secondary syphilides arise from nummular papules. Generally isolated and not numerous, they occur on the nape of the neck, thorax, or face and assume the shape of distinctly circumscribed, sometimes crusted, verrucous plaques 0.5 cm thick and 1 to 4 cm wide. Hypertrophic mucous patches are also examples of verrucous secondary syphilides.

Tertiary proliferating syphilides may develop on a variety of ulcerations, especially on the ulcerative nodulonodal type. In these cases, verrucous or fungating growths arise, making a differential diagnosis from verrucous carcinomas difficult.

Tuberculosis

Orificial tuberculosis may be verrucous. Mouth, anus, and vulva are the usual sites.

Tuberculosis verrucosa cutis (postmortem or prosector's wart) occurs characteristically on the dorsa of the thumb or index finger. The lesion is up to 3 cm in diameter. Multiple lesions may be present. Rarely, other areas are affected. There are three zones: a peripheral elevated zone, a purplish or brownish verrucous median zone interspersed with small adherent crusts or small cribiform ulcers from which pus droplets can be expressed, and a central zone studded with gray or yellowish horny verrucosities separated by grooves and fissures. The base has a fibrous induration. After healing, scarring occurs.

Deep Mycoses

An appearance identical with or closely analogous to that of verrucous syphilides, verrucous tuberculosis, and verrucous carcinomas may be produced by blastomycosis, sporotrichosis, and coccidioidomycosis. In India and Sri Lanka, rhinosporidiosis may present verrucous lesions, especially on the face.

Drug Eruptions

Iododermas and bromodermas may start as a purulent bulla with an inflammatory base that becomes verrucous at the center and rapidly extends peripherally. Multiple lesions are often present. The margin may be distinctly pustular.

Miscellaneous

Rarely, hypertrophic lichen planus may present as a verrucous lesion, as may some of the lesions of Darier's disease and psoriasis (Fig. 16.6 A and Fig. 16.6 B).

Hypertrophic or verrucous discoid lupus erythematosus may exist as a diffuse plaque or as isolated verrucous nodules, sometimes resembling keratoacanthomas.

Pemphigus vegetans is basically a bullous eruption of the large articular folds, groin, and about the mouth. Rapidly the bullae become verrucous, erosive, and acquire a foul odor. Serpiginous extension and confluence of the lesions causes the

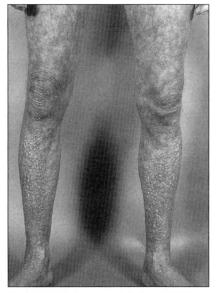

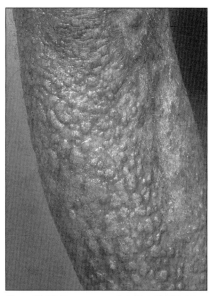

Figure 16.6 A Verrucous paoriasis. Note Cobblestone appearance.

Figure 16.6 B Verrucous paoriasis. Note Cobblestone appearance.

formation of arcuate borders. Frank pustules are common at the periphery. After healing, a brown pigmentation is left.

Verrucous pyodermas are uncommon now, due to effective antimicrobial therapy. These probably are varieties of infectious eczematoid dermatitis (dermatitis vegetans and acrodermatitis of Hallopeau). I am not convinced that these lesions are truly verrucous to the same degree as the verrucous lesions described in this chapter. Blastomycosis-like pyoderma usually occurs in alcoholic, poorly nourished patients who may have an underlying immunologically suppressing disease, e.g. Hodgkins. Such pyoderma frequently follows some innocent trauma and shows peripherally enlarging circinate plaques healing centrally by scar formation. The borders are elevated, fungating, verrucous, and have a heavy black crust beneath which are numerous small abscesses. They have a foul odor, presumably from superinfection with bacteria of the Escherichia coli, Proteus, or Pseudomonas type. This odor is never present in the verrucous lesions of blastomycosis.

Verrucous change in the skin of all forms of elephantiasis is usual (Fig. 16.7). It appears as a roughened cutaneous surface, mamillated and covered with hyperkeratotic verrucosities. Similar findings may be seen on an amputation stump (see also Chapter 19).

Granuloma inguinale, cutaneous leishmaniasis, and yaws may have verrucous lesions. A febrile disease (Verruca peruviana, Carrión's disease) with anemia, bleeding tendency, and disseminated verruca-like lesions should be considered in those who have visited the Peruvian Andes .

Daniel A. Carrion, 1850–1885, Peruvian Student

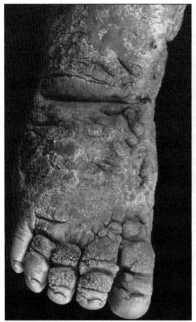
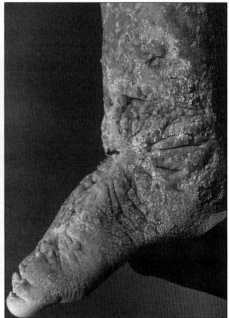

Figure 16.7 A Elephantiasis with verrucous changes, front view.

Figure 16.7 B Elephantiasis with verrucous changes, side view.

Erosive adenomatosis of the nipple is a warty oozing lesion of the nipple.

Warty dyskeratoma is a solitary verrucous papule or nodule usually on the head or neck. Occasionally, capillary or cavernous hemangiomas may be verrucous, especially on the lower legs. They are single as contrasted with angiokeratoma circumscriptum.

There may be a marked verrucous hypertrophy surrounding the various forms of malum perforans. This halo of hyperkeratosis is a common feature of all neuropathic ulcers on weight-bearing areas. At times it is confused with a large fungating wart or with a verrucous carcinoma. It almost never is either.

References

1. Darier J. Textbook of dermatology. Pollitzer S, trans. Philadelphia:Lea & Febiger, 1920.
2. Siemens HW. General diagnosis and therapy of skin diseases. Weiner K, trans. Chicago:University of Chicago Press, 1958.
3. Belisario JC. Cancer of the skin. London:Butterworth, 1959:144–146.

CHAPTER 17

Dyschromias

> *Dyschromia: Abnormal color of skin, hair, nails, or mucosa.*
> *Melanoderma: Secondary post-inflammatory increase in melanin.*
> *Leukoderma: Secondary post-inflammatory decrease in melanin.*
> *Melanosis: Endogenous or primary melanin hyperpigmentation without preceding skin disease..*

Overview

Dyschromia is defined as an abnormal change in the colour of the skin, hair, or mucosae.[1] Erythema is a dyschromia of sorts. For general comments on color in dermatology see Appendix C.

The first point I wish to stress is the mis-use of the term pigmentation. In loose dermatological usage, it covers such colors as the black of some malignant melanomas, the varying shades of brown of some seborrheic keratoses, the brown of stasis "dermatitis", the blue-green of blue nevi, and the slate gray of chloroquine-induced oral mucosal changes. It is obvious that these are all pigmented lesions, but can or should they be grouped all together under the term pigmented? I say no. The actual color seen should be described, not just called pigmented.

The normal skin color is determined by the amount of melanin (brown or red types) and carotene in the skin, the thickness of the stratum corneum, and the amount and degree of oxygenation of the blood.

The color of a skin eruption is composed basically of pigment deposited in the skin and of the color of the blood that fills the cutaneous vessels. So we have to discuss pigments (melanin, hemosiderin, bile, carotene, tattoos, drugs, topical applications, or dirt and debris); intravascular blood (erythema, cyanosis, pallor, and telangiectasia); cells and cellular products (serum, keratinized cells, and cellular deposits), and foreign cells (fungus).

This chapter has been written with emphasis on pigmentation of dermatologic interest. For an encyclopedic listing and discussion of pigmentation of the skin, with stress on pigmentations of general medical interest, see Jegher's article.[2]

Melanin Increase

Localized

Melanin is the most important among the naturally produced pigments and consists of yellow brown granules that accumulate in the cells of the basal layer of the epidermis in the form of supernuclear caps. In fair-skinned races they are less well developed. From here, they go either into the cutis and are picked up by melanophages or are shed from the epidermal surface with desquamation. They give the skin its tan to black (blacks) or yellow (Mongolians) color.*[1]

Freckles (ephelis, ephelides pl.) are small, tan, roundish spots generally under 0.5 cm in diameter (Fig. 17.1). They ordinarily appear in early childhood in areas exposed to sunlight. Extensive freckling is present in persons with red hair. If one wishes, one can restrict the term freckles to the above description only, although there probably is little historical basis for so doing. Duhring in 1876 describes a lentigo as consisting "of pigment deposit, characterized by irregularly shaped, pin-head or pea-sized, yellowish or brownish spots, found usually on the face and backs of the hands".[3] Leider and Rosenblum define a lentigo as "a direct borrowing of the Latin word for a lentil-shaped spot like a freckle".[4]

Portions of the Overview have been taken and modified from Siemens[1] (p. 19).
*Modified from Siemens[1] (p. 49).

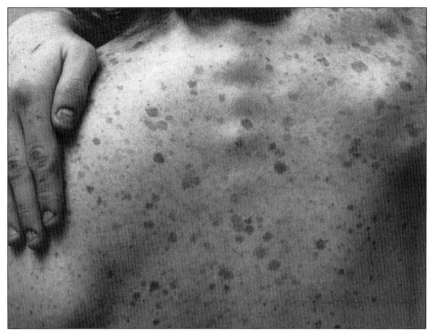

Figure 17.1 Freckles.

In xeroderma pigmentosum, extensive freckling is one of the prominent findings. The freckling is intensive and extensive occurring on such sites as the inner aspect of the arms, forearms, and thighs, where sun freckles are not normally seen. Other findings such as atrophy, telangiectasia, tumor formation and ocular findings, make this condition both a dystrophy as well as a dyschromia.

Large (up to 1.0 cm) irregular stellate black freckles can occur on many areas following extensive use of psoralens and ultra violet light (PUVA) or following massive habitual exposure to sunlight.

The Hutchinson freckle is a multi-hued, brown-black, mottled, irregularly shaped freckle found most commonly on the face of patients over 50 years of age. The pigmentation is composed of fine brown points and irregular length, black or dark brown lines of pigmentation that run throughout the lesion and merge into the normal peripheral skin. In one or several areas, a black papule or nodule may develop, frequently with ulceration. This papulonodular ulcerative lesion developing on lentigo maligna is often a red, in striking contrast to the black or brown color of the freckle. Rarely, Hutchinson's freckle may present as a red patch or plaque similar to Bowen's disease. This has been called an amelanotic Hutchinson freckle.

Solar keratoses frequently have a light brownish color. Although at times this may be from the excess horny layer, in others, it clearly has excess melanin pigment.

Senile ("solar") freckles are 0.5 to 1.0 cm, medium to light brown freckles that slowly increase in size. Their localization is on the dorsa of the hands, forearms, and face. They may or may not be intermingled with solar keratoses and other signs of habitual exposure to sun. They are often associated with seborrheic keratoses, and in fact, most are flat seborrheic keratoses. However, flat pigmented nevi, lentigo maligna, and brown or black macular solar keratoses must be considered in the differential diagnosis. In fact, if all of these are excluded, the entity of senile lentigo may no longer exist.

Junctional nevi in children are often black and nonpalpable. They are often slightly irregular in shape and probably lentigo simplex.

A brown pigmented spot may occur at the site of prior removal of pigmented nevi and malignant melanoma. Nevus spilus, speckled acquired nevus, nevus "en cocarde", halo nevus, and some dysplastic nevi can also present totally, mainly, or partly as a freckle.

Zosteriform lentiginous nevi are freckles arranged in a linear pattern along the lines of Blaschko. They are present at birth and do not change.

Extensive freckling in the vault of the axilla and the torso occurs in individuals with neurofibromatosis.

In the Hutchinson-Peutz-Jegher syndrome small (3 mm) freckles occur on the vermilion area of the lips, on the buccal mucosae, about the mouth, and on the dorsa and sides of the distal portions of the fingers. A similar pigmentary pattern is seen in the Laugier-Hunziker syndrome. A preferred term might be idiopathic lenticular mucocutaneous pigmentation.[5]

In the lentiginosis profusa, or leopard syndrome, there are literally hundreds of irregularly shaped, tan to blackish-brown, pinpoint dots to 5 mm areas. Occasionally, larger lesions may be present. The lesions are most extensive on the face, neck, trunk, and extremities, with fewer on the palms, feet, hands, and in the axillae. The soles and mucous membranes are spared. Scattered tumors (myoblastomas) may also be present. Other general findings such as deafness, ocular hypertelorism, genital hypoplasia, and growth retardation may be present.

Café au lait spots are large (up to 5 cm in diameter), variably shaped, and uniformly light brown or tan. They are usually present at birth and occur anywhere singly or in large numbers. When several of these spots are present, the diagnosis of neurofibromatosis (smaller, regular outline), polyostotic fibrous dysplasia (large lesions, "coast of Maine" outline), and rarely other neurocutaneous syndromes should be considered.

There is an irregular macular pigmentation on the shoulder, anterior chest, or scapular region in the Becker's nevus (pigmentia hairy epidermal nevus). It may be as wide as 20 cm. with thick, dark hairs presenting irregularly through the macular pigmentation. Towards the center, the skin texture becomes thickened and corrugated.

Urticaria pigmentosa is characterized by spots or elevations that are not very prominent, from pinhead to fingernail sized, and of a dusky or tawny color. From a dozen to a couple of hundred spots, the lesions appear mostly on the trunk, but

W. Hunziker
Herald Jos. Jeghers, 1904– U.S. Gastroenterologist
P. Laugier
John Law Augustine Peutz, 1886–1957, Dutch Physician

sometimes on the head and extremities. The pathognomonic sign of urticaria pigmentosa is that these spots become congested, swollen, firm, and distinctly urticarial on active scratching or pressure with a blunt instrument (Darier's sign). Most arise in childhood and disappear by puberty. There are several variations. In some, the lesions may be papular and rarely nodular; in these patients, the lesions are usually less numerous. A solitary nodular type, which when traumatized forms a bulla followed sometimes by a generalized flush or erythema lasting 5 to 10 minutes, has also been recorded. The multiple papule and solitary nodular varieties may also become bullous. The palpable varieties tend to be a lighter shade of brown. In telangiectasia macularis eruptiva perstans, the lesions are macular, light brown, telangiectatic, and less well demarcated. This usually occurs in adults.

The differential diagnosis of urticaria pigmentosa (apart from the characteristic urticaria following trauma), includes (1) with macular type — incontinentia pigmenti (irregular map-like confluent dark brown patches sometimes with whorling), postpyoderma brown staining (larger circular lesions, less brown color), postinflammatory purpuric and nonpurpuric eruptions (syphilitic roseola, lichen planus, post erythema multiforme); (2) with the papular and nodular type — mainly xanthomas (which are corn yellow); and (3) with the solitary type — xanthoendothelioma (more yellowish hue, rougher surface), juvenile melanoma (more reddish and telangiectatic, usually on the face). The urticarial and bullous features may sometimes be quite prominent, and conditions where these are the primary lesions must be considered in the differential diagnosis.

Acanthosis nigricans is a diffuse, brown, velvety verrucosity or fine papillomatosis in the axillae or other body folds. A juvenile variety associated with endocrine abnormalities, a form occurring in the obese, and an adult form frequently associated with an internal adenocarcinoma are the three types (see also "Verrucosities", Chapter 16).

Rarely an irregular freckle may be seen on the hard palate in patients with cutaneous dysplastic naevi.

For papulonodular pigmented black brown tumors, including nevus spilus, see Chapter 11.

A condition called reticular pigmented anomaly of the flexures (Dowling-Degos disease) consists of numerous small (2 to 5 mm), discrete, round or oval, pigmented macules. The vault of the axilla, the genitocrural fold, and scrotum are sites of predilection. The color change is symmetric, progressive, often extensive, asymptomatic, and persistent. Sometimes a lace-like pattern is observed.

Melanoderma

In a sense, melanin hyperpigmentation can be considered the equivalent of a scar after superficial injuries (excoriations, burns) heal without scarring. I call these secondary postinflammatory increases in melanin pigmentation melanodermas, to contrast with the opposite change called leukodermas, which designates secondary decreases or loss of melanin pigmentation following inflammation.

Robert Degos, 1904–1988, French Dermatologist, Paris
G. Dowling, English Dermatologist

Melanoderma occurs following all sorts of cutaneous reactions. It is caused by an increased production or retention of melanin in the skin. A common example is the tanning that develops following a sunburn. In patients with dark skin (brown or black hair), melanodermas develop quite frequently and after seemingly trivial inflammatory reactions. One feature common to many melanodermas is an inflammatory process that severely disturbs the epidermal-dermal junction, e.g. lichen planus, discoid lupus erythematosus, lichenoid drug eruptions, and incontinentia pigmenti. These melanodermas may last much longer (up to 1 year) than other melanodermas, e.g. eczema, dermatitis herpetiformis, impetigo, and psoriasis (which usually last a few months).

Other physical agents causing melanoderma are chronic scratching or rubbing, excoriated acne, ionizing radiation and sequelae to chemical, thermal (including erythema ab igne), and ultraviolet burns.

Not all are described, especially where the color change is not a major part. The color is discussed in the description of many of the other diseases. This description will not be repeated.

Toned Stern

This is a horseshoe-shaped band of light brown pigmentation about the buttocks, occurring in those who sit for prolonged periods on toilet seats. Some underlying disease (e.g. non-tropical sprue) causing malnutrition is often also present.

Incontinentia Pigmenti

There are three stages of incontinentia pigmenti. The first stage is an extensive vesiculobullous eruption arranged in groups and lines, located mainly on the extremities. There is an inflammatory base to many of the blistering lesions. The second stage consists of numerous keratotic, conical shaped, 1.5 cm nodules, usually on the extremities and often on areas of trauma such as the heels. The third stage consists of roughly linear patches and strokes of light slate gray to brown skin pigmentations, any with bizarre patterned edges. Many partial circles and whorls are also present. A few of the areas of pigmentation may be slightly thickened and scaly. The classical V over the spine, the S-shaped arrangement on the abdomen, the inverted U on the upper arm and adjacent chest wall, and the linear arrangement on the extremities all indicate that incontinentia pigmenti follows the lines of Blaschko.

Berloque Dermatitis

This is a browning of the skin of the neck at the sites of application of certain photosensitizing aromatic oils present in perfumes. The sides of the neck are common locations. Perioral brown pigmentation may have a similar cause.

Vagabond's Disease

Infestations with body lice of long standing may produce changes known as vagabond's disease. The skin becomes brown, dry, and scaly, with considerable traumatic eczema, scattered patches of thick crusts, and innumerable new and healed excoriations. This condition is most frequent among street people.

Reticular Pigmentation

This is a type of brown to black, gross, reticular pigmentation occurring in palm-sized areas.[6] The back, nuchae, and clavicular areas are favorite locations. The pigment is melanin. This may follow papular urticaria, late x-ray sequelae, and pigmentation from antimalarial drugs.

Macular amyloid has brown macules with a rippled appearance. It is common on the back.

Melanosis

It would seem appropriate to call the endogenous and primary hyperpigmentations that develop without preceding skin disease melanoses. This includes some conditions where melanin increase is not the cause of the browning.[1]

Primary adrenocortical insufficiency or Addison's disease is a good example of melanosis based on an endocrine disturbance. The browning is strikingly accentuated in areas of the body exposed to the sun, body folds, and at sites of pressure and trauma.

Melanoplakia commonly occurs on the oral mucosa, especially in previously traumatized areas in dark-skinned patients.

Severe cachectic states such as starvation, malignant neoplasms, liver failure, and sprue also give an addisonian melanosis.

Pregnancy causes a melanosis of the nipples, genitalia, linea nigra, and pigmented nevi. In addition, blotchy browning on the face (melasma) may appear.

Metabolic disturbances, especially those involving the liver, may be associated with melanosis, e.g. Wilson's disease, von Gierke's (glycogen storage) disease, Gaucher's disease, and Niemann-Pick disease.

Rarely, a generalized dark blue-black melanosis may develop in a patient with disseminated metastatic malignant melanoma.

The pigmentation on the sun exposed areas of pellagra should be mentioned here.

Facial Melanosis

Hypermelanosis involving the face and neck is common and, often, no final diagnosis is possible. Some of the conditions to be considered are:

1. Genetic and racial factors: Dark-skinned persons often show some irregular areas of increased pigmentation;
2. Endocrine: Facial melanosis is a feature of addisonian pigmentation. Melasma shows a brown hypermelanosis on the cheeks, forehead and chin. Oral contraceptives and pregnancy (endogenous estrogens) are the usual cause in women. Interestingly, the pigmentation often fades after pregnancy; it fades much more slowly when induced by birth control pills. It has been reported after phenytoin use.

Thomas Addison, 1793–1860, English Physician
Phillipe Charles Ernest Gaucher, 1854–1918, French Physician
Albert Niemann, 1880–1921, German Pediatrician and Surgeon
Ludwig Pick, 1868–1944, German Pathologist, Berlin
Edgar Otto Conrad Von Gierke, 1877–1945, German Pathologist
William James Erasmus Wilson, 1809–1884, English Dermatologist

3. Ultraviolet light: This, when combined with drugs taken orally (e.g. amiodarone, chlorpromazine) or applied topically (cosmetics such as musk oil or other perfumes), can produce rather bizarre patterns of pigmentation. This probably explains some of the cases of melasma in males, érythrose pigmentaire péribuccale or Brocq's disease, as well as berlock dermatitis and other acute pigmentary eruptions. Chronic or habitual exposure to light causes the erythromelanosis described in the solar dystrophy section. Both poikiloderma of Civatte and Riehl's melanosis probably are mainly sun-induced from habitual exposure. However, one cannot always rule out, and hence one must think of, some topical or systemic photodynamic chemical exposure.

4. Coal tar exposure: Although rare today, this has been reported as causing a melanosis of the face the same way it used to cause melanosis and keratoses on the exposed areas of the forearms.

5. Keratosis pilaris: This condition can have considerable follicular pigmentation on the face. The follicular keratosis elsewhere and the follicular pattern on the arms and thighs usually helps to make the diagnosis.

Blue Lesions

The brown color of melanin becomes visible on the surface only if it is situated in the epidermis or upper dermis. Pigment that accumulates in the deep cutis in melanophores acts like dark background, which appears blue if seen through a cloudy, but still translucent, skin on top of it. This is the same optical scattering phenomenon that causes the sky to appear blue.

The blue nevus is a circular, blue-green-black papulonodule up to 1.5 cm in diameter, occurring anywhere, and usually present by young adulthood. The mongolian spot is a dark, irregular, bluish patch most frequently located on the lumbosacral area of infants of Oriental ancestry. A certain amount of fading of these lesions occurs with age. When this bluish patch occurs along the area supplied by the fifth cranial nerve (including the sclera), it is called nevus of Ota. Rarely, combinations of blue and true (ordinary) pigmented nevi may present as a bluish papulonodule.

Other blue macules include deep decomposed blood pigments, deep-seated black pigments, blue tattoos (ink, cobalt), bites of crab lice (maculae ceruleae), and deep-seated dilated blood vessels.

Achille Civatte, 1877–1956, French Dermatologist
Gustave Riehl, 1855–1943, Austrian Dermatologist, Vienna

Melanin Decrease
Absent

Partial Albinism

Partial albinism or piebaldism is characterized by the following characteristics.

1. A white forelock involves the anterior scalp and extends down in a triangular shape with the apex on the bridge of the nose. On the forehead, the leukoderma is the manifestation of this white forelock.
2. Large, almost symmetrical areas of loss of pigment appear from the mid-leg to the mid-thigh, from the mid-forearm to the mid-arm, and on the abdomen. The degree of leukoderma varies from case to case. In very light-skinned persons, it may be difficult to define clearly the extent of the leukoderma. The border is not arcuate and not more darkly brown than the ordinary skin color.
3. In the areas of leukoderma and on other normally colored areas are varying-sized light or medium, 1 to 2 cm , freckles. These freckles are generally ovoid in shape and seem to be scattered randomly.
4. In the center of the chin there is an area of leukoderma.
5. The leukoderma is present at birth, and usually other members of the family are involved. Usually there is no change throughout life.

Klein-Waardenburg Syndrome

This consists of a white forelock, hypertelorism, and deafness, as well as scattered areas of loss of pigment. This does not have the distribution of that of partial albinism.

Vogt-Koyanagi-Harada Syndrome

The Vogt-Koyanagi-Harada syndrome is characterized by marked bilateral uveitis associated with symmetrical vitiligo, premature alopecia, white eyelashes and brows, and diminished hearing.

Albinism

The albino has pink skin, white hair, and pink eyes. There is marked hypersensitivity to light. The skin rapidly shows the dystrophic changes of habitual exposure to sun. Other congenital ectodermal defects, mental retardation, deaf-mutism, polydactylia, and retinitis pigmentosa may also be present.

Vitiligo

Vitiligo consists of varying-sized, irregular areas of depigmented skin with white hair. It is commonly located in the flexural and acral areas. The skin surface of the lips and the dorsa of the finger tips and perilungual tissues are often involved. The pulps are spared. Occasionally it is linear. Occasionally marginal inflammation is present. The border of vitiligo is arcuate and is more darkly brown than the normal skin. This

E. Harada, 1892–1947, Japanese Ophthalmologist
D. Klein, 1908– Swiss Geneticist
Yoshizo Koyanagi, 1880–1954, Japanese Ophthalmologist
A. Vogt, 1879–1943, Swiss Ophthalmologist
Petrus Johannes Waardenburg, 1886–1979, Dutch Ophthalmologist

dark border is about 3 mm in diameter. Some follicular brown pigmentation may be present in areas of vitiligo. It is acquired, bilateral, approximately symmetrical, and slowly progressive. It most often starts in young adults. In extensive cases in the fair-skinned, it may be difficult to determine which is the normal skin and which is vitiliginous skin. A family history is common. Alopecia areata and vitiligo may occur together.

Vitiligo may occur about pigmented nevi on the torso in teenagers (halo nevi).

Occupational vitiligo has a different distribution, occurring on contact areas such as the hands, forearms, neck and lower legs, and then later on the genitalia and perianal area.[7] In some patients, very widespread involvement may occur.

Also to be considered is the mountain ash (Rowan tree) leaflet hypopigmented areas in tuberous sclerosis.

Partial Congenital Achromia

Partial congenital achromia (achromic nevus, nevus depigmentosis) could be considered as the opposite of a systematized linear hyperkeratotic nevus. These are varying-sized, milk-white, well-defined linear areas on the extremities. Some lines are thick, some thin, some continuous, some discontinuous. S-shaped, whorling, circular, and oval areas are more commonly seen on the flanks and abdomen, V-shaped areas are seen over the mid-line of the back, and segmental lesions are seen from the center of the back to the flank. The eruption is permanent and nonchanging, is present a birth or early in life, and has no hyperpigmented border around the achromic area. Any hair in the involved area is white. In general, the lines represent those of Blaschko. The skin at the edge of these areas contains the normal amount of pigment. Among the linear lesions there are some islands of normally colored skin.

Leukoderma

Transient secondary depigmentation may also follow a variety of dermatoses such as syphilis or psoriasis. Secondary depigmentations are called leukodermas. In these conditions—as is sometimes the case in primary depigmentations—the pigment is only diminished and not entirely absent. The leukodermas should not be confused with such areas of normal skin which, in the case of widely distributed eruptions, have remained clear. Conversely, the remnants of normally pigmented skin in generalized depigmentations should not be mistaken for hyperpigmentations. In tinea versicolor and other scale-producing dermatoses, sun tanning is locally inhibited by the presence of scale or fungal products. These nontanned areas therefore appear as hypopigmented spots against a generally tanned background[1]*

Lack of pigment, like an excess of pigment, may occur as a "scar equivalent" after superficial injuries to the skin.

---

*Modified from Siemens[1] (p. 21).

Postinflammatory hypopigmentation (leukoderma) is often a curious alternative to melanoderma, and frequently, both occur simultaneously and are called leukomelanoderma. In such cases, the pigment is decreased or absent in the center and increased at the periphery. Two conditions in which this is seen are arsenical melanosis and solar dystrophy.

Atopic Dermatitis

Hypopigmentation following or occurring as a part of the eruption of adult atopic dermatitis is common. Hypopigmentation may also occur in the childhood variety. Often the hypopigmentation occurs in the flexural areas, e.g., elbows, knees, neck, and wrists, at the sites of pre-existing dermatitis. The amount of lichenification, excoriations, and erythema may at times be surprisingly minimal. There may be more pronounced changes at the periphery. There is usually no problem making a diagnosis in these cases.

A diagnosis may be difficult if the hypopigmentation occurs in the outer aspect of the upper arms, upper back, posterior thighs and legs, and cheeks (see pityriasis alba). In these areas, there is a very light, nondescript, branny scale and almost no lichenification. The hypopigmented patches are usually multiple, blotchy, up to 5 cm in diameter, and reasonably, but no sharply, demarcated. Most lesions are basically circular in shape. The border shows a rather quick transformation from the hypopigmentation area to the adjacent normally colored skin. There is no peripheral brown hyperpigmentation. There is no elevated peripheral border.

Hypopigmentation following atopic dermatitis is more common, but less noticed in those of fair skin, and of course is exaggerated by the presence of a suntan in the adjacent skin.

Pityriasis Alba

This is a whitish, hypopigmented, scaly eruption occurring on the cheeks of children. The lesions are up to half-dollar-sized (2.7 cm diameter), are not sharply demarcated, and may number one, two or three on each cheek. Many clinicians believe that pityriasis alba is, in many cases, just a phase of atopic dermatitis. Others consider it a hypopigmentation from a minor external irritant dermatitis.

DIFFERENTIAL DIAGNOSIS

Discoid lupus erythematosus shows, in addition to whitish atrophy, some areas of carmine color, follicular plugging, and an infiltrated border.

Some cases of nonblistering tinea may have a pale center, but there is more scale, especially at the periphery, and the lesion is very well demarcated. Usually a dirty gray brown occurs in the center.

Miscellaneous

Other conditions commonly causing leukoderma are secondary syphilis, pinta, and indeterminate and tuberculoid leprosy. Also, anything that destroys melanocytes will produce leukoderma, e.g., scars and chronic radiodermatitis. Macerated keratin may be whitish, especially between the toes and on the hot sweaty foot.

Yellowing Conditions

In a variety of pathologic conditions, large amounts of bile pigment may enter the circulation, and from there reach the skin and mucosae (conjunctivae) causing a characteristic yellowing (icterus). Rarely, from an intra-abdominal biloma (a collection of bile), the abdominal skin may be stained bile yellow.

The normal pigment of the fat may become visible as a yellow discoloration of the skin. In the xanthosis of small children overfed with carrots or spinach, very large areas of the skin may become yellow due to excessive build-up of carotene. The palms and soles show this particularly well. Localized yellowish areas may be caused by accumulations of lipid or lipid-like masses in or under the translucent epidermis (superficial cysts, enlarged sebaceous glands, sebaceous adenomata, xanthomas).[1*]

The differential diagnosis of yellowish skin papules can be found under xanthoma in "Papular Deposits" in Chapter 11.

Foreign Pigments

Tattoos

Changes in the color of the skin may also be caused by foreign pigments. Best known are the blue patterns of tattoos, which are produced by, for example, the introduction of black india ink into the cutis. The blue color results from the same optical phenomenon that causes deep-seated skin pigment and blood extravasations to appear blue. For the same reason, green patterns evolve from the introduction of blue particles of pigment. Cinnabar and carmine are used to produce red tattoos. Cadmium is used to produce yellow tattoos; cobalt for light blue tattoos. Unintentional tattoos may be caused by gunshot wounds, dirt and debris from mine or mortar explosions, or by abrasions acquired in areas where there is much carboniferous material.[1†]

Drugs

Drugs causing pigmentations can be covered under four headings.[8]

First, some pigmentations are due to actual deposits of the metal or drug. Gold may produce a permanent diffuse blue-gray pigmentation limited to the exposed areas. A faint purplish gingival discoloration may also be seen. Bismuth rarely produces a generalized blue-gray pigmentation (like argyria) and a blue- black bismuth line on the marginal gingiva. The lead line on the gums should also be mentioned. Argyria is the deposition of silver in the dermis and in the mucosae usually after prolonged treatment with silver compounds such as silver nitrate drops or spray. The mouth shows a diffuse slate-gray pigmentation of the gingivae and oral mucosae. The skin assumes a bluish-gray color with accentuation on the exposed areas and over the cartilaginous areas on the head, e.g. nose and ears. The pigmentation is more pronounced on the face, hands, conjunctiva, and fingernails. Cyanosis may be simulated.

---

*Modified from Siemens[1] (p. 24).
†Modified from Siemens[1] (p. 24).

Mepacrine stains all tissues, sweat, and tears a yellowish brown. The sclera are not stained.

Second, some pigmentations are due to overproduction or underproduction of normal body pigments. Trivalent inorganic arsenic (As_2O_3) causes an overproduction of melanin. There is a diffuse hyperchromia predominating in normally colored areas, scars, or cutaneous regions subject to pressure, or it may present as pigmentary spots, which enlarge and become confluent. The color is iron gray, bronze, or even black. The uncovered areas and the mucous membrane are not usually involved. The total body may be darkened with white raindrop areas (leukomelanoderma), or there may just be raindrop dark areas. These are especially noticeable on the torso.

Localized areas of blue-black pigmentation may be produced by any of the antimalarials. It stains positive for both melanin and hemosiderin. These spots are located on the pretibial areas, the face, hard palate, and subungual regions. On the shins, it occurs as irregular patches of varying size. Early lesions resemble ecchymoses. Transverse bands of pigmentation may be seen on the fingernails. Sometimes the lesions of discoid lupus erythematosus become pigmented when they are treated by these drugs. Pigmentation decreases after the drug is stopped.

Melanin deposition is increased as a sequela to fixed drug eruptions. Melasma may be produced by hydantoin and oral contraceptives. Hypermelanosis has also been reported following the use of some anticancer drugs (busulfan, cyclophosphamide, and bleomycin). With bleomycin, peculiar linear brown streaks can occur on the torso. Chlorpromazine and related phenothiazines in large doses produce a purple color, most pronounced on the areas exposed to sun: the face, neck, and hands. Mild pigmentation may also occur on the lid closure line on the cornea and conjunctiva. The pigment is melanin or a close relative thereof. A similar finding can occur from desipramine in normal doses. Adrenocorticotropic hormone may produce pigmentation of an addisonian pattern. Amiodarone can produce a blue-gray pigmentation.

Any lichenoid drug eruption, as from arsenic trioxide or antimalarials, may cause or result in postinflammatory hypermelanosis.

Some drugs may cause a decrease or loss of melanin pigment, e.g. occupational (hydroquinone) vitiligo.

Third, some changes in color are caused by a change in the circulating hemoglobin. Dapsone (diaminodiphenylsulfone), for example, changes hemoglobin to methemoglobin, producing a cyanosis-like color. Carbon monoxide inhaled forms carboxyhemoglobin that gives a cherry red color on the exposed lips.

Fourth, medicaments may, of course, also stain the skin from without. This discoloration is very characteristic of numerous dermatologic preparations such as tars, silver nitrate, anthralin, gentian violet, and potassium permanganate. Repeated topical applications of mercury-containing ointments may give rise to gray-brown pigmentation at the site of application.

Miscellaneous

The cause of taches bleues (maculae cerulea) in infestations with pubic lice is probably hemosiderin. The basic lesion is a macule from 1 to 2 cm in diameter, ovoid in shape and grayish-blue or cyanotic in color. There is no loss of hair, no change in the epidermis, and no palpable change. The lesions are located mainly on the center of the back of the torso, but occasional lesions are present on the front of the torso. They may occur in association with pubic lice on the eyelashes of children.

Some color changes are due to the metabolic production of colored products. Ochronosis shows a bluish-black discoloration in the cartilage of the ears, with thickening. The ear wax is black. Arthropathies and darkening of the urine on standing are also present.

Dirt and Debris

Blackening of horny masses may be caused by their saturation with dirt, as, for example, in the cracks of callouses on the hands and feet. Brownish-black or dirty-gray adherent scales may be seen on the clavicular area, sides of neck, malar and infra-orbital areas and in the scalp of those who do not bathe frequently and with vigour. Also, this "terra firma" may include accumulations of topical medicaments as well as stratum corneum.[9]

Cell and Cellular Products

Cells and cellular products, besides pigments and blood, may also determine the color of pathologic changes in the skin.* Thus the conglomerations of lymphocytes, giant cells, and epithelioid cells that occur in lupus vulgaris appear under glass pressure as a dusky amber color (so-called apple jelly nodule). Cells also cause the purple-red color of lymphomas of the skin and the cooked-ham or copper-colored palmar and plantar lesions of secondary hues. On the other hand, the red spots of lupus erythematosus, the papules of eczema, and wheals disappear completely under glass pressure. Keratinized cells have the brownish yellow color of horny substance (callus, corn, verruca), which color also becomes visible in dried blister tops (sago-grain blisters of tinea pedis). After a prolonged time, keratinized cells may take on a greenish-black color, e.g. Darier's disease and ichthyosis. This gray-brown or black pseudopigmentation of the horny layer is not caused by melanin, but is actually the color of the cells after dehydration. This pseudopigmentation should be distinguished from the various melanodermas. The cause of the black color of the tips of comedones is due to excess production of melanin or oxidation changes in the keratin-sebum, and not due to dirt or other exogenous pigments.

If horny layers are loosely held together, air easily enters and causes a silvery appearance by reflection of light from the separated horny plates (psoriasis). If the horny layer is soaked and waterlogged, it is thrown into coarse folds and finally becomes turbid and white (washerwomen's hands, macerated soles due to hyperhidrosis). On

*Portions have been taken and modified from Siemens[1] (pp. 31, 32, 33, 34).

the mucosae, which normally lack a horny layer, maceration of the upper epithelial layers may create the same milky turbidity (opaline plaques of syphilis). Adherent, persistent masses of pathological cornified epithelium tend to take on a yellowish-white color (leukoplakia). A milky white appearance with more bluish hues may be created by thickening of the granular layer (Wickham's striae in lichen planus and lichen planus of the mucous membrane).

Nonpigmented and scantily vascularized scars show the white color of the connective tissue of the cutis. If, however, the elastic tissue of the cutis has degenerated in a certain way, it may become visible and show a distinct yellow color (pseudoxanthoma elasticum, cutis rhomboidalis nuchae). If the skin is very thin (senile atrophy, acrodermatitis chronica atrophicans), the yellow tendons may be readily visible along with the prominent blue veins.

The yellowish color of serum, like the color of blood, may become noticeable if it leaks from the vessels, as in eczemas.

Foreign Cells

The color of lesions may be influenced by foreign cells attached to the skin externally. This is the case in superficial fungus diseases and is exemplified by the mealy white scales of the *Microsporum* and the lemon yellow accumulations in the scutula (little shields) of favus. Another example is the black silver nitrate-like patches produced by the *Cladosporium werneckii* in tinea nigra on the palms.

Mixed

The presence of a combination of pigments is not rare, and of course complicate evaluation of the dyschromias. For example, in the sequelae of chronic stasis about the ankle, increased melanin and hemosiderosis may occur, and this along with the varying red changes of passive erythema and telangiectasia, and perhaps the yellowish hue of topically applied iodochlorhydroxyquin (Vioform®), may make a most complicated dyschromia.

Table 37: Mucosal Pigmentation

Pigmentation of the Mouth without Skin Pigmentation

1. *Metals:* Lead, bismuth, silver, mercury, copper, and zinc are usually present as a metallic sulfide line on the gums near the teeth. Occasionally, it is more diffusely spread out. Amalgam can present as several dark blue areas usually on or near the alveolar ridge.
2. *Tobacco stains:* Fingers and nails are also usually tobacco stained in most cases.

Pigmentation of the Skin without Pigmentation of the Eyes

1. Carotenemia.
2. Mepacrine pigmentation.

Pigmentation of the Eye Without Pigmentation of the Skin

1. Blue sclera of osteogenesis imperfecta.
2. Kayser-Fleischer ring of Wilson's disease.
3. *Pigmentation of chromium workers:* A band shaped area of brown color is seen in the superficial layer of the cornea, confined to the palpebral aperture.
4. *Copper pigmentation:* A green and reddish brown discoloration of the cornea occurs either from copper injury to the eye or following prolonged copper ingestion (therapeutic).
5. *Siderosis bulbi:* The presence of a particle of iron from outside for any length of time causes a rusty-brown or greenish discoloration of the iris and lens, occasionally in the cornea; in the lens, there is a characteristic rusty deposit in the form of a circle just beneath the anterior capsule.

References

1. Siemens HW. General diagnosis and therapy of skin diseases. Weiner K, trans. Chicago:University of Chicago Press, 1958.
2. Jegher H. Pigmentation of the skin. N Engl J Med 1944; 231:88–99, 122–136, 181–189.
3. Duhring LA. Epitome of diseases of the skin. Philadelphia:Lippincott, 1886:61.
4. Leider M, Rosenblum M. A dictionary of dermatological words, terms and phrases. West Haven, CT:Dome Laboratories, 1976:179–180.
5. Gerbig AW. Idiopathic lenticular mucocutaneous pigmentation or Laugier-Hunziker syndrome with atypical features. Arch Dermatol 1996; 132:844–845.
6. Nagashima M, Ohshiro A, Shimizu N. A peculiar pruriginous dermatosis with gross reticular pigmentation. Japan J Dermatol Series B 1971; 81:38–39.
7. Malten KE, Seutter E, Hara I, Nakajima T. Occupational vitiligo due to paratertiary butylephenol and homologues. Tran St Johns Hosp Dermatol Soc 1971; 57:115–134.
8. Drug-induced pigmentary changes: quarterly review. Br J Dermatol 1973; 89:105–112.
9. Duncan WC, Tschen JA, Knox JM. Terra firma–forme dermatosis. Arch Dermatol 1987; 123:567–568.

CHAPTER 18

Cutaneous Atrophies, Scleroses, and Dystrophies

Atrophy: Diminution in the number or volume of the constituents of the skin, in particular the elastic tissue; it is often associated with sclerosis.

Sclerosis: A condensation and/or overproduction of connective tissue with or without other morphological changes such as atrophy and telangiectasia.

Dystrophy (literally fault of nutrition): A variety of atrophy that may have certain combinations of findings making diagnoses clear.

Overview

Scars, atrophies, and dystrophies in and of themselves may be diagnostic. Consequently, I will spend some space outlining the various findings of morphological significance (Table 38).[1,2]

Although atrophy and sclerosis constitute different and in some respects opposite conditions, they are sometimes difficult to distinguish clinically; they are often combined or associated or follow one another. Therefore it seems sensible to study the diseases in which they occur in the same chapter.

Table 38: **Some Recognizable Patterns of Atrophy**	
Primary Atrophies	Simple Congenital
	Senile
	Striae
	Anetodermas
Secondary Atrophies	Drug
	Post-traumatic-sclerotic atrophy
	Postulcerative
	Postinflammatory
Variegated Atrophy (Poikiloderma)	

Cutaneous sclerosis is a condensation of the skin components. The sclerotic skin may be thickened or normal or even thinned; in the latter case it seems to be atrophic; but it is always more firm, less depressible, generally difficult to fold, and often adherent to the subjacent tissues.[1]

Cutaneous atrophy is a disturbance of the skin in which there is a diminution in the number or volume of its constituents, the elastic tissue in particular. The atrophic skin is more supple, more easily folded, and often thinner than the normal skin. Its color is usually altered, being either pinkish or pearly white. Sometimes, as in certain linear atrophies, the skin seems to be thickened on inspection, while remaining soft, depressible, and easily folded.

A cutaneous dystrophy consists of a combination of findings, including varying degrees and types of sclerosis and atrophy, with other morphological abnormalities. It seems to me this chapter is a logical place to include them as sclerosis and atrophy are prominent features of any dystrophy.

A scar consists of newly developed tissue that has replaced tissue destroyed by a variety of external conditions (e.g. wounds) or diseases (e.g. infections, tumors, inflammations). This new tissue is most often fibrous in nature, but the reconstruction of the skin is imperfect.

In scars, the normal arrangement of the collagen fibers is lost, they can go every which way, the normal papillary arrangement of the upper dermis is destroyed. The latter results in a loss of the normal rete ridges with a corresponding thinning and smoothing out of the epidermis. Histologically, the collagen is more dense than normal and relatively acellular.

The elastic tissue fibers are absent or decreased and are not arranged in a regular organized manner. This, of course, results in a loss of elasticity.

Portions of the Overview have been taken and modified from Darier[1] (p.334) and Siemens[2] (pp. 87–98).

The blood vessels that regenerate in a scar are lacking in regular arrangement and number, with a resulting pale color typical of a scar. At times though, there is an increase in size of some of the superficial vessels.

The pilosebaceous units and the sweat glands may also be damaged, distorted, or destroyed.

In summary, scars consist of rarefied, thinned epidermis over cutis without papillae, hair follicles, or glands. They are poor in blood vessels and elastic fibers. Scarred skin has no surface relief, which is normally formed by follicle openings as well as the furrows corresponding to the papillae and rete ridges. Hence scars are smooth and glossy. A scar may therefore be a secondary sclerosis and a cutaneous atrophy at the same time.

In contrast to spots of leukoderma, where surface relief and follicular pore pattern is normal, scars are completely devoid of follicle openings, or, when present, these are distended into flat, hairless pits. If one tries to pull together the skin of some scars between thumb and index finger, fine, crisp, glossy wrinkles like those of crushed cigarette paper become apparent, because the epidermis is thin and dry. At times, these wrinkles may be particularly fine. In some cases, the epidermis is so tightly attached to the underlying fibrous connective tissue that wrinkles can hardly develop. The scar character of such a lesion can be recognized from the fact that reliefless epidermis can no longer be wrinkled over its dense, immovable, underlying tissue. In this case, a combination of epidermal atrophy and cutaneous fibrosis exists, called a sclerotic or fibrous scar.

If the scarring process involves only the follicles, the result is follicular pits, which are of varying size, some being quite large, deep, and funnel-shaped. These are called follicular scars. They should not be confused with enlarged follicular openings, which, in some persons, occur on the nose, cheeks, and forehead and have a much more uniform appearance (megaloporia). If the follicular scar pits are so dense that they merge, the skin takes on a worm-eaten (vermicular) appearance. Very large, round pits with sharply outlined steep edges may follow necrotic vesicles or necrotic pustules (varicella). They were especially characteristic of smallpox (variola), which explains the term varioliform scars. In general, they are not follicular, but they may also be seen after necrotizing follicular inflammations (acne necrotica). Remnants of destroyed follicles and displaced epithelium may give rise to scar comedones, double comedones, or giant comedones. After an ulcerative breakdown, the skin edges may join together in irregular fashion, forming coarse linear bundles (hidradenitis) or delicate skin bridges (acne vulgaris).

At first, the color of scars is red, but, in the course of months, they grow paler. Finally, the color may become white because the connective tissue, which has lost most of its blood vessels, reveals its own color through the thinned epidermis. Sometimes this connective tissue, by degeneration, takes on a yellow hue. The pale color of anemic connective issue is especially conspicuous because, in general, the epidermis is thinned and no longer forms melanin pigment. Nevertheless, irregularly distributed hyperpigmented spots and halos are found in scars and in their immediate vicinity.

Since lengthened and widened blood vessels (telangiectases) frequently develop in the cutis, which otherwise has very few blood vessels, a characteristic dappled picture may develop. This triple-colored, dappled appearance is composed of the brown of hyperpigmentation; the white of depigmentation, thinned epidermis and sclerotic dermis; and the red of telangiectases. This combination, with a certain degree of atrophy and sclerosis, is called poikiloderma (from poikilos, Greek for "varied, irregular") or variegated atrophy. It may occur as an independent disease entity, but it is typical of x-ray and radium scars as well as xeroderma pigmentosum, in which, because of a certain hereditary sensitivity, ordinary sunlight causes the same effects in the skin (variegated atrophy, later carcinoma formation) as are normally produced only by x-ray and radium exposure or very severe prolonged sun exposure in fair-skinned individuals. Thus xeroderma pigmentosum represents what might be called poikiloderma solare.

Mutilations are caused by the destruction of deeper structures. They may be seen on the fingertips in Raynaud's disease. In epidermolysis bullosa dystrophica, loss of nails, subcutaneous tissue, and bone can occur. It is characteristic of lupus vulgaris that it destroys the skin and cartilage of the nose, leaving a tipless or "worn off nose". Nasal involvement in syphilis is mostly localized in the bony parts, causing the bridge of the nose to collapse, but leaving the tip relatively intact (saddle nose).

Scars may be hypertrophic (raised above) or atrophic (below the level of the skin) (Fig. 18.1). The hypertrophic scar bulges like a tumor and really is a fibroma poor in blood vessels, nuclei, and elastic fibers. It is covered by thinned epidermis without

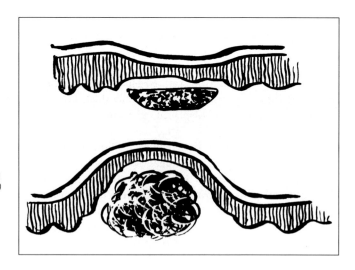

Figure 18.1
Atrophic *(Upper)* and
Hypertrophic *(Lower)*
scars. Redrawn after
Siemens.[2]

rete ridges or appendages. If the scar is very pronounced and exceeds the traumatized area, then characteristic bizarre stripes and oblong extensions develop, suggestive of the claws of a crayfish. The appearance explains the name keloidal scar (Greek, chele, "crayfish claw") given to these lesions. If such fibromas develop without preceding injury, one uses the term genuine or spontaneous keloid. In most cases, it cannot be determined with certainty whether insignificant trauma, e.g. a suppurative folliculitis, might have preceded the keloid. For this reason, the distinction between keloidal scars and true or spontaneous or idiopathic keloids is vague.

In extensive scars, both atrophy and hypertrophy may coexist side by side. Often a scar is first hypertrophic, then flattens in the course of months and years, assuming an atrophic character, a development which is cosmetically desirable and can be enhanced by cautious ionizing radiation or intralesional triamcinolone acetonide.

The smooth glossy surface of scars is subject to various changes. Sometimes remnants of the rhomboidal skin relief may be retained, and scales resembling ichthyosis form. In other cases, keratin formation may become so pronounced that yellow horny masses pile up. Sometimes flaccid blisters filled with serous or hemorrhagic fluid form. Scars can tear forming painful fissures. In other scars, especially those under tension or pressure over bony prominences (as in amputation stumps), areas of necrosis may develop, followed by slow-healing scar ulcers. Shrinking or contraction of scar tissue, after considerable time, may also cause disturbances of motility and various disfigurements (ectropion, pterygium or web formation, microstomia, arm and leg contractures).

It is difficult to define the distinction between an atrophy and an atrophic scar. Primary atrophies are caused by a regressive process without preceding inflammation or other pathologic change. The best-known example is senile atrophy of the skin. In old age the entire skin may become atrophic, i.e. smooth, glossy, largely hairless, excessively easy to shift, and, because of this latter quality, wrinkled like crushed cigarette paper. As always, when large skin areas become thinned, the blue deeper veins and the yellow tendons may become more or less faintly visible. There are histological differences between the primary atrophies and the scar atrophies, although clinically they may have the same degree of smoothness, glossiness, and wrinkling.

If marked degenerative changes occur in the dermal elastic fibers, areas of defect develop into which the palpating finger falls. If such gaps are small and round, they give a feeling similar to that of the button-hole sign of neurofibrometous. There is a round center which can be easily pushed below the level of the surrounding skin. This primary atrophy involving the elastica (anelasty) is termed anetoderma (slack skin). It is true that this anomaly often affects the epidermis also, which becomes extended and loses its rete ridges. Thus, the anelastic foci acquire a great similarity to ordinary atrophies, their surface being smooth and glossy and easily thrown into wrinkles, which, however, bulge a little. The best-known examples of anetodermatic atrophy are the striae of pregnancy, which may occur as long bands as well as diamond-shaped figures. Sometimes the affected areas of the skin look somewhat depressed; sometimes, if the skin has lost its normal tension, they bulge out and form something like a hernia. At the start, their color is erythematous, livid red or bluish; later this is changed, usually to an iridescent white. Occasionally, if other primary atrophies occur in the subcutaneous fat, deep indentations covered with a taut epidermis and dermis may be seen.

Secondary atrophies (Fig. 18.2) can be externally (post-traumatic) or internally caused. These internally caused atrophies can be postulcerative (pyoderma gangrenosum) or postinflammatory (discoid lupus erythematosus).

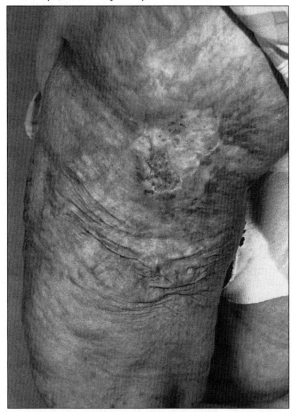

Figure 18.2 Secondary atrophy in thermal burn scar with partially healed ulcer.

A surprising degree of secondary atrophy can occur in this postinflammatory type. At times, it is hard to believe that there was not a preceding ulceration.

As an aside, it is interesting that some dermatoses (e.g. psoriasis, erythroderma) never form scars, even though there may be much visible pathology and even shedding of hair and nails.

The same interstitial processes that cause secondary atrophies (e.g. late radiation sequelae, scleroderma) occasionally lead to a fibrous toughening and hardening or sclerosis. In this case the skin, as in sclerotic scars, is difficult to fold and is immobilized, boardlike, and firmly fixed to its base. In these cases, atrophy and sclerosis may occur next to each other and in the same area successively or next to each other at the same time.

Poikiloderma

Poikiloderma is three-colored, with the brown hyperpigmentation, the white of depigmentation and anemia, and the red of telangiectasis, and always has a certain degree of atrophy, and sometimes sclerosis. If the sclerosis predominates, the condition could be classified as sclerosis.

X-ray poikiloderma is limited to areas exposed to ionizing radiation (Fig. 18.3).

Poikiloderma solare may occur from habitual exposure to sunlight. Poikiloderma congenitale consists of xeroderma pigmentosum, Rothmund-Thomson disease, Bloom's disease, and older patients with Cockayne's syndrome. I suppose extensive varieties of neonatal lupus erythematosus might be considered poikilodermatous. Changes in these diseases are limited to areas exposed to the sun's rays.

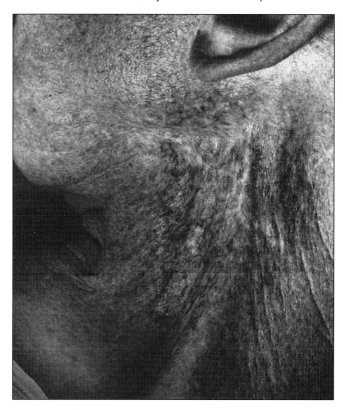

Figure 18.3 Late radiation sequelae.

Poikilodermatomyositis is usually most well developed on the chest, not necessarily limited to those areas exposed to sun. Some areas may assume the morphology of *atrophie blanche*. This condition may be a collagen disease, but may also be a pseudocollagen disease, i.e. as a reaction to an internal cancer. This was Jacobi's original case (poikiloderma vasculare atrophicans). Poikilodermatous changes can also be seen in systemic lupus erythematosus in sclerodactylia (scleropoikiloderma), and mycosis fungoides.

Other sclerosing and atrophying diseases occasionally present poikilodermatous change, perhaps most often seen in lichen sclerosus et atrophicans, rarely in atrophic lichen planus, discoid lupus erythematosus, morphea, or acrodermatitis chronica atrophicans.

Poikiloderma as a stage of parapsoriasis en plaques (mycosis fungoides) has already been described. These lesions tend to be well demarcated, more common on the torso, ovoid, and often preceded by a psoriasis-like (parapsoriatic) eruption. The localized nature of these patches is in distinct contrast with the Jacobi type which tends to be a confluent eruption.

In poikiloderma of Civatte, atrophy and sclerosis are so minimal that the eruption would be better classified as poikiloderma solare. Riehl's melanosis is most likely the same condition. See "Solar and senile dystrophy" later in this chapter for details.

Stasis "dermatitis" (sequelae) with its sclerosis (dermal and hypodermal) and epidermal atrophy, in conjunction with its areas of brown pigmentation, atrophie blanche, and atrophie rouge, may at times be considered a poikiloderma.

Occasionally the sequelae of widespread itchy dermatoses such as lichen simplex chronicus are mottled brown and white with occasional telangiectatic blood vessels. The amount of atrophy is not great, and often there is lichenification rather than sclerosis.

Atrophies
Acrodermatitis Chronica Atrophicans

The basic lesion of acrodermatitis chronica atrophicans consists of atrophy, primary in some cases or else preceded by a red edematous doughy infiltration of firm consistency.[3] From the hands and feet, this scleroedematous infiltration that deforms the fingers and toes invades the forearms and legs, forming ulnar and tibial bands with redness.

The atrophy is red or rose colored, slowly extending, and permanent. The thinned-out skin through which can be seen the venous network and tendons is nearly bald, slightly squamous, and puckers like tissue paper. On touch, the skin is soft.

Fibrous subcutaneous nodules may appear in the extensor surfaces of the elbows, knees, and dorsa of the hands. They may be single or in groups and have a yellow or yellowish white or cyanotic red color.

Eduart Jacobi, 1862–1915, German Dermatologist

Scleroderma-like changes, with whitish-yellow skin that is firmly indurated with indefinite borders, fade gradually into reddish-blue atrophic skin through which veins are visible and prominent. Occasionally, torpid ulcers are present.

A deforming rheumatoid-like arthritis with bone atrophy may be present in the hands and feet. Atrophy of mucous membranes (tongue and nose) and macular atrophy with ballooning on the torso may also be present.

Facial Hemiatrophy of Romberg

Romberg's disease consists of a very marked thinning of the skin of one half of the face, without sclerosis or adhesion. It covers the corresponding half of the palate, the velum, and sometimes the tongue. The prominences of the bony framework are likewise reduced. The skin is white, the sensitivity is intact, but anhidrosis and alopecia are present (cf. coup de sabre, linear scleroderma later in this chapter).

Striae

These scars have been described in the "Overview". They occur in pregnancy, in growing pubescent boys, and in those who do very vigorous physical activity, e.g. wrestling and weight lifting. Also in the axillae and groin, striae may develop following prolonged use of potent topical corticosteroids.

Macular Atrophy

In macular atrophy, there are discrete, multiple, 1 to 2 cm, oval, skin-colored or dirty-brown areas of skin in which it is possible to feel a depression as if there were no corium. The upper torso is the site of predilection. Sometimes there is actual herniation or ballooning out of the atrophic skin. In some cases, the fat may herniate into the atrophic area.

In the anetoderma (slack skin) of Schweninger-Buzzi, the condition is completely noninflammatory; in the anetoderma of Jadassohn, preceding erythematous macules later become atrophic with or without bulging; in the rare Pellizari form, the preceding lesion is an urticaria weal. Rarely, macular atrophies may follow secondary syphilis.

In the macular atrophy following morphea, the truncal areas are larger (up to 4cm across) and not necessarily oval in shape. This is probably the so-called atrophoderma of Pasini and Pierini. In some cases, the atrophy develops in areas where there has been no obvious sclerosis. Considerable brown gray pigmentation may be present. The combination of linear scleroderma, morphea, and atrophoderma of Pasini and Pierini is not uncommon. Herniation is not usually present. Macular atrophy has also been reported in patients who have discoid lupus erythematosus and acrodermatitis chronica atrophicans. Patients with acne vulgaris may develop post acne anetoderma-like scars on the upper back.

Fausto Buzzi, 1890–
Augustin Pasini, 1875–   Italian Dermatologist, Mailand
Pietro Pellizari, 1823–1892, Italian Dermatologist, Florence
Luigi E. Pierini, 1899–1987, Buenos Aires
Moritz Heinrich Romberg, 1795–1873, German Neurologist, Berlin
Ernst Schweninger, 1850–1924, German Dermatologist, Berlin

362 *Morphological Diagnosis of Skin Disease*

Perilesional atrophy of epidermis and dermis has been seen about psoriatic plaques on the buttocks or lower back treated by repeated and frequent applications or injections of potent fluorinated corticosteroids.

Focal Dermal Hypoplasia of Goltz

The lesions are present at birth as irregular linear streaks of telangiectasia, atrophy, and pigmentation on the trunk and limbs. Widely distributed groups of soft nodules are reddish yellow subcutaneous fat herniated through defects in the dermis. Papillomatous lesions may be present on the lips. The nails are dystrophic. Many other skeletal abnormalities also occur. The linear streaks follow Blaschko's lines.

Ehlers-Danlos syndrome shows skin that is easily stretchable but returns to normal. Easy bruising and atrophic patulous scars are often seen on the knees and elbows.

Fat Atrophies

Insulin lipodystrophy presents as a few to numerous localized areas of atrophy of the fat as manifest by depressions in the skin at sites of prior injection of insulin. The size is up to 2 cm. There is no change in the overlying skin. The anterior aspect of the thigh is the usual site.

Progressive lipodystrophy, a very rare disease occurring in women, is symmetrical, starts on the face, and proceeds downward to the lower torso. It is manifest by large, irregular areas of loss of fat tissue and fat pads. This gives the patient a peculiar cachectic appearance from the hips upward with an obesity from the hips down and especially in the thighs.

Miscellaneous

Annular atrophic plaques of the skin occur mainly on the faces of elderly caucasian men. Multiple large (5 to 10 cm) irregularly shaped sclerotic and atrophic plaques with irregular whitish scar-like borders are present. The differential diagnosis includes atypical solar elastoses akin to the pseudocicatrix of Colomb, morphea, discoid lupus erythematosus and lichen sclerosus et atrophicus.[4]

A marked atrophy, particularly of the epidermis and dermis, occurs on the forearms and hands in those with severe crippling rheumatoid arthritis and following prolonged use of systemic corticosteroids. Certain hereditary and congenital syndromes of premature ageing e.g. pangeria (Werner syndrome), agrogeria (Gottron), metageria, total lipodystrophy, Rothmund's syndrome, and progeria (Hutchinson-Gilford syndrome) show extensive atrophy. Very rare linear nevoid atrophy of the epidermis and dermis has been reported. Congenital ectodermal dysplasia of the face is a familial condition that shows areas of atrophy in the temporal regions. In addition, other linear areas of atrophy may be present in the central forehead. Deficient eyebrows, multiple rows of eyelashes, a fleshy nasal tip, and a chin furrow can be present. Diabetic dermopathy presents as discrete varying

Hastings Gilford, 1861–1941, English Physician
C. W. Otto Werner, 1879–1936, German Physician

sized brown atrophic areas on the shins of older diabetics. They are probably post traumatic. Interestingly, it does not occur with necrobiosis lipoidica diabeticorum. Aplasia cutis congenita is a deep defect area, usually on the vertex, present at birth, which heals leaving a white deep sclerotic scar. There are many varieties.[5]

Linear perilymphatic atrophy may be seen following intralymphatic injection of radioactive materials. Penicillamine dermatopathy lesions are characterized by asymptomatic violaceous friable hemorrhagic macules, papules, and plaques that are most commonly located over bony prominences and sites subject to pressure or trauma. Minor trauma often results in ecchymoses or bleeding. Bulla formation has also been observed. Many of these lesions subsequently develop numerous cream-colored milia over their surfaces. Rarely, plaques of lichen planus may show atrophy.

Scleroses

Hypertrophic Scars and Keloids

A description of these two conditions has been given in some detail in the overview for this chapter and is not repeated.

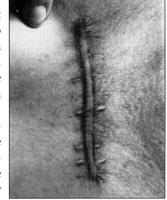

A useful distinction between the two is that hypertrophic scars (Fig. 18.4) are limited in extent to the site of the preceding injury or disease; whereas a keloid characteristically extends beyond these borders. Continuous pressure on an area may prevent the development of a hypertrophic scar (e.g. a belt on an abdominal scar).

Keloids, which may be familial, may occur anywhere, even on the sole of the foot, but they are most commonly seen on the upper torso and deltoid area. Although with treatment they may be flattened out on the upper torso and deltoid, they tend to reform, presumably due to continual tension or from a low-grade underlying grumbling acne.

Figure 18.4 Hypertrophic scar.

DIFFERENTIAL DIAGNOSIS

The differential diagnosis is mainly with malignant fibrous tumors such as dermatofibrosarcoma, although occasionally a recurrent fibrotic amelanotic malignant melanoma presents a similar picture.

Necrobiosis Lipoidica Diabeticorum

This is a brownish or brownish yellow telangiectatic dermal sclerosis with atrophic epidermis. This sclerotic plaque may have a yellowish hue in the center with a violaceous component. Later on it may be darkly pigmented brown. After the lesion has been present for some time, the central atrophy becomes more obvious with a definite central depression and sometimes scaling. Prominence of the hair follicle orifices may be noted. Ulcerations of varying size and extent may be present. There may be a peripheral ridging with a central depressed area. The lesions commonly are located on the shin and present as several, 4 to 5 cm plaques, which may coalesce, or one large long plaque. At times there may be many smaller lesions on the legs, arm, and back. Rarely, they occur on the forearms and temple. In the latter location, it is very similar to the so-called actinic granuloma.

DIFFERENTIAL DIAGNOSIS

The major differential diagnosis includes localized scleroderma, radiodermatitis, sclerosing basal cell carcinoma, granuloma annulare, and sarcoidosis. (For a detailed description of the differential diagnosis, see "Nodular plaques on the shins" in Chapter 12.)

Sclerotic Radiation Sequelae

A typical example might appear on the lower back as four basically rectangular areas of hypopigmentation, the largest being 1.5 by 4 cm. These areas show irregular, dark brown borders surrounding white skin with areas of prominent telangiectasia, especially at the periphery. The epidermis is atrophic with loss of hair and pilosebaceous orifices; there is an underlying sclerosis of the dermis; and the tissue may be fixed to the underlying structure. In some cases, especially following megavoltage radiotherapy (as from cobalt[60]) a marked fibrosis of the skin and subcutaneous tissue may be the major feature. The involved area corresponds to the treated area, and is usually circular or rectangular.

An unusual finding is the development of the clinical and histological sclerotic changes of morphea or lichen sclerosis et atrophicus following radiotherapy, usually for breast cancer. These diseases may be limited to irradiated areas, but may also extend to the non-irradiated skin of the chest, shoulder, flank, and back. Clinically these sclerotic changes have to be distinguished from sclerotic and erysipeloid breast cancer and from radiation sclerosis.

Following radium treatment, the lesion tends to be more sclerotic and adherent with loss of the hypoderm.

Bony malformations due to irradiation of growing bones may be present. In severe cases, noninflammatory ulcerations with a dry yellowish sclerotic base appear. Large ulcerative defects may appear if any of the underlying fat, bone, muscle, or other tissues have been destroyed and sloughed out.

With lower doses, which produce sequelae, basal cell carcinoma may occur. With higher doses, squamous cell carcinoma may occur. Basal cell carcinoma occurs frequently at the border of previously irradiated areas.

Radiation sequelae may also be classified as a dystrophy.

White-Spot Disease

In my opinion, white-spot disease is almost always lichen sclerosus et atrophicans. The basic lesion is an irregular, flat-topped papule, whitish or yellow in color. Delling and follicular plugging are present. There may be peripheral browning. Later, atrophy and plugging become more evident. There may be no scar, but white parchment-like tissue may develop. On the semimucosa of the vulva extending onto the perineum and perianally, a considerable atrophy may occur with all sorts of telangiectatic vessels. Minor bleeding may occur with minor trauma. Lesions are also seen on the surface of the torso (especially on the breast, beneath the brassiere strap on the shoulder), on the groin, or on the back.

DIFFERENTIAL DIAGNOSIS

In very occasional cases, classic buccal mucosal or wrist lesions of lichen planus may also be present. Rarely, atrophic and sclerosing lichen planus (lichen planopilaris) may show scarred areas beside typical lichen planus papules. This is often associated with a scarring alopeia of the scalp and pubic area. Malignant atrophic papulosis of Degos should be considered in the differential diagnosis. I doubt the existence of the entity called guttate morphea. A full description of lichen planus and lichen sclerosis et atrophicus is found in Chapter 11.

Idiopathic guttate hypomelanosis is represented by small, angular depigmented macules with some evidence of epidermal atrophy in some of the lesions. They are most common on the sun-exposed areas of the extremities in both blacks and whites.

Sclerema Neonatorum

Occurring in the newborn, the skin is of a yellowish white color, giving the appearance and impression of soft wax. The feel of the skin and flesh is hard and resisting, but not edematous. The skin is fixed in such a manner that it will not slide over the subjacent muscles, not even on the backs of the hands, where it is normally very loose and pliable. This structure often extends over the whole body, but the skin is particularly rigid in the parts about the face, and on the extremities (see also in Chapter 13).

Scleredema Adultorum

In scleredema adultorum, which is more common in women, one sees and feels swelling and induration of the dermis and hypoderm. The skin is hard, does not pit on pressure, and cannot be picked up. The epidermis and its appendages are not affected. The induration is mainly on the face, neck, and shoulder. There is a mask-like appearance of the face.

Systemic Scleroderma

In systemic scleroderma, the skin of the face, upper trunk, upper limbs, dorsal surfaces of the hands and fingers, and to a lesser extent, the lower trunk, hips, thighs, and legs, show a diffuse thickening, induration, decreased mobility, and obliteration of normal skin lines. There is a mask-like appearance of the face. The mouth shows restriction of opening and of pursing the lips. The hands and fingers are held in a semiflexed position with shortening of the terminal phalanges and increased longitudinal curvature of fingernails. Small pitted scars are present on the tips of the fingers, tip of nose, and rims of ears. More extensive scarred areas are present over the bony prominences of the interphalangeal and metacarpal joints, elbows, and bony prominences of the shoulders. Ulcerations frequently occur in these scars. A profuse arborizing and mat-like telangiectasia is seen on the upper trunk, face, and palms. The scrotal skin is thickened, with partial obliteration of the skin folds and linear areas of telangiectasia also present. There is thickening and sclerosis of the oral mucosa. A mottled light-brown pigmentation is present, especially on the upper torso and upper extremities. In some cases this pigmentation is perifollicular. All terminal hair is sparse. The facial, torso, and limb lanugo hair is absent.

A scleroderma-like syndrome consisting of fasciitis, myositis and eosinophilia (Shulman's syndrome, eosinophilic fasciitis), should be distinguished from systemic scleroderma.

Sclerodactylia

Sclerodactylia (acrosclerosis) is a sclerosing process involving mainly the fingers. They become stiff and semiflexed because of shrinkage of the skin. There is marked board-like induration of the terminal phalanges. The tips of the fingers are round or tapering. Ulceration may occur with the formation of stellate scars. Deformed and stunted nails also are present. The extent of the sclerotic induration decreases proximally from the fingers to the hands, wrists, forearms, and elbows.

Table 39 lists most of the sclerodermoid conditions.

Morphea

Morphea begins as a more or less thickened and indurated, lilac or purplish dermal plaque that slowly increases in size. In a few months, the center is pale and indurated, light brown, from 1 to 20 cm in diameter, of basically oval (but irregular) shape, of whitish or yellowish color and waxy texture. Rarely, the central areas are spotted with pigment, mottled with telangiectatic vessels, or scaly. It is bordered by a zone of mauve or purplish color 0.5 cm in width, the so-called lilac ring. The plaques are of hard or woody consistency; sometimes they are closely adherent to the subjacent layers (bones and muscles). Alopecia, diminished secretions, and decreased sensibility are noted. Rarely, the plaques may be bullous. After a variable course, the lesion stops growing, the lilac ring disappears, the center shrivels, becomes supple, and leaves behind an area of localized brown-colored atrophy. Not all cases appear to go through all phases and not all lesions show a lilac ring. Rarely, morphea may be widespread and also rarely subcutaneous. The pansclerotic type of disseminated morphea may simulate systemic scleroderma, but the fingers and toes are not involved. Nodular or keloidal scleroderma occurs as many bound-down flesh-colored nodules on the torso and upper extremities. It may be a variety of morphea or may be a part of systemic scleroderma.

Lawrence Shulman, 1919–   U.S. Rheumatologist, Baltimore

Table 39: **Sclerodermoid Conditions**	
Genetic	Phenylketonuria
	Progeria
	Werner's syndrome
	Rothmund-Thomson syndrome
	Congenital fascial dystrophy (stiff skin syndrome)
Occupational	Vibration syndrome
	—jackhammer
	—chain saw
	Polyvinyl chloride
	Silicosis
	Epoxy resins
Metabolic	Congenital porphyria
	Porphyria cutanea tarda
	Primary systemic amyloidosis
	Hashimoto's thyroiditis
	Diabetes, childhood, digital sclerosis
	Poems syndrome
	Carcinoid syndrome
	Necrobiosis lipoidica diabeticorum
	Scleromyxedema
	Acromegaly
Immunologic	Chronic graft versus host disease
	Adjuvant disease following cosmetic injections, mammoplasty and rhinoplasty with silicone, paraffin, or other injections
Chemical	Polyvinyl chloride
	Bleomycin
	Isoniazid
	Pentazocaine
	Valproate sodium
	L-5 hydroxytryptophane and carbidopa (1980)
	Epoxy resin vapor
	Vitamin K_1 (locally) phytonadione injection
	Organic solvents
	Nitrofurantoin, hydantoin
	Spanish rapeseed oil disease
Malignant	Carcinoid syndrome
	Metastatic melanoma
	Bronchoalveolar carcinoma
	Paraneoplastic
	Morpheaform basal cell carcinoma
Post-infection	Scleredema
	Acrodermatitis chronica atrophicans
	—Lyme disease
	Partial lipodystrophy
	Hypodermatitis sclerodermiformis (chronic indurative cellulitis)
Neurologic	Dermal fibrosis in spinal cord injury
	Limb immobilization
Post-treatment	Radiation sequelae

Hakaru Hashimoyo, 1881–1934, Japan

Scleroderma-like fibrosis occurs in patients with carcinoid syndrome, in which the fibrosis starts in the feet, ankles, and legs, and then spreads into the thighs and abdomen. There is little epidermal change, and the appendages may be normal.

Scleroderma-like changes in the hands, forearms, and face can occur in porphyria cutanea tarda.

Pseudoscleroderma of the legs due to chronic gravitational edema may resemble the sclerosis seen in the legs in patients with generalized morphea. This has been called chronic indurative cellulitis or lipodermatosclerosis (see under "Stasis Dermatitis Sequelae").

Scleroderma In Bands

Scleroderma may appear in linear bands of approximately 2 to 5 cm in diameter, from the shoulder to the hand, from the pelvis to the heel, or around the torso, usually first obvious in childhood, spreading for a number of years, and then burning itself out to present only as atrophic dirty brown colored bands. Lilac rings are rarely present. The first lesion is commonly the largest, the most sclerotic, and the most deeply pigmented. Pre-pubertal lesions may interfere with growth and function, especially on an extremity. Frontal scleroderma *(coup de sabre)* from the superior orbital foramen across the forehead to the anterior fontanelle is a type of scleroderma in bands. It occurs in a younger age group and should be distinguished from types of facial hematrophy. There is no relationship between the distribution of the bands of scleroderma and the distribution of the cutaneous nerves. The bands follow the lines of Blaschko. Rarely, band-like scleroderma and lichen sclerosus et atrophicans may co-exist. Rarely discoid lupus erythematosus and lupus erythematosus profundus may co-exist.

Annular Scleroderma

Very occasionally, a band of scleroderma may cause an annular or semiannular groove around a limb or around a finger. The stricture may produce edema and elephantiasis below it.

This is to be distinguished from ainhum, a spontaneous amputation of the toes, which is endemic in Negroes in tropical countries and begins in adult life, almost invariably at the little toe, which it strangles and finally separates.

Also different are congenital amputations. This is observed in all races, affects the limbs at any level, and is attributed to an intrauterine constriction by amniotic bands. Separation is incipient at birth and may become complete in a few weeks or years.

Table 40 lists the forms of localized scleroderma.

Table 40: **Localized Scleroderma**	
Morphea	Plaque Guttate Profundus Nodular or keloidal
Linear Scleroderma	En coup de sabre With facial atrophy: Romberg's disease With arthritis, myositis, growth defects of bone
Generalized Morphea	Pansclerotic With lichen sclerosus et atrophicus Pre-systemic scleroderma Atrophoderma of Pasini and Pierini

Morpheaform Basal Cell Carcinoma

The basic lesion of this disease is a sclerotic, poorly demarcated, infiltrating, waxy yellow plaque, with a smooth shiny surface indicating epidermal atrophy. Central ulceration may be present. Numerous telangiectatic blood vessels may traverse the lesion. Almost all lesions are located on the head and neck. Morpheaform basal cell carcinoma is to be distinguished from some other basal carcinomas that have a moderate degree of fibrosis either spontaneously or as a result of treatment. The true morphea type of basal cell carcinoma does not have a pearly border.

Other basal cell carcinomas with fibrosis include the grass fire (or flat cicatricial), the basal cell carcinoma over dermatofibroma and in burn scars. See also Table 33 in Chapter 12.

Other benign and malignant tumors may undergo self-healing with resultant sclerosis. Such healing occurs in basal cell carcinoma and malignant melanoma commonly, and rarely in squamous cell carcinoma. Other tumors, such as seborrheic keratoses and Bowen's disease, may have areas of apparent self-healing, but in these cases, rarely is there scarring. I suspect that the absence of growth is from noninvolvement of certain areas, rather than a true self-healing process.

DIFFERENTIAL DIAGNOSIS

The differential diagnosis includes morphea, discoid lupus erythematosus, and necrobiosis lipoidica diabeticorum.

Carcinoma en Cuirasse

Carcinoma en cuirasse (forming a breastplate) is an erythematous, infiltrating plaque with papules, nodules, and ulcerations. The borders are poorly demarcated with some areas of finger-like projections. At times, portions may look like morphea. Telangiectases and lymph vesicles may also be seen (telangiectatic carcinoma).

Dermatofibrosarcoma

This may present as a very sclerotic nodular tumor.

Stasis "Dermatitis" (Sequelae)

Numerous findings may be present, but the first thing to say is that the word dermatitis is incorrect: late stasis sequelae would be a much more appropriate term, as in many cases there may be no dermatitis.

Sclerosis is a cardinal sign and consists of a dense dermal or hypodermal fibrosis involving the lower leg and ankle areas. The border is reasonably well defined. The inverted milk or champagne bottle leg is a result of this fibrosis.

Epidermal atrophy with smooth shiny skin and loss of appendages is present over the sclerotic areas.

Varying degrees of brown or brown-black pigmentation are usually present. In some cases, this pigmentary change may be so marked that one has to consider the pigmented purpuric eruptions, especially if the fibrosis is not marked.

Edema of the ankles, lower legs, or ankle area is almost always present.

These four findings (sclerosis, atrophy, browning, and edema), really are the basic lesions of late stasis sequelae without which the diagnosis of stasis sequelae should not be made. Many other lesions that can be seen are described below.

The overall picture produced by the sclerosis, atrophy, pigmentation, and edema can be quite variable depending on which element predominates. At times, it can closely resemble cellulitis or erysipelas; at times, it can present with morphea-like sclerosis; at times, it can be bilateral; and at times it can have sharply defined borders. This has been called chronic indurative cellulitis, sclerosing panniculitis, or lipodermatosclerosis.[6,7]

Atrophie blanche consists of white, irregular, slightly depressed stellate or circular scars. They are quite common as part of stasis sequelae and in large vessel ischemic disease. They are called atrophie rouge if they are red. Sometimes these conditions may be present alone, and this represents a variety of purpuric vasculitis (see Chapter 3).

Atrophie blanche or rouge is to be distinguished from round larger atrophic scars formed by healing of stasis ulcers.

Ulcers occurring in stasis sequelae are round or oval, of varying size, usually with a clean base, and have sharp, straight, but not undermined edges. Some extend deeply and look anemic. They are located in the previously described areas of sclerosis. Ischemic or hypertensive ulcers usually occur higher on the leg, are smaller, have a more punched-out appearance, and appear dry and blanched. In some cases, mixed types may occur (see Chapter 14).

Varying numbers and sizes of venous stars, telangiectasis, and external varicose veins may be present.

Varying degrees of eczematous dermatitis (eczema) may be superimposed on the above changes. There may be oozing, crusting, excoriations, and lichenification.

DIFFERENTIAL DIAGNOSIS

Stasis on the legs and ankle can confuse and complicate the diagnosis of such easily diagnosable conditions as lichen planus, granuloma annulare, and morphea, when they occur in an extremity stricken by stasis.

Erysipelas (sometimes recurrent) and occasionally chronic lymphedema as from long-standing stasis or lymphatic obstruction (as in stasis "dermatitis" legs and postradical mastectomy upper extremity swelling) may be nonpitting and occasionally confused with the sclerosis of stasis (cf. Chapter 19).

Acro-angiodermatitis of the feet is an unusual manifestation of severe venous stasis of the legs.[8] What is seen is a combination of dilated capillaries, purpura (and its subsequent hemosiderosis), sclerosis, white atrophic areas, and numerous crescentic shallow ulcerations on the inner dorsal aspect of the first and second and second, and third toes. All of these lesions occur on the extensor surfaces, particularly on the first and second digits, but all digits may be involved as well as the adjacent areas on the dorsa of the feet. The sides of the toes may also be involved. Edema of the feet and ankles is usually present. Rarely, the lesions have an angiomatous component resembling Kaposi's sarcoma.

Dermatofibroma

Usually only one lesion is present in dermatofibroma. The basic lesion is a papule, which rarely is over 1.0 cm in diameter. Rarely, they are giant (over 5 cm). The papule is adherent to the overlying epidermis, but free of deep fascial attachment. The covering epidermis does not wrinkle when the lesion is compressed (Fig. 18.5). Rarely, the lesions appear as livid brown or red firm puckering of the skin. There may be pseudoatrophy of the epidermis with superficial scaling, or the papule may have a smooth surface. The color varies from normal skin color to light-brown and occasionally bluish-black, yellow, or purple. The lesion is most commonly located on the shin, thigh, or forearm. Recurrence after surgical excision may occur. Rarely, picking or digging by the patient may produce a crusted ulcer or healing erosion on the surface.

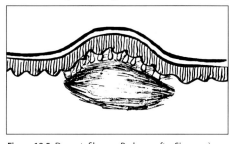

Figure 18.5 Dermatofibroma. Redrawn after Siemens.[2]

Rarely, multiple elongated 5 by 2 mm firm dermal fibrous tumors may be seen all over the torso in the wrinkle lines. This has been called dermatofibrosis lenticularis disseminata.

Generalized eruptive histiocytoma has a more brown granulomatous color and some lesions may spontaneously disappear. This is probably a variant of systemic histiocytosis.

DIFFERENTIAL DIAGNOSIS

The differential diagnosis includes xanthoma (when yellow), malignant melanoma (when dark brown or black), and keloid (when red). Occasionally, a small wen or a secondary tumor deposit may resemble a dermatofibroma.

Other rare fibromatoses may also be seen.[9] The rare connective tissue nevus should be included here as a possibility.

Knuckle Pads

Numerous fibrous thickenings of variable dimension (up to 1.0 cm in diameter) occurring on the extensor surfaces of the proximal area and distal interphalangeal joints of the fingers are known as knuckle pads. Up to a dozen may be present; they are permanent; their surface may be hyperkeratotic; and they are freely movable over the bone, but are firmly embedded in the skin. These thickenings do not occur on the thumbs. Often, they are associated with Dupuytren's contracture of the palmar fibrous tissues. The lesions occur mainly in young adults. The knees and heels may also be involved.

DIFFERENTIAL DIAGNOSIS

The differential diagnosis includes ganglion, xanthoma, reticulohistiocytoma, gouty tophus, rheumatic node, Heberden's node, traumatic lichenification ("gnaw warts") and pump bump.

Mondor's Phlebitis

Thrombophlebitis of the veins in the pectoral region that produces knot-like cords of subcutaneous veins 3 to 5 mm in diameter extending along the anteriolateral thoracic wall like strings of spaghetti is Mondor's phlebitis. Tenderness and slight pain may be present.

Miscellaneous

Lymphangitis dorsalis penis manifests itself as cord-like linear subcutaneous swellings in the postcoronal or dorsal regions of the shaft of the penis. The cords are single, bilateral, or multiple.

Familial cutaneous collagenoma is an inherited condition characterized by multiple, skin colored, dermal nodules symmetrically distributed on the trunk, arms, and neck. The upper two-thirds of the back is the site of greatest concentration and where the lesions are largest and often confluent. There is at times a Christmas tree-like arrangement on the back. Individual lesions are oval, firm to indurated with peau d'orange change in the overlying epidermis.

Shagreen or collagenous patches or plaques may be seen in tuberous sclerosis.

Dermatitis artefacta, particularly on the face may produce a bizarre type scarring at times resembling the end stage of severe scarring discoid lupus erythematosus. Linear scarring is a feature of long-standing hidradenitis suppurativa, especially in the axilla.

Lichen planus can scar. There is much sclerosis in some patients with balanitis xerotica obliterans.

(Le Baron) Guillaume Dupuytren, 1777–1835, French Surgeon
William Heberden, 1710–1801, English Physician
Henri Mondor, 1885–1962, French Surgeon, Paris

Dystrophies

Xeroderma Pigmentosum

This rare disease has clinical findings mainly on the sun-exposed areas of the skin and eyes, but neurological abnormalities, short stature, and immature sexual development may also be present.

In infancy there may be an acute sensitivity to sun as manifest by prolonged erythema, edema, and blistering on minimal sun exposure. In early childhood, freckles develop on the sun-exposed areas, rapidly becoming innumerable. The freckles vary in size from 1 to 10 mm. They have indefinite borders and tend to merge one with another, interspersed with similar-sized leukodermic spots. Each freckle is of the same color throughout, but the color of different freckles may be any shade of brown or black. Hutchinson's freckles (lentigo maligna) may be present.

The skin becomes dry and scaly. Telangiectasias and small areas of hypopigmentation develop. In many cases before puberty the skin becomes atrophic, especially in the leukodermic areas. This atrophy plus the widespread admixture of leukodermatous and brown-black spots and the telangiectatic spots make a poikiloderma solare. The overall appearance of these changes, plus the coarse wrinkling and the yellow-brown old leather look, makes this condition closely resemble skin damaged by habitual exposure to sun.

Solar keratoses, basal and squamous cell carcinomas, and malignant melanomas may also be present. Blepharitis, atrophy of the lower lid, conjunctivitis, and corneal opacities may be present, especially in severe cases.

DIFFERENTIAL DIAGNOSIS

The differential diagnoses of xeroderma pigmentosum are habitually sun-damaged skin, late radiation sequelae, and arsenical melanoderma.

Solar and Senile Dystrophy

I realize that some of the conditions described in this section have been described in other areas of this text. They are included here again because they form an important part of the dystrophies and it would be tiresome and confusing for the reader to be continually referring to other areas.

Changes Caused by Aging and Habitual Exposure to the Sun

Most skin changes can be seen by the time a person reaches the age of 60 years; therefore the term elderly is used to mean 60 years of age and older.[10] Like all biological changes, skin changes vary considerably as to the time of onset and the speed of development. Some appear early, some much later, and all take a number of years to develop fully.

Habitual exposure to sunlight means frequent day-by-day exposure, continuing over a number of years. Exposure may result from an outdoor occupation, as in the case of a farmer or rancher, or it may be recreational. Exposure may be more on some days than others and is usually greater in areas with sunny climates such as Texas or Australia.

Changes from sun damage are more pronounced on the sun-exposed areas of the head and neck. The dorsa of the fingers, hand, forearm, and the upper V of the chest may be involved to a lesser degree. All the sequelae of habitual exposure to sunlight may be seen in xeroderma pigmentosum (in which the changes start earlier in life and are more severe) and in radiodermatitis (in which the changes are restricted to the areas treated by ionizing irradiation, whether sun-exposed or not). The skin beneath the chin is rarely affected by the sun and can, therefore, serve as a basis of comparison to determine if the visible change is caused by age or sun (Table 41).

Summary and comparison of skin changes visible in the elderly and in persons habitually exposed to sunlight is provided in Table 41.

I prefer the term dermatoheliosis (originally proposed by T.B. Fitzpatrick of Boston) to describe all the changes caused by habitual exposure to sun.[11]

The skin changes described for the elderly are not nearly so marked in nonwhite persons. Black residents of the southern United States show few or none of the clinical or histological changes from habitual exposure to sunlight. White persons usually consider sun damage in estimating age, and this probably is why most of them have difficulty judging the age of black persons. Among persons of the white race, sun damage is most extensive in those with blue or green eyes, blond or red hair, and fair complexions—often characteristic of people of northern European, Irish, or Scottish ancestry.

Table 41: **Comparison of Senile and Sun-Damaged Skin**

Structure	Senile Skin	Sun-Damaged Skin
Epidermis	Thin	Keratosis formation
Dermis	Thin, inelastic; wrinkles	Leather-like
Hypoderm	Fold formation	—
Blood Vessels	Ectasias, purpura, venous stars	Diffuse telangiectasia, erythromelanosis colli
Sebaceous Glands	Oiliness of head and scalp	—
Hair	Gray, alopecia	—
Brown Pigmentation	Senile lentigo	Brown, leather color
Eccrine and Apocrine Glands	Dry skin	—
Nails	Dystrophic changes	—
Miscellany	—	Pseudociatrix de Colomb, collagenous plaques, nodular cutaneous elastoides, colloid pseudomilium, disseminated superficial actinic porokeratosis, and stucco keratosis

Colomb

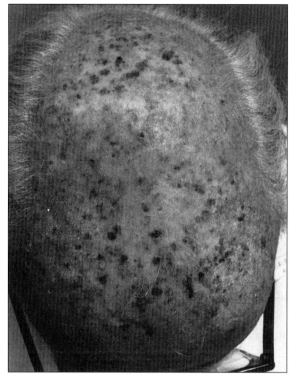

Figure 18.6 Solar dystrophy of the bald pate.

Epidermis

By the time a person reaches the age of 60 years, a general thinning of the epidermis has occurred. This is especially noticeable on the dorsa of the hands, where prominent blue veins and yellow tendons may be seen through the semitranslucent skin. The vulvar skin and adjacent semimucosa show atrophy.

In the habitually sun-exposed skin, numerous sharply demarcated dirty grayish thickenings of the horny layer are common (Fig. 18.6). These horny thickenings (solar keratoses) may vary from an atrophic, telangiectatic, slightly scaly surface to a central keratotic horn. The skin surface of the upper lip is a common location for this kind of lesion especially in women. These lesions always are more easily felt than seen. The scale is extremely adherent and forced removal causes bleeding from the small capillaries. Sometimes large areas of sun-exposed skin (for example, the cheeks) may be involved in this keratotic process. In some patients with severe sun damage, there is a widespread atrophic epidermal change, which results in an overall superficial tightening of the facial skin, resulting in ectropion. The lower vermilion lip may show wrinkling, fissuring, and scaling.

Dermis

In the elderly, all of the skin is thin and inelastic (especially noticeable on the dorsa of the hands) and shows decreased tone. Excessive wrinkling on the forehead, around the eyes (especially the lateral angles), around the mouth, and on the cheeks and neck may result in dermatochalasis, in which the skin hangs in folds. The lips become thin and the vermilion area becomes smaller.

The changes brought about by sunlight are thickening, excessive pebbling, corrugation, wrinkling, and coarse rhomboidal cross-hatching, with a flattening out of the intervening skin line. There very well may be some variation in the degree of telangiectasia. Individuals over 80 years of age seem not to have telangiectases. This is most fully developed on the nape of the neck (cutis rhomboidalis nuchae). The skin feels like leather and has a pale yellow, straw brown, or old ivory color. Pale yellow dotted areas are easily seen on the mustache area, on the temple, and lateral portions of the forehead (where the skin is thinner) and these yellow dots become confluent (solar elastoides). In the center of the forehead and extending down on to the bridge of the nose, in a V shape, this change is not seen.

In the large creases of the forehead and on the posterior aspects of the sides of the neck, linear ridges of yellowish papules can be seen.

Hypoderm

There is considerable loss of subcutaneous fat in the elderly, causing a tendency to skin fold formation in the periorbital, preauricular, circumoral, and neck areas. The sun has no effect on the hypoderm.

Blood Vessels

In the elderly, bright red angiomas up to 5 mm in diameter, usually compressible, are scattered mainly on the torso (senile ectasia, cherry angioma, Campbell de Morgan spots). On the scrotal skin, if keratotic, they are called angiokeratomas. Purplish angiomas of similar size occasionally are seen on the vermilion of the lip and on the pinna. Blotchy areas of hemorrhages of varying sizes produce the usual colors of a bruise (Bateman's or actinic purpura). These are particularly noticeable on the areas exposed to trauma such as the backs of the forearms and arms and on the sun-damaged skin of the V of the neck, especially in females. Venous stars may be particularly evident on the thighs and around the ankles. Pulsating vessels often are seen or can be detected in the temporal area, at the antecubital fossae, on the posterolateral aspect of the hand, and on the sides of the neck. Varicose veins of varying sizes may be present in the lower extremities.

Sun-damaged skin often shows symmetrical diffuse telangiectasia, particularly prominent on the cheeks, sides and wings of the nose, and the neck. Sometimes, amid the telangiectatic areas, are areas relatively free of telangiectasia. On the posterior half of the side of the neck, and involving less of the upper portion than the lower portion, a telangictatic browning occurs in which follicular prominence is marked (erythromelanosis colli). The telangiectatic portion often has an anteroposterior linear aspect. Near the root of the neck, the browning and telangiectatic portions decrease and a semilinear arrangement of the pinhead-sized yellowish dots representing solar elastotic papules is seen. Erythromelanosis colli is probably the same as poikiloderma of Civatte.

Two conditions like erythromelanosis colli, but probably related to a pigmentary photoeruption are Riehl's melanosis, in which pigmentation is brownish-grey and located mainly on the forehead and temples, and Brocq's érythrose péribuccale pigmentaire in which color is mainly peri-oral and central facial.

Another condition closely resembling erythromelanosis colli is the facial follicular inflammatory and atrophic variety of keratosis pilaris. The latter almost always shows keratosis pilaris lesions elsewhere and is more common in the young.

Still another condition in which pinhead-sized dots of pilosebaceous units are found in blacks on the lateral forehead region and sides of neck and nose, is linear papular ectodermal-mesodermal hamartoma.[12]

Other facial melanoses include melasma, pigmenting photo-eruptions (berlock), ashy dermatosis of Ramirez, and the post-inflammatory brown pigmentation following many conditions such as impetigo.

Sebaceous Glands

In the elderly, sebaceous glands may be patulous and overactive on the bald pate, causing oiliness. An oily scaliness may occur in the retroauricular folds, on the glabella, and in the nasolabial folds. On the face and elsewhere, the skin is dry or xerotic, particularly on the lower legs. Yellowish translucent perifollicular papules up to 3 mm in diameter, with central umbilication at each follicular orifice, are frequently present on the forehead and cheeks (senile sebaceous adenoma, senile sebaceous hyperplasia).

Sun damage produces no visible changes in the sebaceous glands. The dryness of aged skin is caused by damage to the epidermis and decreased function of the eccrine and sebaceous glands, attributable to the aging process. Occasionally, prominent blackheads are present on the temples. Large (up to 1 cm) blackheads/cysts sometimes are present on the abdomen and back.

Hair

Usually, by age 60 years, the hair turns gray, particularly on the scalp. Frontotemporal and occipital nonscarring alopecia occurs more prominently in men than in women (male-pattern alopecia). Fine, lanugo-like hairs may persist in these areas, but eventually the loss of hair is complete. Localized areas of alopecia occur on the outer aspects of men's legs. In both sexes, the eyebrows become bushy and ear and nasal vibrissae are more prominent. In women, the facial hair (particularly in the mustache area) becomes more prominent. The sun has no effect on the hair roots.

Melanocytes—Brown Pigmentation

In the elderly, numerous brown and tan freckles of varying size appear on the dorsa of the hands and forearms and on the face (senile lentigo). On the lower legs and ankles, as a result of minute interstitial hemorrhages, large, more or less distinctly

Oswaldo Ramirez, 1924–1985, Salvadoran Dermatologist

outlined spots of a mottled brown and reddish brown color often are present. There are numerous circular or ovoid papular lesions, varying in size from 0.5 to 2 cm in diameter (seborrheic keratoses). These papules are firm, raised, light tan to pitch black in color, and have a verrucose, greasy, fissured, or pitted surface, with a well-defined border. The lesions have a "stuck-on" appearance. Large lesions may be polypoidal in shape. They are commonly seen on the face (especially the temple) and the back. Multiple flabby, light brown, usually small (1 to 2 mm) pedunculated tumors occur on the sides of the neck, in the axillae, and in the genital region (papilloepitheliomata). Occasionally, pea-sized or grape-sized lesions are seen with a seborrheic keratosis-like surface.

Chronically sun-damaged skin may be a diffuse brown leather color or may show light brown freckling amid areas of hypopigmentation.

Eccrine and Apocrine Glands

These glands are decreased in number, size, and function in the elderly, causing dryness. They are not affected by the sun.

Nails

The toenails of the elderly may be thickened, yellow, brittle, and occasionally, long and curved (onychogryphosis). Longitudinal ridges on the fingernails become coarsened, and splitting occurs at the bed or nail plate free margin. Exposure to the sun causes no changes in the nail.

Miscellaneous

Stellate and oval and round scars may be present on the dorsa of the hands and forearms both in the elderly and in those who have sun-damaged skin (pseudocicatrix de Colomb) (Fig. 18.7). These scars often are seen with actinic or Bateman's purpura.

Special Changes from Habitual Exposure to Sunlight

Collagenous plaques on the hands, at sites of trauma, occur in outdoor workers in sunny climates. They consist of small warty papules, yellowish or skin colored, extending in a narrow band, sometimes telangiectatic, at the junction of palmar and dorsal skin from the tip of the thumb around the web to the radial side of the index finger. The ulnar portions of the hand also may be involved. This is very similar to keratoelastoides marginalis of the hands. Other possibly related conditions are acrokeratoelastoidosis and focal acral hyperkeratosis.[13]

Nodular cutaneous elastoides with cysts and comedones (nodular elastosis of Favre-Racouchot) are accumulations of numerous small nodules, usually surmounted by comedones and disordered pilosebaceous elements, resulting in follicular cyst formation. The nodules are yellowish, translucent, and cystic, with dilated hair sacs and atrophic sebaceous glands. They are seen mainly about the orbits, extending to the temporal and zygomatic areas. Usually there is yellowish

M. J. Favre, 1876–1954, French Physician and Dermatologist
J. Racouchot, 1908– French Dermatologist

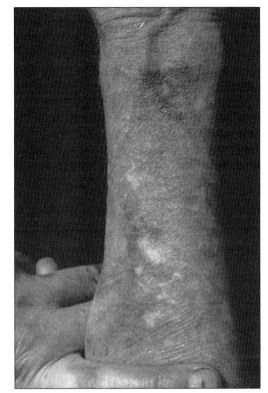

Figure 18.7 Pseudocicatrix and Bateman's (solar) purpura.

leathery skin on the chin. I have seen black follicular lesions on the dorsa of the fingers between the knuckles in severely sun-damaged skin. A related condition is the actinic comedonal plaque.[14]

Colloid pseudomilia (colloid degeneration of the skin, hyaloma, colloid milium, elastosis colloidalis conglomerata, and miliary colloid degeneration of the cutis) are translucent, soft, yellowish, waxy papules, ranging in size from that of a pinhead to that of a pea, disseminated or conglomerated, on light-exposed areas, especially on the upper one-third of the face around the orbits, but also on the dorsa of the hands and forearms, the helixes of the ear, and the neck. A rare type, with nodules and plaques up to 5 cm in diameter and usually with telangictasia, is present on the facial skin.

Disseminated superficial actinic porokeratosis has, as its early or primary lesion, a tiny conically shaped papule, 1 to 3 mm in diameter, usually follicular in location and topped with a small keratotic plug. It is usually brown or brownish red. The plug sometimes falls out, leaving a minute central depression. The papule then enlarges centrifugally, usually leaving a somewhat depressed or atrophic area surrounded by a slightly raised, hyperkeratotic, sharply defined ridge. Sometimes the central area remains pigmented, erythematous, or both, and often it is separated from the border by a hypopigmented zone; some lesions show keratotic papules with delling. Usually, the center is devoid of hairs. The lesion gradually enlarges, making a round or oval shape with a peripheral ridging of brownish-gray color, from 0.5 to 1 cm. Disseminated superficial actinic porokeratosis occurs only on sun-exposed areas, especially on the anterior portion of the legs and outer portion of forearms and arms in women of Celtic ancestry.

Stucco keratoses are grayish-white, brownish-gray, or dirty gray in color, usually found about the ankles, on the dorsa of the feet, and on the outer aspects of the arms and forearms. As with other other keratotic lesions, some are more easily felt than seen. Stucco keratoses are from 2 to 5 mm in diameter, oval or round, with a hard, rough, dry surface. If the keratotic portion is scratched off, there is no bleeding, but a fine scaly collarette is left. The skin in the area is usually dry and wrinkled.

Elastotic nodules of helices and anti-helices are bilateral, semitranslucent whitish to skin-colored nodules, which are about 2 to 4 mm in diameter.[15]

References

1. Darier J. Textbook of dermatology. Pollitzer S, trans. Philadelphia:Lea & Febiger, 1920.
2. Siemens HW. General diagnosis and therapy of skin diseases. Weiner K, trans. Chicago:University of Chicago Press, 1958.
3. Asbrink E, Brehmer-Andersson E, Hovmark A. Acrodermatitis chronica atrophicans—a spirochetosis. Am J Dermatopathol 1986; 8:209–219.
4. Ramos-Caro FA, Podnas S, Ford M, Mullins D, Flowers FP. Annular atrophic plaques of the skin (Christianson's disease). Int J Dermat 1997; 36:518–520.
5. Frieden IJ. Aplasia cutis congenita: a clinical review and proposal for classification. J Am Acad Dermatol 1986; 14:646–660.
6. Ormsby O, Montgomery H. Diseases of the skin. 8th Ed. Philadelphia:Lea & Febiger, 1954:542.
7. Jorizzo JL, White WL, Zanolli MD, Greer ICE, Solomon AR, Jetton RL. Sclerosing panniculitis. Arch Dermatol 1991; 127:554–558.
8. Mali JWH, Kuiper JP, Hamers AA. Acro-angiodermatitis of the foot. AMA Arch Dermatol 1965; 92:515–518.
9. Fleischmajer P, Nedwich A, Reeves JRT. Juvenile fibromatoses. Arch Dermatol 1973; 107:574–579.
10. Jackson R. Solar and senile skin. Geriatrics 1972; 27:106–112.
11. Fitzpatrick TB, Elsen AZ, Wolfe K, Freedburg IM, Austen KF. Dermatology in general medicine textbook and atlas. 3rd Ed. New York:McGraw Hill, 1987;150.
12. Butterworth T, Graham JH. Hamartoma moniliformis. Arch Dermatol 1970; 101:191–205.
13. Rongioletti F. Marginal papular acrokeratodermas. Dermatologica 1994; 188:28–31.
14. Eastern JS, Martin S. Actinic comedonal plaque. J Am Acad Dermatol 1980; 3:633–636.
15. Shbaklo Z, Kibbi AG, Zaynown ST. Multiple harartomas of the ears: A report of a case. J Am Acad Dermatol 1991; 24:293–295.

CHAPTER 19
Hypertrophies

> *Persistent, localized, extensive thickening of all or many layers of the skin.*

Overview

In this chapter I deal with conditions characterized by a persistent increase in the thickness of the skin as a whole. Thickenings of a portion of the skin, e.g. epidermis (keratosis) and dermis (sclerosis), are dealt with elsewhere. Fibrous or fatty thickening of the hypoderm likewise is discussed under the nodal lesions.

Hypertrophies are usually regional, rarely extensive.[1] The boundaries are indistinct. In addition to a variable degree of thickening of the whole skin, there is a change in the consistency. The skin tends to be woody, firm, unyielding, and leaves no dimple on finger pressure. The thickened skin cannot be decreased in size by pressure, it cannot be raised in a fold, and it usually adheres to the subjacent tissues. Occasionally, the consistency is softer and more elastic. The condition of the surface and the color of the affected regions varies greatly.

There are three related processes that must be distinguished from cutaneous hypertrophy. The confusing factor is that these three related processes may precede or become part of the cutaneous hypertrophies. First, inflammatory cellular infiltration is due to multiplication of fixed tissue and circulating blood cells with edema and sometimes damage to lymphatics. Inflammatory edema is frequently the start of cutaneous hypertrophy. Second, fluid exudate that infiltrates the tissue is called edema. It is depressible, plastic, retains the imprint of the finger, and is entirely reducible by compression en masse, even in chronic cases. Edema due to mechanical causes— systemic (cardiac or renal), or local (tumorous lymph glands in the groin)—rarely causes hypertrophies. Various patterns and degrees of facial edema can rarely be seen following acne vulgaris and rosacea. Also rarely seen, is indefinite eyelid and malar edema in hypothyroidism. Third, tumors are circumscribed, heterotopic or hyperplastic, new growths. The distinction between tumors and cutaneous hypertrophies is not always easy, e.g. unilateral elephantiasis of a vulva may resemble a myxoma.

Lymphedema is swelling as a result of obstruction to the outflow of lymph; no matter what the cause. After a long duration, the area becomes enlarged and has a brawny induration which is irreversible and does not pit on pressure. I have used this word interchangeably with elephantiasis.

Descriptions of the nonlymphedematous cutaneous hypertrophies are given as they are discussed.

Scars of certain sorts may be considered as cutaneous hypertrophy, but often the overlying epidermis is atrophic; because of this, scars are considered in Chapter 18.

Lymphedema

The clinical diagnosis of lymphedema (elephantiasis) of the lower extremity is based on (a) exaggerated and deepened skin creases, due to thickened skin and subcutis; (b) a diffuse keratotic change; (c) papillomatosis; and (d) the inability to pinch a fold in the skin at the base of the second toe.

Portions of the Overview have been taken and modified from Darier[1] (pp. 360, 361).

The lower limb, a common site for lymphedema, takes on the appearance of a column or an elephant's leg. The skin is enormously thickened and adherent to the deep tissues. The skin's consistency, which is that of a doughy firmness at the thigh, usually becomes harder and more resistant as it approaches the malleoli, where it is woody. The surface may be smooth and normal color or purplish or brownish; again, it may be covered with laminated scales or cracked hyperkeratoses. In the majority of cases, it is covered by more or less conglomerated verrucosites, rounded, of unequal size from that of a millet-seed to that of a cherry pit. The verrucosities may be pinkish or white, slightly reducible, and translucent like vesicles; in such cases, they are due to lymphangiectases or lymphatic varicosities, which can be pricked with a needle and yield a profuse, prolonged flow of lymph (lymphorrhea). In other cases the verrucosities are hard, polygonal through mutual pressure and are often covered with a hyperkeratotic layer, of dry or oily consistency, that is a dirty gray or blackish color. Under the crusts, as well as in the grooves, a macerated and fetid epidermis is exposed and sometimes ulcers having an irregular outline and a floor with a bloody discharge are present.

On the legs, elephantiasis is unilateral or bilateral. When it is caused by a local lesion, such as an ulcer of the leg, the pachydermia develops below this lesion on the foot. When the causative lesions are situated higher up, the elephantiasis is contrarily often limited by the malleoli and shoe pressure, forming an enormous cushion separated from the foot by one or several deep grooves. The foot may retain its normal volume, but is usually swollen and verrucous in its dorsal region, chiefly near the toes and above the heel. The thighs are invaded from below upward.

Rarely, the elephantotic skin develops palm-sized or larger areas of superficial erosions from which serum exudes. If the leg is elevated consistently, the erosion will heal.

Elephantiasis of the external genital organs constitutes the second seat of election of elephantiasis. In men, hypertrophy of the sheath of the penis may transform this organ into a pear-shaped mass 20 to 40 cm in length. When the scrotum is the seat of elephantiasis, it may become as large as or larger than an adult's head, engulfing the penis. Its surface is smooth or verrucose.

In women, various portions of the vulva, especially the labia majora and minora, or only one of these, assume an enormous size. The condition may simulate a myxoma.

The upper extremities appear transformed into monstrous sausages, constricted at the elbows and wrists (Fig. 19.1). Verrucous changes are less common than on the lower extremities and scrotum.

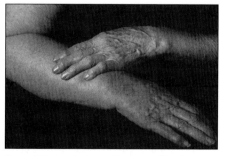

Figure 19.1 Lymphedema of forearm and hand following surgery and ionizing radiation to the axilla.

In the face, elephantiasis generally appears in the form of permanent bloating, a flabby but nonplastic edema, usually consecutive to recurrent erysipelas. Lymphedema may occupy the entire face and be accompanied by lymphatic varicosities of the mouth. In other cases, it predominates in a given region, for example on the ears. The eyelids, especially the lower lid, may become the seat of a smooth pseudomyxomatous globular swelling. On the lips, nose, and chin, elephantiasis may be secondary to the lesions of leprosy, or especially sclerogummatous syphilides; the resulting facies is called leontiasis.

In all kinds of elephantiasis, several territories may be invaded at once or consecutively. At the borders of the elephantiastic regions, the transition into the normal condition is always gradual; the intermediate zone is edematous and soft.

The causes of lymphedema are any disease that destroys lymphatics and/or blocks the outflow of lymph. Some common causes today are (1) longstanding stasis sequelae on the leg and foot, usually with repeated ulcerations; (2) obstruction of outflow by carcinomatous deposits in lymph vessels and lymph nodes that drain the extremities, e.g. groin; (3) obstruction of outflow following extensive surgical removal of lymphatics and lymph nodes; (4) obstruction of outflow following deep radiotherapy with subsequent damage to the lymphatic system; (5) recurrent streptococcal infections, e.g. ear and eyelid, either by themselves or in combination with some of the above conditions; and (6) trauma especially to the pinna in professional boxers.

More unusual causes now are sclerotic and gummatous tuberculosis and syphilis especially involving the lymph nodes and rarely, filiariasis.

In most cases, the morphological diagnosis is obvious and often so is the cause. Of special note is postmastectomy lymphangiosarcoma occurring in the lymphedematous arm or forearm following extensive surgery and radiotherapy for carcinoma of the breast with axillary gland involvement.

Some forms of lymphedema may resemble cutaneous myxedema.

Note that although the changes of stasis may occur with lymphedema, many cases of lymphedema have no stasis sequelae as manifest by dermal sclerosis, epidermal atrophy, browning, and pitting edema. Also, stasis changes rarely occur on the dorsum of the foot where lymphedematous changes are common.

The Melkersson-Rosenthal syndrome consists of a grossly lymphedematous lip (or lips) associated with recurrent facial swellings and paralysis as well as a scrotal tongue. Histologically, it shows a granulomatous inflammation.

Hypertrophies Secondary to Vascular or Neural Malformations

Congenital macroglossia (Table 42) is usually due to a diffuse lymphangioma or cavernous angioma. The same conditions may cause a grossly enlarged lower lip.

Congenital or prepubertal lymphedema may occur due to aplasia or hypoplasia of the lymphatic system, e.g. Milroy's disease. Other causes of congenital or prepubertal lymphedema include diffuse angiomas and lymphangiomas (Fig. 19.2),

William Forsyth Milroy, 1855–1942, U.S. Physician, Omaha, NE

Table 42: **Macroglossia**		
Diffuse		
	Congenital	Down's syndrome
		Beckwith's syndrome
		Cretinism
		Hurler syndrome
		Hunter's syndrome
	Secondary	Acromegaly
		Amyloidosis (primary systemic)
		Melkersson-Rosenthal syndrome
Localized		
	Lymphangioma, cystic hygroma	
	Hemangioma	
	Neurofibromatosis	
	Blockage of the lymphatics with cancer of tongue	

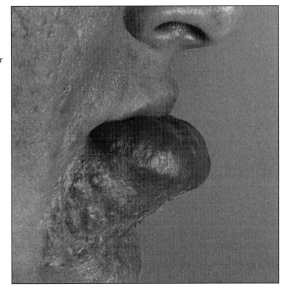

Figure 19.2 Hypertrophy of the lower lip due to a lymphatic and angiomatous malformation.

and sometimes combinations of them both; lymphatic edemas due to tumors or malformations; and neurofibromas or diffuse fibromatosis.

Acromegaly may show a deepening of the lines on the face.

Hypertrophic osteoarthropathy produces clubbing of the distal phalanges and nails. Obesity could be considered a hypertrophy.

Leontiasis (face of a lion), as caused by leprosy, lupus vulgaris, gummatous syphilis, mycosis fungoides, and some lymphomas, presents as nodules arranged in parallel above the brows, down the nose, over the cheeks, the lip, and the chin. Thus the brows deeply overhang the sockets, the eyelids show stasis, and the lips part.

John Bruce Beckwith, 1933– , U.S. Pediatric Pathologist
John Langdon Haydon Down, 1828–1896, British Physician
C. Hunter, 1873–1955, Canadian Dermatologist
Gertrud Hurler, 1889–1965, Austrian Pediatrician

Rhinoscleroma

This is a rare hypertrophy of the nose and upper lip. There are solid elevations on the septum of the nasal fossa or at the columnella and the upper lip, with a smooth tense epidermis of a red-pink or pale color, which develops into a tumor of cartilaginous hardness, resembling a keloid. Scarring and stenosis may occur.

Dermatolyses

These are malformations, usually congenital, consisting of thickening and well-marked loosening of the skin in certain regions of the body. The relaxed skin forms large, thick, and flabby folds, which are dragged down by their own weight so as to cover subjacent parts.

Cutis laxa is a good example of dermatolysis. In cutis hyperelastica (Ehlers-Danlos syndrome) the skin is not distended or loosened, but is of a soft doughy consistency. The skin and joints are very hyperextensible. The skin is fragile and forms of atrophic scars, especially on the knees, elbows, and shins. At the site of traumatic hematomas, there is development of pseudotumors, which are soft and bluish pigmented and present a wrinkled surface. In some cases, small hard subcutaneous nodules form at points of fat necrosis. Some clinicians have suggested that the last two conditions be classified as an atrophy.

Cutis verticis gyrata has furrows in the scalp, over the crown and back of the head, which present a surface which roughly suggests the convolutions of the cerebrum. There may be a few to twelve, fifteen, or more furrows in a particular case.

Pregnancy, senility, or severe weight loss are not true dermatolyses.

The huge plexiform neuromas of neurofibromatosis must be mentioned here because they can present with a gross hypertrophic appearance.

Myxedema

General

The skin is swollen, waxy white, dry, scaly, indurated, and does not retain the imprint of the finger. The hairs fall out, the sebaceous and sweat secretions are decreased. There is also a bloated full-moon face, hanging cheeks, large nose, and swollen and open lips. The buccal mucosa may be swollen and waxy. The palms and soles are dry and fissured.

Localized

The skin shows single to multiple, thick, firm, nonpitting, indurated plaques or nodules situated usually in the pretibial area, but sometimes on other sites such as the dorsum of the feet. The nodules may be up to 5 cm in diameter. The surface is tawny and resembles pigskin. Hair is tawny and resembles pigskin. Hair is sparse in the lesions. Very rarely, these lesions may occur elsewhere on the body.

Reference

1. Darier J. Textbook of dermatology. Pollitzer S, trans. Philadelphia:Lea & Febiger, 1920.

CHAPTER 20

Folliculoses

Supperative, acneform, and keratotic eruptions that primarily involve the pilosebaceous unit..

Overview

The pilosebaceous unit, including the hair follicle, can react to disease in a variety of ways. Follicular eczemas, purpuras, pustules, atrophies, and keratoses are some examples.[1]

In adults, pustules are commonly related to hair follicles and in infants to the openings of eccrine sweat glands. If the process of suppuration takes place in a hair follicle, the pustule and the surrounding infiltrate are raised and resemble a cone or a blunted pyramid (Fig. 20.1). This, plus the pattern of follicular involvement, makes it easy to distinguish follicular and nonfollicular pustules. A hair can often be detected in the center of a follicular pustule. If the lower or lowest portion of the follicle is involved, the conical shape is not so obvious.

The acne papule is a special type of follicular lesion. In this lesion, the hair follicle is closed by a horny plug. Rupture of a sebaceous gland causes a cellular inflammatory exudate. In the early stages, papule formation dominates the picture, later the pus, which has been forming as a small abscess in the perifollicular cutis, appears as a pointed pustule on the surface. Frequently, perforation does not take place in the center, which is plugged, but somewhere at the side. Pathologically, the acne papule/pustule is a small perifollicular abscess often with associated foreign body granuloma formation, whereas clinically, it is a combination of papule and pustule.

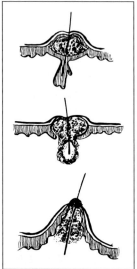

Figure 20.1
Upper: Osteofolliculitis.
Middle: Deep folliculitis.
Lower: Acne pustule.
Redrawn after Siemens.[1]

If a severe inflammatory process involves the follicle more deeply and causes necrosis and separation of the dead central core, we are dealing with a boil or furuncle (Fig. 20.2).[2] The furuncle is a deep, necrotizing type of folliculitis. When several adjoining furuncles coalesce to form a single focus, the condition is called a carbuncle.

I have included the scarring depilating folliculoses under "Alopecias" in Chapter 21. It seemed to be easier to consider all of the diseases producing alopecia in one place.

Follicular keratoses are part of the folliculoses. They frequently have a keratotic character, i.e. they form hard granules that cannot be easily removed from the skin. This is certainly true of diseases in which comedo-like, pinhead-sized or larger, brown to black, horny plugs fill the follicles (pityriasis rubra pilaris) or protrude as dark granules or little balls from the follicles (discoid lupus erythematosus). The latter eventually drop out, leaving pitted follicular scars. Sometimes the skin between the follicles is covered with a whitish, chalk-like to blackish scale. If one carefully lifts this

Portions of the Overview have been taken and modified from Siemens[1] (pp. 53, 114).

coherent scale cover, small pointed horny pegs corresponding to the follicle openings may adhere to the undersurface of the scale. This type of scale is characteristic of lupus erythe-matosus, the so-called "carpet tack" scale. In some nonscarring conditions, they are of lighter color and more spiny, so that an area of the skin in which all follicles are involved feels like a grater (keratosis pilaris). If the follicular scales are still thinner, they may be found in each follicle as short, whitish filaments sticking out from the surface more or less perpendicularly (lichen spinulosus). If they are not pointed, but rather roundish, they may look like hard papules (keratosis follicularis,

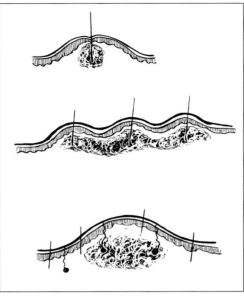

Figure 20.2 *Upper:* Furuncle. *Middle:* Carbuncle. *Lower:* Hidradentis. Redrawn after Darier.[2]

Darier's disease). All these plugs, spines, and filaments may take the place of hairs, or such horny elements may be present beside hairs (scarring alopecias, lupus erythematosus).

Acute Suppurative Folliculitis

Sycosis Simplex

Acute suppurative staphylococcal folliculitis of the hairy regions affects the mustache, beard, pubic area, axillae, and in children, the hairy scalp. The basic lesion is a peripilar pustule beginning deep or becoming so later. The lesions are scattered irregularly or they may be grouped or clustered. Suppuration is usually primary and early, but sometimes the lesions start as deep follicular papules or even extensive tender tight soft elevations and suppurate only secondarily. The hairs can be pulled out easily and their roots are surrounded by a gelatinous translucent sheath. This finding distinguishes a follicular from a nonfollicular pyoderma.

Other follicular staphylococcal disease may also be present in the nasal fossae and styes may occur on the eyelid margins.

There may be basic underlying causes such as seborrhea on the face and torso (follicular seborrhea), pediculosis on the scalp, and scabies in the pubic area.

Stye

A stye (hordeolum) is staphylococcal folliculitis of the eyelash follicle on the eyelid margin. An erythematous tender follicular papule, which may be topped by a pustule, develops. The perifollicular tissue is edematous and inflamed. Multiple lesions may be present. Other associated pyoderma lesions may be present. Chronic seborrheic blepharitis may also be present.

Furuncle

A furuncle (boil) is a massive staphylococcal folliculitis with an acute inflammatory course and much necrosis. A boil starts with a red pointed elevation with a hair in the center, the two essential features being induration and pain. There is often considerable edema and a varying degree of erythema. In 3 to 5 days, the growing protuberance has assumed a purplish, later pustular, apex. Then the boil softens, opens, and discharges pus. The core or slough of necrotic tissue infiltrated with pus, is eliminated. The pain subsides when the pus drains out. Boils leave a scar unless they are aborted by early systemic antibacterial therapy. They may occur at any site, but the nape of the neck, the back, the buttocks, the nares, and the thighs are commonly involved areas. Interestingly, skin areas that often contain staphylococci are common sites of boils, e.g. the external auditory meatus, the upper lip (from nasal vestibule), and the perianal area. Regional adenitis and fever are uncommon.

DIFFERENTIAL DIAGNOSIS
A furuncle differs from ordinary suppurative folliculitis by the severity of the inflammatory reaction, the induration of the tissues, the pain, and the presence of a central core of slough. Other conditions to be considered in the differential diagnosis are oriental boil (cutaneous leishmaniasis), myiasis, hidradenitis suppurativa, and deep nodular acne. Rarely, anthrax should be considered.

Carbuncle

The inflammation of a furuncle almost always remains globular, definitely circumscribed, with a follicle in the center even though the inflammation may extend into the hypoderm. In a carbuncle, the infection spreads into the hypoderm and then laterally and toward the surface to appear as a group of secondary furunculoid elevations. A carbuncle therefore has several openings from which pus can be expressed. The local and systemic effects are much greater in a carbuncle than a furuncle and it always leaves considerable scarring. The nape of the neck is a common site. Carbuncles are more common in persons with decreased immunity.

All forms of staphylococcal folliculitis are now rather uncommon probably because of the efficacy of topical and systemic antibacterial therapy. Also, I suspect the extensive use of ordinary and antibacterial soaps and general cleanliness have played a role in the diminution. Certainly, the chronic scarring forms are rarely seen now except in persons debilitated by disease of immunosuppressive therapy. Job's syndrome is a state of recurrent staphylococcal infections with only minimal reactive inflammation. It usually occurs in red-haired females with atopic-like features.

Job – Successful farmer from the land of Uz (Edom), c. 1000BC, Holy Bible, Old Testament

I want to re-emphasize the difference between acute staphylococcal and acute streptococcal infections of the skin. Staphylococcal infections are characterized by a tendency to localization, extensive pus formation, pain, and lack of systemic reaction. Streptococcal infections are characterized by the tendency to a spreading erythema with lymphangitis and lymphadenitis, relatively little pus, and fever and chills.

Acute Trichophytic Folliculitides

Acute fungal (trichophytic) folliculitides (kerion) are peripilar pustules, with a fairly intense inflammatory zone and a rapidly swelling base; they become agglomerated into sharply demarcated, livid red, raised, boggy, circular, edematous masses from which pus escapes through numerous orifices on pressure; sometimes a purulent slough occurs. Patches gradually extend peripherally and new lesions at a distance may occur. The first lesions are the biggest (up to 7 cm in diameter) and most inflamed. Later lesions at a distance (sometimes in bomb-explosion pattern) are smaller and less inflamed. The hairs in the middle of the patch easily come out with forceps and are lustreless. The lower portion is covered by a white gelatinous sheath. Regional adenitis is common. The skin between the lesions is normal. Some scarring and alopecia may occur. There may be various degrees of inflammation with red circles or arcs and peripheral less suppurative follicular papules.

The eruption of the lichenoid follicular trichophytids consists of small perifollicular and follicular, skin-colored papules and is located mainly on the chest, abdomen, and back. It is usually associated with a kerion of the hairy parts of the scalp or beard area.

The following names have been used for this condition: sycosis trichophytica barbae (beard area), kerion celsi (hairy scalp of children or adults), and folliculitis agminata (smooth parts such as the wrists, forearms, legs and neck).

The main differential diagnoses are the pyogenic folliculitides, which do not form as distinctly circumscribed round areas and are more apt to be disseminated. The pyogenic folliculitides are usually smaller lesions. They are common on the upper lip where kerion is rare. Furuncle and carbuncle have a more pronounced and extensive inflammatory edema, are more deeply infiltrated, and much more painful.

Trichophyton Granuloma

Trichophyton granuloma lesions (Majocchi's granuloma, granuloma tricofitico) consist of inflammatory, sometimes crusted, follicular papular granulomas often interspersed and surrounded by a superficial scaly dermatitis. Parts of the border may be arcuate. Sometimes the granulomas become soft and break down, discharging a small amount of serosanguineous fluid. The lesions are usually solitary and are commonly located on the shins of women. Non-blistering tinea is often present on the soles and in the toenails.

Psoriasis is the most common differential diagnosis.

Herpetic Sycosis

Occasionally, recurrent herpes simplex in the beard area of men may be extensive and of follicular localization. The presence of blisters and groupings in some areas confirm the diagnosis. Viral infections due to the herpes zoster and molluscum viruses have been reported with a follicular distribution on the beard area, chest, back, and neck.[3]

Acnes

Acne Vulgaris

The acnes form a rather complicated morphological picture with many different lesions and many different combinations of lesions.*[4] Some have been separated from acne vulgaris and given special names, e.g. acné excoriée des jeunes filles and acne conglobata. The various lesions seen are described and occasionally special types referred to.

Comedones are pinpoint- to pinhead-sized, brown to black, follicular plugs scattered on face, scalp, neck, upper back, and upper chest (Table 43). By applying pressure, they can be squeezed out in the form of a firm yellowish mass with a blackhead, followed by a white unctuous filament resembling vermicelli or a blackheaded worm. Closed comedones are cream colored. Sometimes double comedones are encountered, meaning comedones situated very close together with a communicating base. The comedo results from an osteofollicular hyperkeratosis; its configuration is that of a small cylinder formed by concentric horny lamellae. The exposed surface is colored, not by a deposit of dirt, but through oxidation of the keratin itself and from melanin pigmentation.

Table 43: **Occurrence of Comedones**
Acne vulgaris
Dermatoheliosis
Acne venenata, tars and oils, pomade or cosmetic acne
Giant torso comedones
Acne conglobata
Ionizing radiation reactions
Nevus comedonicus

Numerous, conical, erythematous, well-defined papules, usually about 2 mm in diameter, are present on the face and back. These are confluent in many places. Some are pericomedonal.

Follicular and pericomedonal pustules of 1 to 3 mm in diameter with an erythematous halo of 1 to 2 mm also are present.

*An interesting report of a Consensus Conference on Acne Classification has appeared.[4] Two points of note. Acne vulgaris was classified into inflammatory and noninflammatory. The authors point out that "a strictly quantitative definition of acne severity cannot be established because of the variable expression of the disease."

Acne venenata can be caused by the repeated application of oils and tars and can present basic lesions identical to these three acne lesions: comedones, papules, and pustules. With crude (black or black-green) coal tar, the eruption is more folliculopustular than comedonal. Also, of course, these eruptions occur at sites of exposure, e.g. legs, forearms, where vulgar acne does not occur. Pomade acne, cosmetic acne, and chloracne are other names given to acne produced by the application of the named agent.

Dermal erythematous nodules are about 1 cm in diameter, with a firm consistency and tenderness, sometimes fluctuant, not fixed to deeper underlying tissue; these are relatively few in number and scattered over the upper chest, back, neck, and outer aspects of the arms. Sometimes, these acneform lesions are pseudocystic containing a seropurulent material; sometimes; they are tender and surrounded by a 1 to 2 cm area of erythema; sometimes, they are quite firm, having a fibrotic consistency; sometimes, they are dark bluish in color. They may occur in hairy facial moles. They are common after the age of 20 years, especially on the chin in women. Amazingly, recurrence at the same site is not unusual.

Sometimes there is dark brownish black extensive crusting on the upper chest and upper back, beneath which there are irregular, well-defined shallow ulcerations (formed from confluent lesions in some cases) varying in size from 1 cm to several centimeters (Fig. 20.3). The edges are shaggy and the defect contains yellow pus. This ecthymatous acne rarely occurs in the face or neck and can be distinguished from true ecthyma by the presence of other acne lesions and by its distribution. This has been called acne fulminans or acute febrile ulcerative conglobate acne with polyarthralgia.

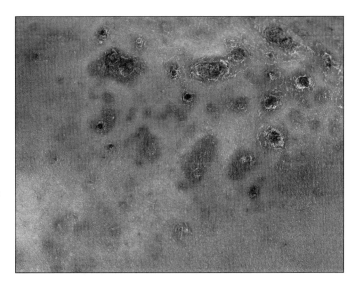

Figure 20.3
Ecthymatous acne.

Enlarged pores (megaloporia, patulous orifices) are especially common in the infra-orbital areas and are commonly associated with a reddish brown color and seborrheic scale. These patients are usually rosaceous (i.e., they flush and blush easily).

Skin-colored 1 to 2 mm pits may be seen on the cheeks; some pits have straight walls, others have sloping sides. These are the follicular scars of acne. Other scarring lesions of acne are as follows (Table 44). On the upper chest and back

Table 44: **Types of Acne Scars**
Pitted (ice pick)
Atrophic
Hypertrophic
Scars from trauma to acne
Keloidal
Associated with sinuses and fistulae
Acne keloidalis
Scars of acne conglobata
Varioliform
Scars with altered color
Treatment scar
Scars with calcification

there are some oval-shaped, erythematous, 1cm long, well-defined atrophic areas with a loss of elasticity in underlying tissue. The epidermis shows cross-striations. Scar tissue bridges and varioliform scars may also be present. At times, dome-shaped, round, 1.0 cm, hypertrophic scars are found on the upper chest or back, presumably at the site of prior lesions. This is not acne keloidalis. In some severe acnes, all sorts of scarring may occur as well as keloid formation, e.g. linear scars on the face and true keloids on the chest. Dermal, bluish firm papules, 1 to 2 mm in diameter, may be seen scattered randomly over the cheeks in those who are scarred by acne. These calcific or ossific deposits can be extruded by incising the overlying skin. The bluish color is probably caused by deposition of tetrcycline. The scarring of discoid lupus erythematosus must be distinguished from the scarring of acne.

Rarely, on the cheeks, confluence of many deep cystic granulomas can cause intercommunicating sinuses and fistulae. Pressure on one portion may cause discharge of a foul-smelling serosanguineous or cheesy material.

Acné excoriée des jeunes filles is commonly seen. Basically it is a polymorphous acne (papules, pustules, blackheads, acneform granulomas, megaloporia, follicular pitted scars), which has been traumatized by squeezing, picking, rubbing, or too strong or overenthusiastic cleansing. The tops are off the pustules and papules and replaced by small bloody or serous crusts. Light brown hyperpigmentation is a common sequela. In some cases, every lesion has been traumatized and if the acne has involved the outer aspects of the arms and the upper back it may be difficult to find the basic acne lesion. In these cases, one should consider neurotic excoriations and dermatitis artefacta.

Actually, any type of acne may have a superadded traumatic factor (acne mechanica). When the monomorphous granulomatous type is repeatedly squeezed, the lesions have an irritated appearance, last longer than normal, scar more, and have a residual brown pigmentation. The skin is also thickened. These findings are particularly common on the ear lobes and in the retroauricular fissures where repeated squeezing is the rule rather than the exception.

Varying-sized cystic structures from a pinhead-sized milia to a grape-sized wen may also be present. The level of the wens in the skin is quite variable—some are just covered by the epidermis, others are hypodermal.

You will notice that I have kept two terms (cyst and granuloma) to describe the deep dermal or dermal subcutaneous nodules, abscesses, or cysts. A few words of clarification on these terms is needed.

1. The basic or onset lesion in all these lesions is a rupture of the pilosebaceous unit with release of sebum, which causes the development, histologically, of a granulomatous reaction. This is manifest clinically by a dermal inflammatory nodule of varying size and varying depth. When the lesion is small it tends to be quite firm with an accompanying inflammatory red color. As it gets bigger the nodule tends to grow darker red and has a feel of containing some fluid material. Actually, it contains a mixture of blood, serum, inflammatory cells, giant cells, and pus cells. Histologically this is a granuloma or a granulomatous abscess. These are the terms that I have used in this text—to wit—acne granuloma or granulomatous acne.

2. Non-inflammatory, lined, varying sized, cystic structures containing cheesy keratinous material can also be seen in some patients with acne, usually after many years of acne when the acute inflammatory lesions have long gone. These are cysts and should be so called.

3. The use of the term cystic acne is not correct. The lesions are granulomas, and if large enough and somewhat fluctuant, they are abscesses. To use the word cyst for these lesions is incorrect. There is such a thing as cysts in patients who have acne, but the inflammatory lesions are not cysts either clinically or histologically.

Varying degrees of dry and oily seborrhea are often present with a greasy nasolabial erythema, a diffusely scaly scalp, and oily hair. This must be distinguished from psoriasis and from seborrhea due to parkinsonism-inducing psychotherapeutic drugs. Occasionally this seborrhea is aggravated by light.

Polymorphous acne especially in blue-eyed fair-skinned individuals may be associated with an increased tendency to flush and blush, megaloporia, and central facial brown erythema. I call this rosaceous acne. Permanent erythema and telangiectatic blood vessels are not features of this rosaceous acne and thereby distinguish it from acne rosacea, as also does the presence of comedones.

Neonatal acne can be present at birth usually with blackheads, pustules, and milia. In prepubertal children occasionally polymorphous acne complete with blackheads, pustules, cysts, dermal nodules, and scarring may be present. Infantile acne always occurs in the face, particularly the cheeks.

Some drugs (especially testosterone, but also iodides, phenytoin, bromides, systemic steroids, lithium carbonate, and isonicotinic acid hydrazide) may produce all or some of the features of acne as described above. However, there is usually some history or findings of pre-existing acne so that these drugs are aggravating rather than causative. The clinical features often include extensive deep cystic disease. Of course, mixtures of all the eleven features outlined may occur. Also, many cases will present with one of the eleven features predominating. In addition, some may show one type predominantly on the face and another on the upper torso.

The localization of acne is usually innate or individualized and may be determined by the sun (back and forehead), by irritation from tight hat bands, turtle neck sweaters, and sports gear such as football helmets and shoulder pads, and as a sequelae of cobalt60 irradiation for systemic cancer. Scalp lesions are usual.

Hot humid climates may also severely aggravate acne (acne tropicalis, Mallorca acne). A rare sequela of severe inflammatory acne is chronic facial edema.

DIFFERENTIAL DIAGNOSIS

Rosaceous acne has been described in detail in Chapter 1 "Erythemas", under Rosacea.

Persistent perioral dermatitis is an erythematous small papular and papulopustular reaction in the perioral area that occasionally extends to the nasolabial folds and onto the glabella. Comedones are not present. This dermatitis responds to the treatment of rosacea, but unlike rosacea rarely recurs. Other nonspecific facial eruptions may have an acneform appearance.

Some other conditions to be considered in the differential diagnosis have already been mentioned in the text. Occasionally discoid lupus erythematosus, especially if excoriated, may present a problem, as may micropapular rosacea and, rarely now, follicular tuberculides (acnitis). Follicular pustules rarely may be caused by gram-negative or Candida organisms. Ingrowing hairs especially on the sides of the neck of the black race may present as follicular granulomas and pustules.

Acne Conglobata

I define acne conglobata as a scarring dermal or hypodermal nodular eruption with abscess and sinus formation. It occurs in the axillae, groin, genital, and perianal areas, as well as on the buttocks, with occasionally other lesions on or under the breasts, nape of the neck, and torso. Band-like scarring is present, as are huge and double comedones.

The nodules increase and decrease in size, becoming tender and somewhat fluctuant, discharging a bloody, foul-smelling, purulent material and then flattening down again.

Vulgar acne, seborrhea, and a pilonidal sinus also may be (or have been) present.

If the lesions are mainly restricted to the apocrine gland areas, this condition is called hidradenitis suppurativa. On the face in young women, this may be the same condition as pyoderma faciale or rosacea fulminans.

Rarely, severe familial and early appearing acne conglobata may be associated with multiple, life-threatening verrucous, scarring squamous cell carcinoma.

Mallorca (A Mediterranean island)

Acne Keloidalis Nuchae

Acne keloidalis nuchae (dermatitis papillaris capillitti) is a hypertrophic scar induced by acne granuloma formation tending to form a thick band on the nape of the neck in dark-skinned patients. The lesions are sometimes inflamed and tender. A hair is often incorporated into the hypertrophic scar.

Suppurating and Cicatrizing Folliculitis of the Scalp

These lesions are characterized by the presence of small to grape-sized, dermal or hypodermal, purplish, semicystic papulonodules. From these papulonodules, sinuses develop and spread directly out to the skin, but also laterally. Pressure on the papulonodules results in the appearance of frank pus, seropurulent material, or a bloody liquid from the orifices of the sinuses or fistulae. Associated with all of this is a tremendous amount of reactive fibrosis, fibrosis plus edema, and fibrosis plus inflammation. The discharging fluid is often very malodorous. Epidermal inclusive cysts and epidermal bridges may also be present. Secondary scarring alopecia is often present.

The relationship between this condition and acne conglobata and hidradenitis suppurativa is very close. These have been grouped under the term follicular occlusion triad. When these lesions exists on the scalp, the term used is suppurating and cicatrizing folliculitis; when on the face or back, acne conglobata; and when in the axillae or groin, hidradenitis suppurativa. Sometimes, however, all areas may be involved. On the scalp, the fibrosis tends to be more prominent.

I do not know if folliculitis decalvans is a minor variety of this condition. I think not.

DIFFERENTIAL DIAGNOSIS

The differential diagnosis includes chronic staphylococcal folliculitis, which shows more of the features of an acute pyogenic infection (pus formation, tenderness, and regional adenitis). Other noduloulcerative lesions must also be considered.

Acne Necrotica

The basic lesions is a small, follicular, vesiculopustule that dries with a biconvex, brownish yellow crust. The adherent crust is embedded in the skin and takes a long time to fall off; then it leaves a depressed round scar. The eruption occurs in crops. The forehead, the borders of the scalp, the sides of the scalp above the ears, and the nape of the neck are the common sites. Many are excoriated. The dramatic response of this type of acne to oral tetracycline suggests acne necrotica is a peculiar type of scarring acne, or if you will, seborrheic perifolliculitis. The importance of picking by the patient in producing scars should not be underestimated. In fact, if early and adequate treatment with oral tetracycline is given, there may be no scarring. Recurrence is prompt after cessation of treatment.

Comedo Nevus

This is a type of localized linear malformation characterized by the presence of closely set, slightly elevated papules that have in their center a dark, firm, hyperkeratotic plug resembling a comedo. Small yellowish inclusion cysts may also be present as may an atrophy of the dermal tissues with an irregular overproduction of fatty material, which appears as dermal or subdermal nodules. Face, neck, and upper torso are the sites of predilection. these lesions are of varying length (from 3 to 4 cm to the total length of an upper extremity). They follow the lines of Blaschko. Some are present at birth, most develop before 20 years of age. There is little continuing extension.

The lesions are of lifelong duration.

Nodular Cutaneous Elastosis with Cysts and Comedones

Solar comedones are large open comedones that aggregate on various areas on the face, commonly lateral to the orbit and on the cheeks. They occur mainly in middle-aged and elderly white men or women whose skin has been damaged by excessive habitual exposure to sun. This is probably an incomplete variety of nodular cutaneous elastoides with cysts and comedones (Favre-Racouchot syndrome[5]). They may also be present on the dorsa of the fingers in the inter-knuckle spaces.

Nodular cutaneous elastosis with cysts and comedones are accumulations of numerous small nodules, usually surmounted by comedones and disordered pilosebaceous elements, resulting in follicular cyst formation. The nodules are yellowish, translucent, and cystic, with dilated hair sacs and atrophic sebaceous glands. They are seen mainly about the orbits, extending to the temporal and zygomatic areas. Usually there is yellowish leathery skin on the chin. This is one of the manifestations of dermatoheliosis.

Follicular Keratoses

A listing of follicular keratoses and a summary of their characteristics is provided in Table 45.

Table 45: **Follicular Keratoses**
Perforating folliculitis—thighs; young men.
Perforating granuloma annulare—usual lesions of granuloma annulare, only some lesions show central dell especially on sides of fingers.
Kryle's disease—rather large lesions on legs and about knees.
Uremic follicular keratoses—many lesions of varying size and some may resemble prurigo nodularis, keratoacanthoma; location is on the thighs, legs, and dorsa of the hands.
Elastosis perforans serpiginosa—arcuate clusters of keratotic papules; sides or back of neck; central keratotic plug.
Keratosis pilaris—arms, thighs, brown-red color, rarely scarring; familial.
Lichen spinulosis—children; hair-like spiny extensions from follicle; torso.
Darier's disease—greasy papules; erosions; odor; symmetry on torso; both follicular and nonfollicular areas involved, e.g. mouth; nicking of distal nail plate; acrokeratosis verruciformis on wrists.
Pityriasis rubra pilaris—red orange; follicular; torso; orange keratoderma; dorsa of the fingers; clear areas.
Follicular atopic dermatoses—torso; children; dark-skinned races.

Pityriasis Rubra Pilaris

The basic lesion of pityriasis rubra pilaris is a squamous follicular keratotic papule.[6] At the base of each broken or dystrophic hair, a little conical papule is seen from which the hair escapes at the summit. Each little pyramid is isolated from neighboring bulbs by an area of healthy skin in such a way that on the affected parts, the skin presents an appearance that has been called "chicken flesh". On the summits of the conical elevations, small, hard epidermal lamellae are partly free and partly adherent so that when one rubs the skin, it conveys the sensation of a rough rasp.

These papules multiply and become agminate, the intermediate skin becomes reddened, and there follow thickened plaques of all dimensions of a yellowish pink covered with a branny, psoriasiform, or granular scale, dotted with horny points, and lichenification. The lichenification is remarkably symmetrical, with parallel lines being present on the anterior aspect of arm and forearm forming a T-shirt pattern on the anterior shoulder. The borders are, as a rule, irregular, dentate, and surrounded by characteristic peripilar papules. Koebnerization can occur.

The eruption of pityriasis rubra pilaris is distinctly symmetrical. The scalp has a diffuse, thick, branny, white scale with no loss of hair. On the face, no pilary cones are seen, but rather a diffuse scaly redness with tension of the skin, even ectropion with greasy crusts on the eyebrows and the nasolabial grooves; on the elbows and knees, orange yellow patches are seen with thick adherent roughened scales, less sharply limited than those of psoriasis. The dorsal surfaces of the phalanges usually, but not always, show red papules agglomerated in patches or blackish horny cones at the piliary orifices. The nails are striated. Palmar and plantar regions are of an orange-yellow color with a thickened horny layer, fissured at the fold, sometimes desquamating with a gradual imperceptible transition into healthy skin. The limbs, and often also the trunk, are the seat of more or less grouped, acuminate papules and patches or thick and scaly surfaces, which may cover large stretches, almost the entire body, although a few localities at least are always exempt. The healthy spaces are angular and limited by concave borders. Exfoliative erythroderma may occur, and the follicular papules disappear, but islands of sparing persist.

In children, the eruption is often not as complete as described above. It may be limited to symmetrical orange-yellow colored, squamous, follicular plaques over the elbows and knees and more or less thickened squamous plaques on the palms or soles, or all of these may be absent and the disease manifest by disseminated to half-dollar-sized (2.7 cm diameter) plaques of follicular squamous papules, some appearing flat-topped. Hypopigmented areas may be present in these patches. Very occasionally, the lesions are not follicular.

Occasionally when the condition is seen very early, it may have an appearance resembling an allergic follicular eczematous dermatitis or a follicular atopic dermatitis. At times early on, it may have features of an acute seborrhea on the scalp and/or acute eruptive psoriasis. As time passes (2–3 months), the true scaly follicular papules and yellowish-brown color appear.

DIFFERENTIAL DIAGNOSIS

Pityriasis rubra pilaris must be distinguished from the following conditions.

Keratosis pilaris consists of follicular accumulations of horny material, usually without a definite scale, and light-brown or purplish perifollicular coloring. This eruption is located primarily on the outer aspects of the arms and thighs.

Lichen planopilaris (follicular lichen planus, Graham Little disease) is lichen planus involving the hair follicles, producing spinous follicular lesions. It may be associated with patchy, noninflammatory, cicatricial alopecia of the axillary or pubic regions and other typical cutaneous and mucosal lichen planus lesions. Atrophic cutaneous lichen planus lesions may also be present.

The erythrodermic type of pityriasis rubra pilaris should be distinguished from (1) erythrodermic psoriasis, where the basic lesion is a dark red squamous erythema, the nails show pitting and subungual keratosis, normal islands of skin are rare and do not have concave borders, the palms and soles are frequently clear, ectopion is rare, the scale on the scalp is whiter and more mica-like, and regional lymphadenopathy is more often present, and (2) erythrodermic lichen planus.

Kyrle's Disease

The basic lesion of Kyrle's disease (hyperkeratosis follicularis et parafollicularis in cutem penetrans) is a horny follicular papule with a central, slowly tapering, pointed keratin core. The core occupies over two-thirds of the center of the top of the lesion. On removal of this tightly adherent core, portions of the core are seen to have penetrated into the central portion of the papule. After forcible removal, a small crateriform defect is seen with some small amount of bleeding. The keratin core itself is of tough consistency, grayish white in color. The outside of the core is composed of skin-colored tissue. The whole lesion is sharply marginated and varies in size from 2 to 20 mm in diameter. Amid varying-sized lesions, there are circular or ovoid, 1 to 3mm pits with straight sides and flat bottoms. These are areas where previous lesions have existed.

The sites of predilection are the axillary or pubic regions, abdomen, upper and lower extremities, upper portion of the abdomen, and the back. The thighs, buttocks, and extensor elbows are also commonly involved. (See Table 46.)

Perforating Folliculitis

The patient can present with an inflammatory papular follicular eruption on the thighs, buttocks, calves, and occasionally the upper extremities. The size of each lesion is about 2 to 3 mm. Each individual lesion is conical, the top of which is a keratotic plug, which can be pulled out leaving a small indentation with a flat base. No pustulation or definite hairs can be seen protruding from the top of each lesion. There is no overall arrangement: the lesions are scattered.

The differential diagnosis includes keratosis pilaris, which is a teenage or young adult eruption, that in many cases does not have keratoses, but brownish or brownish-red pigmentary changes about a prominent, sometimes patulous, follicular orifice and that may have many more follicular lesions so that almost every follicle is involved. Also, the outer arms are always involved to some degree and occasionally have a nutmeg-grater-type appearance and texture.

In elastosis perforans serpiginosa, asymptomatic clusters of keratotic papules are often arranged in an annular, serpiginous, or arciform pattern. The lesions appear by the age of 20 years and are most often found on the sides and back of the neck. The conical or flat-topped papules, 2 to 3 mm in diameter, contain a central keratotic plug and are light-brown in color. At times, the scars are lace-like, linear, and quite extensive.

Reactive perforating collagenosis shows firm epidermal–dermal papules with a central, firmly adherent, keratin core (see Chapter 11). Perforating granuloma annulare is not follicular. Iododermas and bromodermas produce a more generalized follicular eruption. Kyrle's disease has fewer larger lesions, with a much more prominent central keratin core, usually located on the legs, trunk, or face. Occupational or oil or tar acnes are more pustular, have comedo-like lesions, and occur on the forearms, dorsa of the hands, and sometimes the thighs. Other rare follicular eruptions include lichen scrofulosorum, drug-induced folliculitis (e.g. actinomycin D), and the follicular ids of acute blistering tinea. Pustular bacterial folliculitis are more inflamed and have a central pustule, not central keratosis.

Other lichenoid follicular eruptions should also be mentioned for consideration. These include follicular lichen planus (lichen planopilaris), follicular atopic dermatitis, follicular eczema from colored permapress sheets and nickel sulfate, follicular syphilis, and lichen sclerosus et atrophicus. These entities have been described elsewhere.

Keratosis Pilaris

Keratosis pilaris shows a dryness of the skin with roughening due to more or less marked, acuminate, papular elevations, which are follicular orifices filled with a very adherent grayish horny cone, in which the downy hair is rolled up as a spiral. The color of the integument is sometimes normal; in other cases, of a more severe type, the follicular contents are red or purplish as is the surrounding skin. It may appear cosmetically inelegant. In the course of time, the shrivelled hair disappears and the elevations flatten with possible transformation into punctiform cicatrices. The lesions most often involve outer surfaces of arms and thighs; less often, calves, waist, hips, and outer surfaces of forearms, elbows, and knees. It spares moist regions such as the flexures. It is very common; frequently it is familial. The onset is at age 2 or 3 years, it flourishes between 15 and 20 years, and then becomes less prominent.

Disseminated and recurrent infundibulofolliculitis consists of 1 to 2 mm follicular papules distributed diffusely over the trunk and extremities in blacks. The pattern follows curved lines in the neck and axillae. The flexural and genital areas are spared.

Ulerythema Ophryogenes

Ulerythema ophryogenes are follicular syndromes with inflammation and atrophy. On the eyebrows, forehead, sides of face, and about the mouth, there is a diffuse redness, with a granular surface due to the acuminate elevations of the pilary orifices, from which protrude scanty and deviated hair. Later, the affected surface becomes bald, and the beard especially, grows only very scantily. There is often an anastomotic network of fine scars. Some cases are examples of discoid lupus erythematosus. Keratosis pilaris is commonly present.

Follicular atrophoderma of the face, elbows, and backs of the hands; hair shaft abnormalities; and multiple basal cell carcinomas have been reported in Bazex syndrome.

Phrynoderma

This extremely rare vitamin A deficiency condition (in developed countries) is manifest by dry and roughened skin that contains firm conical and hemispheric brown papules. Horny plugs or spines project from the hair follicles. The normal skin lines are exaggerated and produce a wrinkled appearance. The eruption is widely disseminated. Sometimes the hairs are broken off at the top of the conical papules.

Lichen Spinulosus

This is basically a childhood disease consisting of minute follicular papules each having a projecting horny spine. The horny spines are best seen by side lighting. They measure about 2 mm in length and give the feel of a nutmeg grater. The horny spines can be removed, leaving a small depression. The lesions are grouped and occur on the neck, thighs, buttocks, and other areas on the torso. The face, hands, and feet are clear. The groups tend to be symmetrical. There may be single scattered lesions beyond the grouped lesions.

Similar follicular spines may be seen in association with lichen planus, lichen scrofulosum, and lichenoid syphilides.

Darier's Disease

Keratosis follicularis usually starts on the head and face. The basic lesion is a greasy, firm, brownish-gray papular keratosis, semiglobular in shape, that varies in size from that of a small to that of a large pinhead. They are, at first, discrete and follicular. On close examination, the papules are observed to contain, in the center, a hardened or fatty-looking mass or plug. The disease extends slowly and shows greatest development about the face, scalp, central anterior chest, loins, and genitocrural regions, frequently with keratoses on the palms and soles. Sometimes a true keratoderma is present. On the scalp, there is a thick seborrhea-like coating, but no alopecia.

A. Bazex, 1911–1988, French Dermatologist

Table 46: Differential Diagnoses of Three Follicular Keratoses	
Clinical Features	Histology
Hyperkeratosis Lenticularis Perstans (Flegel) (dyskeratosis psoriasiform dermatosis)	
Chronic multiple discrete superficial keratoses is most prominent on dorsa of the feet and anterior aspect of lower legs. It may involve upper limbs, trunk, palms and soles. The keratoses have a darkish red-brown color in the center; at the periphery there seems to be a collarette of loose scale; about this collarette there may be radiating fine lines in the epidermis. Some of the lesions have a psoriasiform appearance. They have irregular shapes and vary from l to 5 mm in diameter. Lesions are difficult to remove, and when removed, leave a bleeding base but no epithelial invagination (age group 30 to 60 years).	Orthokeratotic or parakeratotic keratoses surmount a thinned malpighian layer and a dense, upper-dermal cellular infiltrate, with a sharply demarcated lower margin. The cells are mainly lymphocytic and capillary proliferation is present within the infiltrate.
Kyrle's Disease (uremic follicular keratoses)	
These lesions are chronic scattered papules with hyperkeratotic cone-shaped plugs which may coalesce into hyperkeratotic verrucous plaques. Sometimes the lesions look amazingly keratoacanthoma-like. Affects lower limbs bilaterally and upper limbs less commonly – palms and soles never involved (age group 20 to 60 years).	Keratotic plug fills an epithelial invagination. Parakeratotic keratinization of all epidermal cells includes basal cells in at least one region deep to the plug; is usually associated with epidermal disruption with keratinized cells in the dermis, accompanied by a granulomatous reaction
Stucco keratoses	
Chronic multiple keratoses (often extremely numerous) often localized to legs and affecting chiefly the posterior aspect, but also the dorsa of the feet and forearms. Lesions are pale in color. Lesions measure from 2 to 4 mm in diameter, mainly round or oval in shape and gradually slope down at the periphery. The lesions have a definite stuck-on appearance. Trunk, palms, and soles are never involved. Lesions are easily scratched off with a fingernail in one block without causing bleeding or exudation of the skin surface, and leaving a scaly collarette surrounding the denuded surface. Dry ichthyotic skin is commonly present (age group 65 to 75 years).	Keratoses are orthohyperkeratotic. There is marked acanthosis and a tendency to papillomatosis, basophilic degeneration of upper dermal collagen, and conspicuous lack of inflammatory infiltrate.

Modified from Raffle EJ, Rogers J. Hyperkeratosis lenticularis perstans. Arch Dermatol 1969; 100:423–428.

When fully developed, the lesions are larger and in some places may be confluent and present an irregular, verrucous or nutmeg-grater-like surface with considerable fissuring. The lesions are of various sizes and shapes: some keratoses are keratosis-pilaris-like, some are larger with firm or fatty central concretions, and a few are rounded or flattened, dull-red to dark- brown papules showing no central opening. Others, especially of an advanced age, are hard and horn-like, of dark-gray or dark-brown color, hemispheric, and project well above the surface. In places with extensive disease, the lesions present an uneven surface and are covered by thick, yellowish or brownish, flattened horny concretions giving a verrucous appearance. Rarely, large (up to 2 cm) horny masses with blunt truncated apices, yellowish in color, of dense consistency, and compactly crowded, can be seen. The masses can be removed with difficulty and have elongated red, moist bases. On some areas, these bases show erosions. Sometimes, secondary pyoderma with a purulent discharge is present. There is often a foul-smelling odor even when no obvious pyoderma is present. Close inspection especially at the beginning shows that the lesions are all follicular. Later, the papules become confluent and it can be seen that the interfollicular area is involved.

Hyperkeratotic and verrucous lesions on the dorsa of the hands and feet (acrokeratosis verriciformis) are sometimes present.

The nails show subungual keratosis and other changes. Small papular lesions may be present on the margins and lateral side of the tongue and on the buccal mucosae. Occasionally Darier's disease may disappear entirely and recur at intervals.

At times, it may be clinically and histologically difficult to distinguish this disease from localized areas of familial benign chronic pemphigus of Hailey-Hailey and transient acantholytic dermatosis (Grover's disease).

Miscellaneous

Rarely, eruptive xanthoma may occur in a perifollicular location. Seborrhea at times and especially on the chest and interscapular areas may have a perifollicular arrangement. This follicular seborrhea may have a superadded follicular staphylococcal pyoderma. Candidiasis on the back of the bedridden may have a follicular pattern. In experimental scurvy, enlargement and keratoses of the hair follicles on the upper arms, back, buttocks, back of thighs, calves, and shins is found. Multiple follicular papular granuloma may occur on the beard area of the neck at the sites of ingrowing hairs; this is particularly common in blacks (pseudofolliculitis barbae).

Eruptive vellus hair cysts show multiple discrete, 1 to 3mm papules with the suggestion of a comedo in the center. They occur on the extensor portions of arms and anterior thighs, and central portion of the abdomen.

References

1. Siemens HW. General diagnosis and therapy of skin diseases. Weiner K, trans. Chicago:University of Chicago Press, 1958.
2. Darier J. Textbook of dermatolgy. Pollitzer S, trans. Philadelphia:Lea & Febiger, 1920.
3. Weinberg JM, Mysliwiec A, Turiansky CW, Redfield R, James WD. Viral folliculitis. Atypical presentations of herpes simplex, herpes zoster and molluscum contagiasum. Arch Dermatol 1997; 133:938–986.
4. Poch PE, Shalita AR, Strauss JS, Webster SB. Report on the consensus conference on acne classification. Washington DC. March 24, 25, 1990. JAAD 1991; 24:495–500.
5. Sanchez-Yus E, del Rio E, Simon P, Requena L, Vasquez H. The histopathology of closed and open comedones of favre-racouchet disease. Arch Dermatol 1997; 133:743–745.
6. Griffiths WAD. Pityriasis rubra pilaris. Clin and Exp Dermatol. 1980; 5:105–112.

CHAPTER 21

Trichoses

Conditions where the abnormality is primarily of the hair itself.

Overview

There are two types of hair. Unmedulated, unpigmented, fine hair less than 2cm in length is called lanugo, perinatally, and later on, vellus hair. Terminal hair may be asexual on the scalp, ambisexual in the axillae, and sexual in the beard.[1]

Hairs are bloodless, insensitive horny structures that do not respond in the same manner as the living integument does. When one examines hairs, one must keep in mind that the hairs of different regions of the body are differently developed and that the different types of hair on the same person may react to a disease in different ways. Therefore, in a hair disease, one should not fail to inspect all hairy regions. If the patient complains about the scalp only, one should also examine the eyebrows and lashes, the beard, the axillary and pubic hair, and the vellus hair on the trunk and extremities. Examinations of the vellus hair should be done under changing angles of illumination, so that small glossy hairs are lit, e.g. tangential light in front of a dark background. The changes to be looked for are: (1) changes in color; (2) increased amount of hair (hypertrichosis); (3) decreased amount or absence of hair (alopecia); (4) changes in shape of the individual hairs; (5) deposits on the hairs, such as deposits produced by the body or deposits of foreign bodies; (6) distribution and extent of the hair changes; and (7) texture.

Color of the Hair

The color of the hair, which shows well-known individual and racial variations, may also change during the course of life (darkening after infancy and in childhood, bleaching by summer sunshine, graying with age). Hair may also become darker or lighter (canities) than other hair in a circumscribed area without affecting the skin. In other cases, the discoloration may also be associated with changes in the skin, such as brown pigmented tumors (nevus pigmentosus), thickening (bathing suit nevus), or depigmentation (vitiligo). In other cases, the skin may show an erythematosquamous eruption (discolored hairs in trichophytosis) or the color change may be associated with the loss and regrowth of hair (white hair in alopecia areata). Pili annulati (ringed hair) shows alternating light and dark bands on the shaft.

Hypertrichosis

Increase in hair growth may affect the fine silky vellus or the stronger terminal hairs. The vellus hair may grow enormously, with failure to develop terminal hairs. This is true, in the so-called "monkey men". In these cases it may be difficult to decide whether the condition should be called a lanugo hypertrichosis or a terminal hair hypotrichosis.

Hypertrichoses may also occur without demonstrable changes in the underlying skin, in a generalized as well as in a circumscribed form (hypertrichosis sacralis lanuginosa, fawn tail, hypertrichosis sacralis terminalis), or they may be associated with a variety of skin changes. These changes may be permanent, such as the pigmen-

Portions of the Overview have been taken and modified from Siemens[1] (pp. 157–167).

tation and thickening of the skin in bathing suit nevus, or they may be transient, like the inflammatory phenomena (e.g. lichen simplex chronicus) that occasionally lead to irritative hypertrichosis.

Alopecia

Decrease in hair amount may come about by neurotic pulling out, by rubbing off (as in the occipital area of infants and in itching eczemas), or by breaking off. The latter may be caused by fungi entering the hairs or it may be due to changes in shape of the individual hairs.

Scanty hair growth may be associated with failure of vellus hair to become thicker after childhood. In such cases, the number of hairs may be normal or decreased. On the other hand, the hairs in scanty growth may be of more or less normal caliber, but deficient in numbers (hypotrichosis). In other cases, the normal terminal hairs may be sparse, thin, and vellus-like (male pattern alopecia).

Hair of originally normal density may become sparser after local inflammations (eczema), after systemic disturbances (fever, post partum), or even from completely unknown causes (cyclical hair loss in middle-aged women—telogen effluvium). If the shedding of hair is very marked, it may lead to complete baldness. Alopecia may be circumscribed, involve the entire scalp, or even the entire body surface. The androgenetic alopecias are patterned.

Certain medical conditions and drugs cause total or partial alopecia (anagen alopecia). In areas where a large percentage of the hairs are rapidly growing (e.g. scalp), there will be much more hair loss than in areas where only a small percentage of the hairs are rapidly growing (e.g. eyebrows). In some patients, this difference may appear to be absolute, i.e. the alopecia may seem to involve only the scalp.

When hairs are absent, the skin may be normal or abnormal. One must first establish whether the follicles are preserved. If so, they can be seen as fine dots, points or pits, as, for example, in alopecia areata. If the follicles have disappeared, atrophy is present, and the skin is smooth, glossy, and lacks surface relief (discoid lupus erythematosus). When such atrophic skin is pinched together between thumb and index finger, it exhibits the characteristic pattern of little folds which is traditionally compared with crushed cigarette paper. If the skin is loose or slack, similar small folds may occur and look like atrophy. In this case, however, the follicle mouths are still visible.

Atrophic skin may also simultaneously manifest whitening and browning, and telangiectases (traumatic scars, scleroderma x-ray atrophy), giving a clinical picture of poikiloderma. Based on the above observations, one should classify alopecias into the scarring and nonscarring types.

In areas of complete loss of hair, the skin may also exhibit features of inflammation, especially erythema or erythema with desquamation. The desquamation may spread diffusely over a large part of the scalp as it commonly occurs in the early stages of seborrhea associated with common baldness, or the scales may be found at the bases of the still existing hairs. The lost hairs may also be replaced by keratinous spines or by carpet tack plugs (discoid lupus erythematosus).

Changes in Shape of Individual Hairs

Curly hair is caused by hair which is elliptical in cross-section. Straight hair has a different shape. Abnormal keratinization of the skin at the mouth of the follicle may prevent emergence of the growing hair from the follicle and force it to roll itself into a spiral beneath the surface and cause an inflammatory nodule containing an ingrown hair. Sometimes these ingrown hairs are visible through the transparent horny layer as little rings (rolled hair). Splitting of the hair at the end is called trichoschisis, splitting within the shaft (trichorrhexis), which may appear as a little gray papule in the hair or often a kink at the site of the split is called trichorrhexis. The impression of a little papule in the hair shaft may be created by actual rolling of the hair into knots (trichonodosis), which may cause the hair to fray and break off. A periodic knob-like thickening of the hair may also be simulated by twisting of the hair around its longitudinal axis (trichokinesis or pili torti). In this anomaly, the very thin hairs are slightly curled and have a peculiar mottled luster due to the altered reflection of light from the twisted hair shafts. Intermittent apparent swellings, which actually result from periodic thinnings of the hair shaft, are found in monilethrix. In this condition, the hairs almost regularly break off near the base at one of the thinnings causing alopecia. There also are small papules on the scalp and nape of neck. Another condition that may present the appearance of swellings of the hair shaft arranged in bead-like fashion may, on closer examination, turn out to be simply white or paler air-containing sections alternating with dark and air-free portions (pili annulati, ringed hair). The dark parts of the hair give the impression of "beads". Most of these changes can be differentiated only with a magnifying glass or microscope.

Deposits

Deposits on the hairs may be foreign or derived from the body. The latter are scales and crusts, including peripilar keratin casts. Scales may be dust-like, small, or larger particles adhering loosely to the hairs, or they may partly sheathe the length of the shaft ("tinea amiantacea") in psoriasis. In the latter case, the hairs may be matted together forming hair tufts. Of course, crusts can cause hairs to stick together and, with neglect, form an inextricable mass of hair, serum, pus, and lice. Such impetiginized types of the pediculosis capitis are now rare.

Among deposits of foreign origin is the light-colored, flour-like coating with which the microsporon fungi cover the hair. Nits, as the eggs and eggshells of head and pubic lice are called, are light-colored, pearly, glossy, discrete structures firmly attached to the hair like little buds. Pubic lice are found in coarse haired areas—pubic and genital areas, axillae, eyelashes, eyebrows, and rarely, the scalp. Head lice are usually restricted to the scalp. Body lice are found on the clothing seams. Only rarely does one see mixed infestations of head, body, and pubic lice. Dark, very hard granules containing fungus spores are found in tropical piedra, whereas in the related trichomycosis axillaris, granules or longer irregular sheaths of yellow to red color surround the hairs. These granules and sheaths consist of concretions of various types of corynebacteria.

Distribution and Extent of Hair Changes

In every case of hair disease, distribution and extent of the morbid process should be considered. A hair disorder may occur in a circumscribed focus or may be generalized, affecting many haired areas. Finally, such hair diseases may be universal, involving the entire body surface. A hair disease may affect all hairs or only terminal hairs (defluvium after typhoid fever). In other cases, the hair changes are regional, involving only certain areas, such as the scalp, bearded area, or axillary region.

Of the greatest practical importance are the diseases of the scalp hair. Diseases are circumscribed, occurring in a confined site; areated, affecting several circular areas (alopecia areata); or diffuse, without sharp borders and covering a large part of the scalp (male or female pattern alopecia). If the scalp hair is completely affected, the condition is called total (alopecia totalis), which differs from universal loss of hair (alopecia universalis). If there are isolated foci, one must distinguish between diseases characterized by large lesions (alopecia areata) and those with small lesions (syphilitic alopecia). It is also important to decide whether the distribution is symmetrical or nonsymmetrical.

Textural Changes

These occur in some endocrinological conditions and in male pattern alopecia.

Hypertrichoses

Pigmented hairy epidermal nevus (Becker's nevus) is a blotchy brown or dark-brown patch occurring on the top of the shoulder and extending onto the deltoid area, characteristically in males. The border is irregular and the nevus often has satellites. Coarse black hairs are usually present, being most numerous and thickest in the central portions. Becker's nevus appears at puberty and darkens with exposure to the sun.

Hypertrichosis lanuginosa is an over-growth of fetal lanugo type hair. There is an acquired and congenital form. Malignant down is the name given to the acquired form occurring in association with an underlying internal malignancy.

Nevoid hypertrichosis may occur as a circumscribed developmental defect by itself or in association with pigmented nevi of all sorts (Fig. 21.1). The sacral area (fawn tail) is a favorite location.

Hirsutism usually refers to the growth, in the female, of coarse terminal hair in part or in the whole adult male sexual pattern. It is caused by androgenic stimulation. The elucidation of the cause is not within the scope of dermatological morphology.

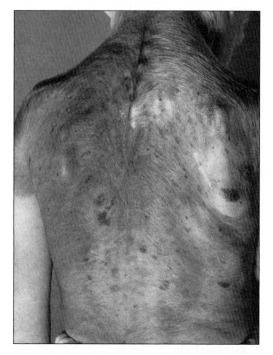

Figure 21.1 Hairy "bathing suit" nevus.

All sorts of miscellaneous conditions have been reported as showing varying degrees of hypertrichosis, e.g. porphyria, epidermolysis bullosa dystrophica, childhood dermatomyositis, and certain congenital states. As they are of no diagnostic importance, they are not described here. Hydantoin, penicillamine, streptomycin, minoxidil, diazoxide, cortisone minoxidal, and cyclosporine may cause hypertrichosis. Localized trauma may also be a cause.

Alopecias

Male Pattern Alopecia

The change in male pattern alopecia is as follows.[2] Each successive generation of hair lessens in diameter, the hirsute growth becoming finer and finer until the follicle no longer produces the hair; progressive immaturity finally ends in atrophy. Although hair becomes thinner in the marginal area, it is never completely lost, and even extreme cases of hippocratic or classical male pattern baldness still maintain a border fringe a few centimeters wide, festooned around the back of the head from ear to ear.

The rate of hair loss varies. In the early stages, many hundreds of hairs may be shed in 1 day. After several months, this may decrease to approximately 30 per day. If half of the hairs are not lost by the age of 30 years, the patient will never suffer from exaggerated alopecia. At first, following excessive loss, there is some regrowth of fine silky hair which never develops into regular terminal hairs.

The temperofrontal areas and the posterior vertex are sites of predilection. This is a patterned, symmetrical, nonscarring type of hair loss.

Seborrhea and "seborrheic dermatitis" are common on the scalp in those with severe male pattern alopecia.

The same type of alopecia occurs in females, usually starting at a later date, progressing more slowly, and rarely causing complete alopecia on the crown.[3] The anterior frontotemporal hair line does not disappear, the loss is more diffuse with less patterning.

Congenital Alopecias

Congenital defect of the scalp (aplasia cutis congenita) is a scarring lesion occurring on the scalp of the newborn. Most defects are located on the vertex, on the sagittal suture line, or over the parietal bones. The lesions are loonie-sized (2.5cm diameter) with map-like, clear-cut borders. No hair grows in these areas. The lesions are depressed below the level of the skin and at times have punched out margins. The lesions are atrophic with varying degrees of loss of skin or subcutaneous tissue. Rarely, there is an underlying boggy fibrous nodal mass with incomplete alopecia in areas not originally involved in the defect.

Patients with congenital ectodermal defects (hidrotic and anhidrotic ectodermal dysplasia) have fragile hair and present with diffuse thinning of the scalp hair and loss of the outer two-thirds of the eyebrows. There are palmar and plantar keratoses (hidrotic form). The nails are short and thick and may be elevated at the tip. The nail plate shows striations. Areas of brown pigmentation are often present. The teeth may be defective in number and form. Some forms have a depressed nasal root bridge, proximal frontal bossing, and thick lips.

Congenital total or partial absence of hair of developmental origin occurs in a bewildering variety of clinical forms either as an apparently isolated defect or in association with a wide range of other anomalies. A detailed account of these anomalies cannot be given here. A useful table for those interested is available.[4] Epidermal or sebaceous nevi of the scalp are often devoid of hair.

Diffuse Nonscarring Alopecia

There are many causes for diffuse, nonscarring alopecia such as endocrine (hypopituitary states, hypothyroidism, pregnancy), severe systemic illness or infection, iron deficiency anemia, chemicals (thallium, antimitotic agents, coumarin, heparin), and severe malnutrition. Diffuse thinning of the hair in middle-aged women is a common complaint. The cause is unknown. Many may represent minor forms of androgenetic pattern alopecia. In secondary syphilis, there may be a diffuse hair loss but more often it is patchy forming – what has been described as "footprints in the snow". Pubic and eyebrow hair may also be lost. At times trichotillomania may be diffuse.

Anagen effluvium of the scalp has the following features: almost complete, immediate onset, quick recovery. Telogen effluvium is less in extent, comes on in about 3 months, and may continue for another 6 months.

Noncicatricial Circumscribed Alopecias

Alopecia Areata

In alopecia areata, smooth, sharply outlined, round or oval spots or patches of variable dimensions are most common on the scalp, eyebrows, eyelashes, and beard areas. Exclamation point hairs are pointed like a wet paint brush, black halfway or in the distal two thirds, very thin, tapering and decolorized toward the root, which terminates in a slight swelling (Fig. 21.2).[*5] There are also numerous hairs broken off about 1mm above the level of the scalp. Exclamation point hairs are only seen in the scalp, and almost always at the periphery of lesions. If hairs with exclamation point features are bent, they fracture at the site of thinning. Fresh patches are rose-colored, slightly edematous, and riddled with dilated pilary orifices. After some time, the spot becomes depressed, ivory white, entirely smooth, soft to the touch, and easily folded (pseudoatrophic wrinkling). Healing proceeds from fine downy hairs, to stronger downy hairs, white terminal hairs, and then ordinary colored terminal hairs. Regrowth may be central, centrifugal, or centripetal. Occasionally the hair remains white. In extensive or universal cases, the nails show dryness, white longitudinal striation, pitting, fissuring, crumbling, and indentation. Alopecia totalis refers to total loss of scalp hair; alopecia universalis refers to loss of all body and scalp hair.

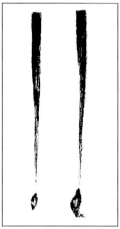

Figure 21.2 Exclamation point hairs.

Ophiasis is alopecia areata extending in a large patch from the nape of the neck, over the ears, above the temples, and to the forehead, i.e. the marginal areas of the scalp.

Trichotillomania

In this traumatic alopecia, there is an irregular partial loss of hair on the scalp, particularly on the crown and occipital area. The amount of hair loss varies; in some there may be almost complete hair loss, with a few obvious short hairs and stubble. Rarely, asymmetric or linear patterns may be seen; rarely, almost the total scalp may be involved. There is no pigmentary change; there is no scarring. Occasionally, other excoriations may be present. Loss of eyebrows and eyelashes may occur with loss of scalp hair or alone. At times both trichotillomania and alopecia areata may be present.

DIFFERENTIAL DIAGNOSIS

The differential diagnosis includes monilethrix, alopecia areata, and tinea capitis. However, the most difficult problem is in distinguishing trichotillomania from hair loss due to head rolling or rubbing the head.

---

[*]All you ever wanted to know about the hair abnormalities in alopecia areata in 6½ pages an be found in Reference 5.

Other traumatic alopecias occur from continual resting of the occiput in one position in the neonatal period; from head rubbing in infancy; from excessive massage; from traction by hair curlers; and from pressure by a circular valve during anesthesia. Certain pre-existing dermatoses, especially pruritic ones, may be associated with some degree of alopecia. The diagnosis is made by the findings of the basic dermatosis, e.g. lichen simplex chronicus on the nape of the neck, psoriasis, or lichen planus.

Circumscribed Hypotrichosis of Men's Legs

Loss of hair on the outer calves and thighs in men, with no other change in the skin is presumably due to trauma of trousers and long socks, although alopecia areata should be considered in the differential diagnosis.

Alopecia Mucinosa

Alopecia mucinosa is a roughly circular plaque or collection of follicular papules, reasonably well circumscribed, that usually occurs on the head and neck area (especially eyebrows and nape of neck) or on the torso or limbs. On the head and neck, the lesions are edematous and most hairs are broken off at the follicular opening. Where present, the hairs are easily epilated with the external sheath clinging to the hair. On the torso, the alopecia is not nearly as obvious. This has been called follicular mucinosis. When squeezed, visible mucous globules may be expressed through the opening of the hair follicle. Some cases appear to occur by themselves; others, in adults, occur obviously as part of the picture of a cutaneous lymphoma. There is no scarring.

Pyodermic Alopecias

Impetigo, furuncles, and suppurations in general, especially on the scalp in children, often leave behind noncicatricial, distinctly outlined, round alopecic spots, the size of a dime (1.8 cm diameter) to that of a silver dollar (3.5 cm diameter), on which regrowth of at first downy hairs then normal hairs may be delayed for several months. A central macule or papule is present. There are no exclamation point hairs, but the hairs may be broken off at the scalp.

Cicatricial Circumscribed Alopecias

Pseudopelade of Brocq

This condition presents as alopecia with cicatricial spots or patches, scattered or grouped on otherwise healthy scalp. The spots have various dimensions and shapes, sometimes rounded and very numerous, sometimes several centimeters in diameter, irregular with geographic outlines. Borders are distinct; the surface is waxy white or faintly pink, perfectly smooth, without scale or broken or lanugo hairs; and even the follicles have disappeared. The scalp never becomes entirely bald and some healthy hair always remains.

Folliculitis Decalvans

I can find only one basic difference between this and pseudopelade. In folliculitis decalvans, inflammatory papules or pinhead-sized pustules can be noted at the border. I suspect some cases are scarring acne of the scalp. The inflammatory process and pus formation is much less in folliculitis decalvans than in suppurating and cicatrizing folliculitis of the scalp.

Discoid Lupus Erythematosus

The findings of discoid lupus erythematosus are the same as those in other areas, viz. carmine telangiectatic areas, follicular plugging, atrophic scarring, and carpet-tack adherent scale. The destruction of the hair follicles and the scarring produce an obvious alopecia.

Miscellaneous

Other causes of this type of alopecia are wounds, burns (including late radiation sequelae), caustics, tineas (including favus and occasionally kerion), scleroderma, necrobiosis lipoidica diabeticorum, cancers (primary or secondary), syphilis (ulceronodular, gumma), tuberculosis (lupus vulgaris), acne keloidalis (dermatitis papillaris capillitii), cystic acne of the scalp (suppurating and cicatrizing folliculitis), acne necrotica, lichen planopilaris (Graham Little syndrome), bullous pemphigoid, and gangrenous herpes zoster. Rarely, some congenital developmental defects may cause cicatricial alopecias.

Dystrophies

Some of the dystrophies of hair have been discussed in the Overview. Figure 21.3 shows a few dystrophies of hair, although there are other structural abnormalities of hair.*[6]

Trichorrhexis Nodosa

In this condition, there is localized splitting of the hair, the fibers become separated and take the form of two brooms pushed into each other. This results in the appearance of white micronodosities at the level where the hair bends and is easily broken off. There may be one or two nodes on each hair. The nodes usually appear near the tip. Scattered isolated hairs may be involved, or circumscribed patches may show this defect. The essential provocative factor is trauma.

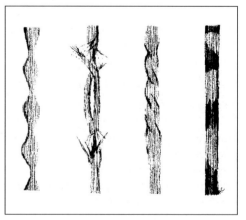

Figure 21.3 *Left to right:* Monilethrix, trichorrhexis nodosa, pili tori, and pili annulati (ringed hair).

*For fine drawings and a more complete review, see Reference 6.

Bamboo hairs (trichorrhexis invaginata) are seen in ichthyosis linearis circumflexa (Netherton's syndrome). Telescoping of the hair occurs before fracture. The telescoping causes ball and cup joints resembling those of bamboo.

Monilethrix

Monilethrix is a developmental defect of the hair shaft which is beaded, brittle, and easily broken. The condition becomes apparent in early childhood. There are small reddish, horny follicular papules on the scalp from which emerge a brittle beaded hair, which breaks before it is 1 or 2cm long. The nape of the neck and the occipital areas are most commonly involved. The keratosis may come before or after the appearance of the beaded hair.

Pili Torti

This condition is a developmental defect in which the hair shaft is flattened and twisted on its own axis. It is first obvious in childhood. The affected hairs have a spangled appearance in reflected light. There may be extensive stubble-like baldness, an irregular and patchy baldness, or a more or less normal scalp in which the affected hairs must be sought. Occasionally other areas are involved. It should be distinguished from ringed hair.

Miscellaneous

Some other dystrophies are trichomalacia (or rolled hairs), peripilar keratin casts, bayonet hairs, kinky hair disease, wooly hair, wooly hair nevus, and trichostasis spinulosa (Fig. 21.4).

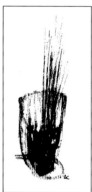

Figure 21.4
Trichostasis spinulosa.

Color Changes

Canities or graying of the hair may occur physiologically or in association with some other diseases, e.g. hyperthyroidism and in some hereditary conditions, e.g. progeria.

Poliosis is the presence of a cluster of white hair. Alopecia areata, vitiligo, and piebaldism are examples. It also occurs in some hereditary conditions. It may develop following zoster or radiation sequelae on the scalp.

Ringed hair (pili annulati) shows regular alternation between normally pigmented bands and light bands each about 1mm wide. The banding may be irregular. The alternate light and dark bands give the hair a distinctive sheen in reflected light.

Pseudopili annulati shows striking bright bands at intervals along the hair; but here, in contrast to pili annulati, the internal structure is normal. The cause is a flattening in cross section and at intervals of partially twisted hairs in two alternating directions. The bright segments represent reflection and refraction of light by the flattened, twisted surface.

Rarely, drugs, metabolic disorders, and local inflammatory conditions may cause a change in the color of the hair. Accidental discoloration (sometimes from therapeutic applications) and cosmetics can also change the hair color.

Parasitic Trichoses

In all parasitic trichoses, final diagnosis rests on the findings of examination by Wood's light (365 nm), KOH examination of the hairs, and culture on appropriate media.

Noninflammatory gray-patch ringworm, as from Microsporum audouinii, usually involves several areas of the scalp, which is scaly. The hair in these areas is full, lusterless, of an ashen gray color, and broken off 2 to 3 mm above the surface of the skin. There are no vesicles. The lesions increase in size by peripheral extension up to the size of a silver dollar (2.7 cm diameter). All parts of the scalp may be involved, but the nape of the neck is a common site. The condition may exist on the glabrous skin. This is basically a disease of childhood.

Inflammatory scalp ringworm as from Microsporum canis is similar in size and shape to the noninflammatory type. There are two differences; one is the presence of small peripheral vesicles, pustules, or crusting with rather more loss of hair; the other is the presence of similar lesions on the glabrous skin. In these cases, definite vesiculation is easily seen. Adult infection is rare.

The black-dot ringworm, as from Trichophyton violaceum or Trichophyton tonsurans, causes basically a scaliness with broken-off hairs or stubs. The patches slowly enlarge forming polygonal or angular areas. The margins may be indistinct, finger-like projections with many areas of normal hair seen within the patch. The black dots are produced by the breaking off of the hairs at the scalp. An inflammatory reaction and scarring may occur. The disease may persist for years. It is present in both children and adults. With marked hair loss, it is easily confused with seborrhea, psoriasis, the scarring alopecias, bacterial folliculitis, and discoid lupus erythematosus. Rarely, the glabrous skin and nails may be involved.

Favus is rare in North America. The characteristic finding is a yellow cup-shaped crust, composed of a dense mat of mycelia and epithelial debris, called a scutulum. The concavity of the cup faces upward and is pierced by a hair around the orifice of which the cup has developed. The cups thicken to form prominent yellowish crusts that are reported to have a mousy odor. Alopecia is not as marked as with other tineas of the scalp, so the hairs may be a normal length and the hair stubs are not a prominent feature. All of the scalp, other areas of the body, and the nails may also be involved. Atrophy with permanent hair loss is common. The hair loss is uneven and patchy.

The differential diagnosis of the fungal trichoses includes the oily scaling of seborrhea, which is diffuse with no alopecia; psoriasis, which has sharply marginated elevated squamous lesions with little if any hair loss; and lichen simplex chronicus.

Piedra is rare in North America. It consists of black or brown, elongated nodules up to 1 or 2 mm in size, which are firmly adherent to the shaft and stony hard. The shaft is undamaged. Piedra occurs in the scalp and beard. The concretions are irregularly located along the shaft and give the sensation of hardness to touch.

Trichomycosis axillaris is an affliction of the axillary and pubic hairs. The hair shafts are covered by discrete, rather adherent, tiny, soft accumulations forming a continuous filmy sheath. The accumulations may be scattered irregularly along the shaft, are often continuous, and are usually golden yellow in color, but rarely, they are red or black. Hyperhidrosis is often present.

References

1. Siemens HW. General diagnosis and therapy of skin diseases. Weiner K, trans. Chicago:University of Chicago Press, 1958.
2. Hamilton JB. Patterned loss of hair in men: types and incidence. Ann NY Acad Sci 1951: 53:708–728.
3. Ludwig E. Classification of the types of androgenetic alopecia (common baldness) occurring in the female sex. Br J Dermatol 1977; 97:247–254.
4. Champion RH, Burton JL, Ebling FJG. Textbook of dermatology. Vol.4. London:Blackwell Scientific, 1992:2579.
5. McCarthy L. Diagnosis and treatment of diseases of the hair. St. Louis:C.V. Mosby, 1940:161–167.
6. Whiting DA. Structural abnormalities of the hair shaft. J Am Acad Dermatol 1987; 16:1–12.

CHAPTER 22
Onychoses

Diseases that affect the nail plate and surrounding structures.

Overview

It is not the purpose of this chapter to give an encyclopedic listing and description of all known and recorded nail abnormalities. Our present state of knowledge of the morphological changes in the nail does not warrant such an approach. Rather, stress is laid on the morphological patterns of response of the nail to many and varied internal and external stimuli. Detailed attention is paid to the differential diagnosis of common nail abnormalities and to abnormalities in which the presence of nail changes may be of help in making a diagnosis.

A large nomenclature of nail abnormalities has accumulated in the literature. Many of these terms mean nothing and add nothing to our knowledge. In many cases, the same word means different things to different authors. I have tried to use as few of these terms as possible.

The living gross pathology of the nails is dominated by the fact that a dead disc of horn forming the nail plate is able to produce a much smaller variety of changes than the living skin (Fig. 22.1).[1,2] Thus, the same disease may manifest itself in different ways at different times and different diseases may produce similar changes in the nails. The reactivity of the nail and nail tissues to systemic diseases is by no means constant. Many so-called characteristic nail findings in systemic disease are inconstant, not at all distinctive, and frequently absent. The diagnosis of a disease usually cannot be made from the findings in the nails alone, although an experienced observer can often hazard a shrewd guess. For example, it is often not possible to distinguish clinically eczema and psoriasis of the nails from the onychomycoses. In this case, a decision about the diagnosis may rest on the presence or absence of fungal elements. Only occasionally is a certain finding in the nails alone highly suggestive of a skin disease, e.g. pitted nails of psoriasis. The general rule to never consider a dermatological diagnosis as definitive without having examined the entire skin surface of the patient is particularly important in the case of nail diseases. By so

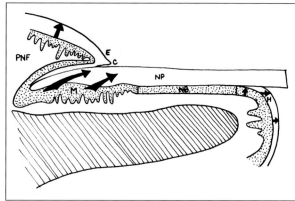

Figure 22.1
Cross section of the nail.
PNF, Prominal nail fold; C, Cuticle;
M, Matrix; NP, Nail plate; NB, Nail
bed; H, Hyponychiun; and
E, Eponychium.
Redrawn from Zaias.[2]

Portions of the Overview have been taken and modified from Siemens[1] (pp. 169–185).

doing, the physician may occasionally succeed in establishing an apparently impossible diagnosis. This is well illustrated by the case of a schoolgirl with chronic subungual keratosis on the thumbnail, the psoriatic nature of which could be assumed when a single, yet typical, psoriasis lesion was discovered in the sacral area.

When examining the nails, one should proceed just as methodically as in the examination of the skin and hair. Failure to do so, invites great difficulty in analyzing the features of an unusual picture crowded into a small field in a tissue with a limited number of reaction patterns. Therefore, the examiner should systematically consider the following details: (1) shape of the nail plate; (2) color and translucency; (3) irregularities of the surface (level differences); (4) changes in texture (scaliness, splintering, crumbling); (5) consistency (hardness and softness) of the nail plate (palpation findings); (6) hyperkeratosis (thickening); (7) atrophy and anonychia (thinning, or complete absence of the nail plate); (8) onycholysis; and (9) distribution and extent of the nail change, such as changes in the tissues surrounding the nail (nail fold, cuticle).

Changes in Shape of the Nail Plate

The nails may be abnormally large or abnormally small. Enlargement may occur with enlargement of the whole finger (acromegaly), or it may be restricted to the tip of the finger. In the latter case, the nail may bulge like a balloon and be excessively curved convexly and longitudinally (Hippocratic nails). This shape occurs in the so-called clubbed fingers that develop as a result of heart and lung ailments (bronchiectases), but it may also occur independently of such ailments.

The nail plate may also be unusually shortened. This may be a hereditary anomaly (especially on the thumbs), or it may be the result of nail biting.

The nail plate may be of normal size but otherwise deformed. In some nails, the normal gentle curvature is absent, which results in a flat, horny disc. Following injury, pathological keratinization, subungual keratoses, or subungual bony exostoses, the nails may appear lifted up like the keel of a ship.

Changes in Color and Translucency

Little white spots (leukonychia punctata, "good-luck spots") exhibited on the nail plate are caused by air penetration between the layers of the nail plate. The spots have a tendency to line up in transverse bands (leukonychia striata). The whitening may become total. A white silvery luster may come about if desquamation or splitting of the nail permits air to invade the nail substance, causing reflection of light in much the same way as happens in the horny layer of the skin.

Thickened nail plates are usually turbid and yellowish or brownish to blackish, the same colors as the color of horny substance elsewhere. Exceptionally, a nail or part of it may be dark brown from melanin pigmentation. Blood blisters under the nails appear dark red to black. A variety of discolorations may be caused by subungual tumors (e.g. angiomas, melanomas, epitheliomas, verrucae).

A striking discoloration of the nails may be caused by foreign dyes contacting the nails either occupationally or as medicaments (e.g. silver nitrate, potassium permanganate). These discolorations travel distally with the growing nail and can be scraped off.

Irregularities of the Surface

The surface of the nail plate may be either smoother than normal or less smooth and show surface irregularities. The former condition, glossy nails, which makes the nails look as if they were polished, is encountered in persons with chronic itching dermatoses who rub their nails continually against the itching skin.

Longitudinal ridges of the nails may occur in the elderly. They may also be associated with grooves, e.g. after injury to the matrix, periungual fibromas of tuberous sclerosis, or ganglions in the nail matrix area. Frequently associated with ridges and grooves are desquamation and splintering (fraying). Transverse ridges are common in onychogryphosis.

More frequently, depressions are encountered in the nail plate. Most remarkable are the numerous, small, sharp-edged pits diagnostic of psoriasis (pitted nails). Sometimes these pits are arranged in longitudinal rows. Sometimes even relatively few typical pits are sufficient to suggest the diagnosis. It is, however, true that similar pits occur in eczemas and other nail diseases, but then they are usually not so regular nor so sharply punched out. Besides such small pits, the nail surface may exhibit larger, trough-shaped, less sharp, sometimes predominantly longitudinal, but more frequently transverse, irregularities or striations of the surface (especially in eczema and dermatomycoses). There may also occur an evenly flat depression of the entire nail, which, because of its appearance, has given rise to the term spoon nail (koilonychia). In this condition, the whole fingertip may be distorted as if it had been pulled up in a dorsal direction.

Transverse arcuate furrows that run across all nails at a similar level and are sharply demarcated are called Beau's lines. They may consist of simple transverse grooves, sometimes with collarette-like scaly edges, or they may also cut transversely through the entire thickness of the nail plate. As the nails grow, the transverse furrows slowly travel distally. They follow a great variety of acute febrile or systemic diseases, and the distance from the cuticle edge permits estimation of the time elapsed since the event that caused their development. In the fingernail, this is 3 to 4 mm per month.

Changes of Texture of the Nail Plate

Either accompanying irregularities of the surface or occurring independently, separation of parts of the nail substance from its base may develop. This may be called desquamation if the detached fragments are not larger than dust or bran. If the parts are larger and peel off horizontally, the desquamation may be referred to as lamellar exfoliation, which represents a minor degree of horizontal splitting of the nail plate into two or more lamellae. Still more common than superficial detachment of scales

Joseph Honoré Simon Beau, 1806–1865, French Physician, Paris

is deep splitting of the nail substance in the longitudinal direction, frequently starting at the free edge. In this case we speak of splintering and brittleness. Splintering, of course, may affect the whole surface of the nail and may be combined with irregularities, longitudinal ridges, and depressions. Splintering may also be very coarse and lead to deep longitudinal tears and splits. The thickened nail plate or parts of it may even break up into irregular pieces and granules, to present a crumbly appearance. Shedding of scales, lamellae, splinters, and crumbs may cause a large part of the nail bed to become bare and thus end in partial or even total absence of the nail (anonychia).

Consistency of the Nail Plate

In examining nail diseases, palpation, compared with inspection, plays a minor role. Nevertheless, there may, of course, exist great differences in the consistencies of nail plates. In onychogryphosis, the nail substance is usually extremely hard. Extreme softness and flexibility of the nail plate are encountered not only in thinning of the nails, but also in marked hyperhidrosis.

Hyperkeratosis

Thickening of the nail plate and hyponychium is not necessarily associated with changes in surface and texture, e.g. enlargement and thickening of the nail in acromegaly. To be sure, discolorations, turbidity, and irregularities of the surface, are, in most cases, at least to some degree, associated with an increase in nail thickness. In some cases, the most thickened extreme portion of the nail appears to be rolled at the edges, making the distal part narrower in width than the proximal part. If the hyperkeratosis of the nail forms lumpy masses or even long horn-shaped excrescences, the condition is onychogryphosis (Greek: grypo, "to bend" or Latin: gryphus, a "griffin"). The surface of such a nail is frequently furrowed in both directions. A more or less columnar central hyperkeratosis of the fingernails and toenails with thickened, wax-colored, opaque, yellowish horny substance is called pachyonychia (Greek: pachys, "thick").

Hyperkeratotic masses may also form under the nail plate. They may grow from the hyponychium and appear as a granular or bulging layer at the free edge. This keratosis of the nail bed or of the hyponychium is termed subungual keratosis. It is mostly dark gray or blackish and occurs in a great variety of chronic inflammations of the nail bed and in diseases of the nails in general. Subungual keratosis may somewhat detach the free end of the nail plate and cause it to bend upward.

Atrophy and Anonychia

Much rarer than thickening is thinning of the nail plate and adjacent structures. This condition can frequently be observed in atrophic states such as x-ray atrophy of the terminal phalanx of a finger, where the surrounding skin also manifests clear signs of radiation injury (atrophic glossiness, crinkled surface, telangiectases). The nail appears shortened because the cuticle usually grows over the nail much farther than is normal. Atrophic nails also generally exhibit exfoliation or splintering from the free edge inward. If there is nothing left of a nail plate except some insignificant lamellous or crumbly remnants, one speaks of anonychia (absence of nail). In this condition, the nail bed may be shrunken down to an irregular depression, or it may be completely gone.

Nail loss or shedding can be mentioned here. Shedding without scarring may be seen from minor trauma, a subungual hematoma, severe onycholysis of any cause, and severe illness. Shedding with scarring is a serious nail finding, occurring in defective peripheral circulation, epidermolysis bullosa dystrophica, or severe trauma.

Onycholysis

A frequently occurring phenomenon is onycholysis or detachment of the nail plate from the nail bed. Often, it starts at the free edge and penetrates more proximally in the center than at the sides, thus becoming crescent-shaped. In other cases, the nail becomes detached at one or both sides. The detached part of the nail appears partly opaque and light-colored because of the reflection of light by air under the nail. The nail plate is usually of normal thickness, but a hyperkeratotic nail may also become detached.

Distribution and Extent of the Changes Within the Nail Plate

Like skin and hair changes, pathological changes in the nails may be disseminated (pits in psoriasis) or diffuse (leukonychia totalis). The changes often have a pronounced tendency to occur in transverse (leukonychia striata) or longitudinal bands (senile ridges). The defects may affect only a part of the nail or the entire nail. Partial changes in a nail may start from the free edge (splintering and onycholysis) or may originate at the root of the nail (desquamation or defect) and slowly shift distally. Changes beginning at the proximal end, of course, always indicate a disturbance of the matrix or of the nail fold (paronychia, tumors, psoriasis, eczema). The number of nail plates involved may be of diagnostic significance.

Changes in the Tissues Surrounding the Nail

A thorough examination of the nails requires attention to the tissues surrounding the nails, especially for skin diseases that invade the nail itself from the nail fold (e.g. psoriasis, eczema) or form a common disorder together with the nail (e.g. x-ray atrophy). It is important to determine if the nail wall is altered, especially swollen, as is the case in eczemas, paronychias, tumors, and "ingrowing toenails". Tumors may be situated at or under the free edge of the nail, as is frequently the case with warts.

Besides the nail wall, the cuticle and eponychium also deserves attention because this structure may be altered in various nail and skin diseases (e.g. ichthyosis, lupus erythematosus, sclerodactylia, hangnail). It may, for example, be widened or cracked. Pterygium formation is a progressive condition usually starting on one nail and extending to others. The eponychium grows forward over the central proximal nail plate to cause complete or partial loss of the nail (e.g. congenital ectodermal defect, severely impaired peripheral circulation, severe lichen planus, epidermolysis bullosa dystrophica).

It should be emphasized that nail diseases may have connections with skin diseases at distant sites (e.g. nail changes in alopecia areata, lichen planus, and psoriasis) and that occasionally they may appear as manifestations of internal diseases (e.g. koilonychia in hypochromic anemia due to iron deficiency).

Diagnosis

Several general statements should be made here. Depending in part on age, the fingernails replace themselves in about 6 months, the toenails in 12 to 18 months. Growth is more rapid in the summer. Congenital nail abnormalities may not be present at birth and permanent deformities of the nail plate can result from long-forgotten trauma to the matrix. Onychomycosis can exist in the nails alone. Nail changes of psoriasis and lichen planus may precede or persist after the other cutaneous or mucous membrane manifestations. Although now very rare, syphilis of the nails should not be forgotten as a possible diagnosis.

It is often useful to consider the four areas of the nail and surrounding tissues to explain the origin of the abnormality. These four areas are matrix and nail plate, nail bed, hyponychium, and the proximal and lateral nail folds (Table 47).

In general, there are six main reactions of the nails to systemic disease. These are onycholysis, nail bed discoloration, longitudinal ridging, transverse depressions, unusual shape of nail plate, and periungual telangiectasia.

Congenital

Describing the wide variety of rare congenital anomalies affecting the nails in many diverse ways is not useful. Many congenital nail anomalies are not diagnostic and must be examined and considered along with other changes in the skin, mucous membranes, teeth, and hair, in conjunction with other members of the patient's family. Also, many vary tremendously in degree and are not always present. In the nail-patella syndrome the diagnostic abnormalities are visible by radiographs of the elbow, patella, and forearm. The nails may show triangular lunulas as well as other dystrophic changes. Pachyonychia congenita is a condition not too rarely seen in which the nail abnormality is reasonably specific.

Traumatic

The Chinese foot-binding syndrome (see Chapter 15) is a major traumatic onychosis.

Damage to the matrix from crushing or cutting or from surgical removal of periungual verrucae may cause permanent abnormalities in the nail plate.

More subtle injuries may often produce most unusual dystrophies, some of which are listed below.

Nail biting generally produces a short, rough-edged nail and usually involves all of the fingernails. Periungual verrucae are common in nail biters. Some children may also tear off their toenails. Frequently, the periungual tissues are bitten and chewed. Occasionally, the whole plate may be bitten or chewed off. Habit tic picking and pulling of the periungual tissues may also be present.

Table 47: Diagnosis of Nail Conditions

	Psoriasis	Lichen Planus	Alopecia Areata	Darier's Disease	Eczema	Fungus Distal Subungual	Fungus ProximalSubungual	Fungus Superficial White	Other Disease and Comments
Matrix Plate									
Pits	x		x		x				
Onychorrhexis* (long)	x	x	x	x					Aged
Beau's lines	x		x		x				Symmetrical = systemic
Leukonychia	x		x	x			x	x	Good luck spots
Onycholysis†	x				x				Demeclocycline photosensitivity Thyroid disease
Erythema lunula	x		x						Dermatomyositis, systemic lupus erythamatosus
Pterygium		x							Trauma, scleroderma Radiodermatitis
Splits		x		**					
Hyperpigmentation		x							Drugs
Onychomedesis‡		x	x		x				Trauma, digit sarcoid
Bed									
Oil drop†	x								
Subhyperkeratosis	x					x			
Onycholysis†	x					x			
Splinter hemorrhage	x								
Atrophy		x							Trauma, radiodermatitis, ectodermal dysplasias
Hypopigmentation		x							
Hyponychium									
Subhyperkeratosis	x				x	x	x		
Nail Plate									
Thinned		x							Radiodermatitis, dysplasias
Thick	x			x	x	x			
Crumbling	x					x			
Destruction	x	x							Trauma
Shiny					x				
Yellowish/white focal	x					x	x	x	
Proximal and Lateral Nail Folds									
Red scaling	x								Candida, wet-trauma
Papules		x							Syphilis, warts

*Onychorrhexis, splitting; ‡ Onycholysis, separation of plate from bed; †Onychomedesis, shedding; **V-nicking.

The habit tic of playing with the nail affects the thumbnails; the patient picks at the cuticle with the adjacent index or third finger. This results in a central depression down the center of the nail with irregular cross-ridges extending from it almost to the edge of the nail.

Overly enthusiastic pushing back of the cuticle can result in transverse, sometimes white, streaks across the nail, as well as transverse ridging.

Median nail dystrophy is a true central longitudinal split through the whole thickness of the nail plate. It is first seen at the cuticle and grows out with the nail until the free margin is reached. The condition usually involves one or both of the thumbnails and all affected patients appear to have very large lunula. It is episodic.

Excessive exposure to water can cause nail splitting (lamellar dystrophy), especially of the tips of the nail plate and especially in individuals over 40 years of age. It is almost always seen in women.

Subungual hematomas occur beneath the toenails from ill-fitting shoes, in addition to other more obvious blunt injuries (Fig. 22.2). The black from the hematoma may extend into the cuticle and adjacent periungual tissues. The other colors of bruising may be present. The problem is distinguishing hematomas from acral ungual and periungual malignant melanoma, as occurs in older lesions. The black from the hematoma takes a long time to grow out and sometimes the original traumatic event cannot be remembered by the patient.

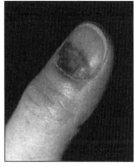

Figure 22.2 Subungual hematoma.

Hangnails are small traumatic tears of the posterior fold and the lateral folds. They are more common in individuals who do manual work. They do not occur in the toes.

In long-standing itchy dermatoses, the free borders of the nails may become concave and worn, their surface being as smooth as a mirror (Fig. 22.3). Loose material is often present beneath the end of the nail plate.

An ingrowing toenail occurs when the edge of the nail plate impinges upon the soft parts in the vicinity and excites the formation of tender ulcerated furrows about which edema, tenderness, and redness occur and from which some pus can be expressed. Proud flesh often grows in this sulcus. Hyperhidrosis, ill-fitting shoes, incorrectly cut toenails, and rubber soled athletic shoes are other contributory factors. I have never seen ingrowing fingernails.

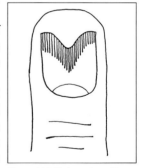

Figure 22.3 V-shaped notching and buffing of distal portion of nail plate seen in patients who have scratched hard and often over a long period of time.

Nails can also be damaged by chemicals in nail polish and other nail preparations.

In the last twenty years or so there has been an increasing emphasis on such activities as cross-country running and skiing, squash, soccer and hiking. These produce frequent, repeated and moderately severe trauma to the nail plates and surrounding tissues. The changes which result can consist of repeated hematomas, thickening and irregularities of the plate, distal subungual keratoses and scarring and compression and flattening of the fourth and fifth toes. I have even seen repeated and severe athletic trauma produce loss of nail plates. The most frequently seen and severe changes are in soccer players. The damage from the sport will, of course, be more severe if improperly fitting shoes are worn. These traumatic lesions may be misdiagnosed as melonotic nail streaking, benign or malignant subungual tumors, and onychomycosis.

Onychomycoses

There are several types of onychomycoses, descriptions of which follow.[2]

Distal Subungual

Distal subungual onychomycoses primarily involve the distal nail bed and hyponychium, with secondary involvement of the underside of the nail plate. First involvement may be seen at the hyponychium or lateral nail fold. At either or both of these places, a thickening of the horny layers with subungual keratosis occurs. This thickening lifts up the nail plate producing a white appearance called onycholysis. As the disease progresses, excessive subungual keratosis can lift the nail plate up to a 45-degree angle. Later, as the nail plate is more involved, it loses its transparency and becomes crumbly and dough-like. Yellow-brown longitudinal streaks or projections of diseased nail plate and underlying adjacent nail bed may develop. The nail plate may be discolored yellow, brown, green, or gray. Finally, the nail plate either crumbles or is traumatically removed. Splinters of nail plate may remain over a thickened nail bed.

Subungual keratosis is the most reliable sign of onychomycosis; however it is by no means diagnostic. Most of the fingernails and toenails are usually involved, although occasionally one or more digits is spared. The rate of involvement and extent of disease of each nail is often not the same.

White Superficial

White superficial onychomycosis appears opaque, white, and well demarcated on the surface of the toenail plates. These islands begin as punctate areas, randomly distributed. They then coalesce and gradually involve most of the surface of the nail plate. Older lesions may have a yellow color. The surface of the toenail is rough and its consistency is softer and more crumbly than the normal nail plate.

Proximal Subungual

Proximal subungual onychomycosis presents as white depressions in the nail plate, extending distally from under the proximal nail bed, confined to the areas of the lunula. One or more fingernails or toenails may be involved. The lesion is in the deeper portion of the nail, which results in the loss of the superficial portions of the nail plate. This loss of nail can be palpated. Rarely, large areas of the nails may be involved as the nail plate carries the disease with it as it grows outwards.

Candidal

Candidal onychomycosis is a candidal infection of the nail plate. It is part of the chronic cutaneous candidiasis syndrome also known as candidal granuloma (it is to be distinguished from candidal paronychia). Other nonwet areas such as glabrous skin and scalp may be involved with concentric, annular scaly lesions. The nails are opaque, noncrumbly, and often have longitudinal white streaks within the nail plate. Nail bed thickening occurs and the distal digit appears bulbous or pseudo-clubbed. Inflammatory reaction with erythema and edema in the surrounding nail tissue may ensue. A variable number of nails may be involved.

Chronic Candidal Paronychia

Chronic candidal paronychia is essentially a disease of women who frequently have their hands in water or who manicure their hands often and vigorously or in men who have wet occupations such as bartending. This paronychia appears as puffy, soft red swellings of the periungual tissues especially about the base of the nail plate. There may be some greenish-black or yellowish discoloration at the lateral nail folds or at the free distal end. Sometimes, a bead of pus may be expressed from the area. The cuticle is gone. Chronic candidal paronychia may affect one or more fingernails. The plate itself may be secondarily involved.

Rarely, the sequelae of chronic candidal paronychia may continue to involve the nail plate after all evidence of the paronychia is gone. This may closely resemble distal subungual onychomycosis.

In onycholysis, the nail bed may become secondarily infected with *Candida* and the nail plate may be infected later.

Dermatoses

Psoriasis

Psoriasis can be involved in several structures of the nails.[3]

Nail Plate

Pits, punctate or irregular depressions up to 2mm in diameter, form a pattern or are randomly spaced on the surface of the nail plate. Pits are more common on the fingers than on the toes. The pits vary in size, depth, and shape. Such lesions may also be seen in chronic eczema, alopecia areata, and in some individuals with no apparent disease.

Furrows or transverse depressions (Beau's lines) may be present and are especially noticeable on the proximal portion of the nail plate.

Nail plates can be seen crumbling on the distal or proximal portions or, in severe cases, all over.

Leukonychia may be present, associated with a rough or smooth surface of the plate. Leukonychia is usually irregular and may be punctate or striate. It is to be distinguished from onycholysis.

Nail Bed

Splinter hemorrhages are commonly seen. They occur longitudinally on the nail plate.

Oval reddish discoloration of the entire or partial nail bed may be present. This, of course, only occurs when the nail plate is not severely damaged.

A horny mass simulating the fallen nail plate may be present in nail tissues severely damaged by psoriasis.

Hyponychium

In psoriasis of the hyponychium, there is accumulated horny debris under the nail plate (subungual keratosis). The amount and color varies. Often it assumes a greasy yellow appearance, or it may be silvery white like the scales of psoriasis. Rarely, great thickening occurs, especially on the toenails.

Onycholysis of the distal and lateral portion of the nail plate may be present and sometimes extends proximally for some variable distance. Complete separation rarely occurs. There is usually a translucent, red-brown line 1mm wide separating the loosened area, which appears white, from the normal nail. This red-brown line is fairly characteristic of psoriasis. A translucent red-brown color may occur from subungual parakeratosis with an overlying relatively intact nail plate (oil drop sign).

There is a yellowish-green-brown discoloration of subungual debris in onycholytic areas.

Every patient with psoriasis of the skin does not automatically have psoriasis of the nails; similarly every psoriatic nail does not have every one of the above described findings; the extent of disease may vary greatly from nail to nail in the same patient. The skin of the proximal and lateral nail folds may have psoriasis, or there may be only minimal psoriasis elsewhere, e.g. on the scalp or perianal area. Arthritis of the distal interphalangeal joints may be present in patients with psoriasis of the nails. Very seldom is onychomycosis found in association with psoriasis. Repeated mycological examinations of the toenail are often necessary to identify the fungus.

Eczema

Eczema of the parts of the finger adjacent to the nails may produce an irregular cross-ridging of the plate, a discolored yellowish hue, splitting, and subungual keratosis formation. Subungual keratosis formation is particularly marked in eczema of the fingertips. The nail plate may be thinned and finally exfoliated. Coarse pitting may occur. The amount of change varies from nail to nail. At first, only the proximal part of the nail plate is damaged. To make the diagnosis of eczema changes in the nails, there must be or have been some peringual eczema, although at times it may have disappeared before the patient complains of the nail abnormality.

Lichen Planus

The commonest change is a deep longitudinal grooving or ridging of the nail plate along with slight depressions on the surface that catch the light when viewed from the side. The ends of the nail are frayed. Transverse ridging is rare. Even more rare is a thinning and loss of the nail plate with an overgrowing pterygium. Atrophy of the nail and absence of the nail plate also is rarely seen. In children, these last two findings may be the so-called twenty-nail dystrophy (Table 48).

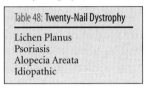

Table 48: **Twenty-Nail Dystrophy**

Lichen Planus
Psoriasis
Alopecia Areata
Idiopathic

Alopecia Areata

In the extensive and generalized forms of alopecia areata, ungual lesions are frequent. The changes consist of dryness, white longitudinal striations, pitting, or of fissuring, crumbling, and indentation.

Pityriasis Rubra Pilaris

In pityriasis rubra pilaris, the nail is thickened, striated, lusterless, and yellowish. There is a hard but porous keratosis of the nail bed. Rarely, pits may be present.

Erythroderma

In severe primary erythroderma, the nails become completely or incompletely detached. When a new nail is formed, it insinuates itself under the remains of the old nail. With the advent of corticosteroid therapy, severe nail changes are now seen infrequently.

Darier's Disease

In Darier's disease, the nails are longitudinally striated, furrowed, and brittle, with occasionally white longitudinal striae and splitting of the free margin of the plate.

Pyococcal

Pus infections about the nail usually occur in the lateral nail fold as a redness, swelling, and tenderness. Later, small, but deep, abscesses may form with the nail involved in extensive chronic pyoderma, although this is now quite rare.

Radiodermatitis

Severe chronic radiodermatitis of the severe type can produce fragmentation, destruction, exfoliation, or even total atrophy. Telangiectasia may also be present.

Syphilis

The nail changes of secondary syphilis include the following.
1. The nail plate may be cracked and brittle at its free end.
2. The nail plate can be detached from below upward with nonpainful redness and desquamation of the bed, and sometimes loss of the nail.
3. The nail may be hypertrophied, thickened, streaked, and blackish without change of its general shape.
4. There may be ulceration with loss of substance, usually oval, crateriform, with lamellar borders. It appears on the lunula and exposes the matrix or the bed of the nail, which is of a grayish pink color.
5. The periungual tissues may become scaly or horny when a squamous papule forms on one of the periungual folds. It may be inflammatory when it consists of a dusky red, very persistent tumefaction. When it is ulcerative, there is a loss of substance with cut out borders, and a bloody floor develops, often as a semicircle on the periungual folds. The extremity of the fingers is swollen and reddened; the nail usually falls out. Several fingers or toes are often attacked at the same time.

Herpetic Whitlow

Primary or secondary herpes simplex infections can occur around the nails (see Chapter 8).

Miscellaneous

The nails may be distorted, becoming thick and opaque in an infection by Norwegian scabies. There may be loss of the nails in epidermolysis bullosa dystrophica and following some severe generalized drug eruptions. The nails may be involved in bullous dermatoses such as pemphigus and dermatitis herpetiformis. Reiter's disease and pustular psoriasis have been discussed elsewhere. The telangiectatic blood vessels, the purplish erythema, and the hemorrhages of subacute or systemic lupus erythematosus should be remembered. In the yellow nail syndrome, the nails become yellowish or greenish, thickened, and may be excessively curved from side to side with the lateral margins of the plate being replaced by soft tissue. The cuticle is usually absent. Fingertip clubbing with associated nail changes is classically associated with lung or heart disease with cyanosis. The nails of old age often are dull, opaque, and have longitudinal ridging. There is an increased tendency to splitting.

All sorts of degenerative changes occur in the fingertips and nails in diseases associated with impaired circulation, e.g. Raynaud's disease, scleroderma, sclerodactyly, and diabetics with arteriosclerosis.

Onychogryphosis

This deformity consists of enormous, very hard thickening with a change in the direction of the nail, which becomes raised and curved on itself. To a minor degree, the nails assume the appearance of very hard, grayish or brownish claws, curved transversely and from front to back and raised from the bed by keratosis. To a higher degree, the nail is entirely deformed, convex, and twisted, resembling a ram's horn. It is implanted almost vertically on its bed, is of a brownish color, and marked at the same time by longitudinally and transversely undulating striae. The nail grows slowly, but as its stony hardness prevents it from being cut, it often reaches from 3 to 4cm length. It is most commonly seen on the toenails, especially on the big toe. The elderly are the usual victims of this condition.

Tumors

Any skin tumor can occur in the skin about the nails. Some benign tumors producing nail deformities are verrucae, periungual fibromas, pyogenic granuloma, myxoid cysts, ganglions, and pigmented nevi. The rare malignant tumors include Bowen's disease, squamous cell carcinoma, and malignant melanoma.

The malignant tumors are easily missed because of their flat, erosive, ulcerative nature. They are slow growing, therefore frank nodular tumor formation is often a very late finding. The friable hemorrhagic tissue and the local destruction of the tissues are the main clues. Acral ungual and periungual melanomas are supposed to show a black pigment spread to the cuticle and periungual tissues (Hutchinson's sign)—but this can also be seen with severe ungual hematomas. Ungual and periungual malignant melanomas can, like other acral melanomas, be without visible black or brown pigment (e.g. amelanotic melanoma).

Dyschromias

Color change (dyschromia) is one way nails respond to stimuli.[4]

White Nails

Terry's nails show an ivory white color of almost all the nail bed (⅛ nails) except for the zone of normal pink near the distal edge (⅛, ⅞ nails). This anomaly occurs in advanced liver cirrhosis.

Leukonychia may be total or partial.[5] If partial, it can be striate or punctate.

Mees' lines are transverse white stripes seen in such conditions as acute renal failure, acute arsenism, and acute thallium poisoning (Table 49).[6]

Muehrcke's lines are paired, narrow white bands that run parallel to the lunula and are separate from one another and from the lunula by areas of normal pink nail. They do not move forward with the nail. The distal band may be slightly wider than the proximal one. These changes are seen in hypoalbuminemia (Table 50).

Severe anemia may cause a pallor of the nail beds.

Trichophytosis can also cause white areas in the nails.

R.A. Mees, 20th Cent, Dutch Physician
Muehrcke
Terry

Blue Nails

The nail bed in hypoxic cyanosis may be a bluish hue. Methemoglobinemia and sulfhemoglobinemia also can cause a pseudocyanosis of the nail bed. In Wilson's disease there may be azure half moons. Among the drugs that can cause bluish nail changes, the following are examples: argyria (blue gray), chloroquine (blue black), phenothiazine (purple), and phenolphthalein-fixed drug eruptions (blue half moons).

Yellow Nails

Nails may have a yellowish color in lymphedema, jaundice, psoriasis, and onychomycoses including favus. In the yellow nail syndrome, the nail plate is yellow and thickened (Table 51). The nail grows slowly, has cross-ridging, and there is loss of the lunulae and cuticles. It occurs in lymphedema and in patients with pleural effusions. Systemic drugs such as demethylchlortetra-cycline and mepacrine may cause yellow nails. Topically, resorcin, chrysarobin, chromium salts, picric acid, dinitrotoluene, iodochlorhydroxyquin, Vioform, and formaldehyde and tobacco can stain the nails yellow.

Green Nails

Pseudomonas and other infections, particularly candidal, can produce a dark green color of the nails.

Red Nails

Polycythemia and carbon monoxide poisoning cause red nails. In congestive heart failure, there may be red half moons.

Brown and Black Nails

Certain tumors such as malignant melanomas (melanotic whitlow) may cause a dark color. Pigmented nevi can present as linear brown streaks. These are especially common (80%) in the black race. Some Proteus infections, and infections due to Alternaria grisea may show dark nails. Systemic infections such as syphilis (amber colored), pinta, and malaria can cause dark nails. Also to be mentioned are gangrene, ochronosis, the freckling of Peutz-Jeghers syndrome, the diffuse melanin pigment of Addison's disease, the transverse brown band of chronic radiodermatitis, and the black of traumatic hematomas and splinter hemorrhages. In chronic renal failure, the half-and-half nail shows a dull whitish proximal zone and a red pink or brown

Table 49: Mees' Lines

Arsenic Poisoning
Carbon Monoxide Poisoning
Chemotherapy Drugs
Hodgkin's Disease
Leprosy
Malaria
Myocardial Infarct
Pellagra
Pneumonia
Psoriasis
Renal Failure
Sickle-Cell Disease
Thallium Poisoning

Table 50: Muercke's Lines

Chronic Hypoalbuminemia
Nephrotic syndrome
Glomerulonephitis
Liver disease
Malnutrition

Table 51: Yellow Nail Syndrome

Features	Associations
Yellow Color	Brochiectasis
Absent Cuticle	Cancer of the Larynx
Transverse Curvature of the Nail	Chronic Bronchitis
Absence of Lunula	Chronic Lymphedema
Onycholysis	Rheumatoid Arthritis
Longitudinal Curvature	Sinusitis
Regular Slight Thickening	Thyroid Disease

distal zone (Lindsay's nails). Many topical agents, such as nicotine, caramel, gold and mercury salts, photography solutions, varnish, some woods, silver nitrate, potassium permanganate, and some nail polishes, may stain the nails. Nails should be scraped with the edge of a glass slide to check suspicions of an external source of the color.

References

1. Siemens HW. General diagnosis and therapy of skin diseases. Weiner K, trans. Chicago:University of Chicago Press, 1958.
2. Zaias PN. Psoriasis of the nail. Arch Dermatol 1969; 99:567–579.
3. Zaias PN. Onychomycosis. Arch Dermatol 1972; 105:263–274.
4. Daniel CR, Osment LS. Nail pigmentation abnormalities. Cutis 1980; 25:595–607.
5. Albright SD, Wheeler CE. Leukonychia. AMA Arch Derm 1964; 90:392–399.
6. Mees RA, Een Verschijnsal BJ. Polyneuritis arsonicosa. Nederl T. Cenecsic 1919; 1:391–396.

Lindsay

CHAPTER 23
Hidroses

Functional or organic disturbances of the apocrine or eccrine sweat glands.

Overview

The term hidrosis can be applied to functional and organic disturbances of apocrine and eccrine sweat glands. In general, I have used the terms anhidrosis and hyperhidrosis to apply only to the eccrine sweat glands.

Anhidrosis

Neurologically, lesions of the hypothalamus, brain stem, spinal cord, or sympathetic nerve fibers (as in leprosy) may cause widespread or local areas of anhidrosis. Drugs that block the autonomic nervous system, e.g. atropine, can produce anhidrosis.

There are numerous cutaneous causes of anhidrosis. Congenital ectodermal defect, localized absence of sweat glands, and many conditions associated with an atrophy of the sweat glands (senile skin, scleroderma, radiodermatitis) can cause eccrine anhidrosis. Sweat retention anhidrosis may occur in patients with dermatitis and other inflammatory skin diseases or it may occur without other cutaneous disease as in miliaria crystallina, rubra, and pustulosa (see below). Skin affected by the lesions of psoriasis, atopic dermatitis, and lichen planus does not sweat.

Hyperhidrosis

Generalized hyperhidrosis can occur from febrile illness, environmental heat, increase in internal heat load, and by stimulation of the hypothalamus. Localized hyperhidrosis may occur on the palms, soles, axillae, and forehead. The sweat may run freely off these areas. On the palms and soles, a cold, clammy effect may be present. Some neurologic disorders of the peripheral autonomic nervous system may cause bizarre patterns of localized hyperhidrosis. Gustatory hyperhidrosis is development of excessive sweating on the scalp and/or face following ingestion of such spicy foods as mustard pickles or chili peppers.

Sharply marginated, burning, purplish-red erythema with hyperhidrosis may exist on the soles (lividity is symmetrical). There are no blisters. In some areas, the lesions look like burns.

In teenage boys who wear rubber soled shoes, have hyperhidrosis, and are physically active, small, solitary, 2 to 3 mm pits or confluent areas of pitting with loss of the uppermost horny layers may be present, particularly on the plantar surface of the heel and beneath the anterior arch. This is called basketball feet or pitted keratolysis. White maceration may also be present with or without the above described pitting (see also Chapter 15).

Miliaria

Miliaria crystallina (sudamina) consists of minute cysts located at the orifices of eccrine sweat glands.

Miliaria rubra (prickly heat) shows clusters or patches of small (1mm) erythematous papules especially on the back and sides of the trunk, the abdomen,

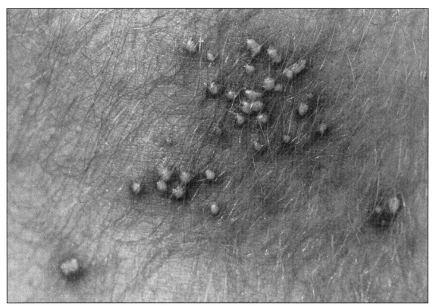

Figure 23.1 Miliaria pustulosa on the thigh of a patient with atopic dermatitis.

and the antecubital and popliteal fossa. It is usually symmetrical. At times, the erythematous element may be quite prominent, as the lesion affects the living spinous layer of the epidermis. The palms and soles are not involved.

Miliaria pustulosa is the pustular form of miliaria. The small pustules are distinct, discrete, superficial, and filled with white purulent matter. Rarely, a central dark dot representing a plugged sweat gland can be seen (Fig. 23.1).

Miliaria profunda presents in patients as a cobblestone appearance with evenly scattered, rounded, flesh-colored papules. The skin is dry. Heat stroke may also be present. This is rare in nontropical climes.

In some cases, more than one type of miliaria may be present at the same time. Miliaria occurs in hot, moist, environments. Occasionally, candidiasis may have a distribution suggestive of miliaria.

Miscellaneous

Granulosis rubra nasi is a localized hyperhidrosis occurring in a prepubertal child on the face, palms, and soles. On the face, there is a maculopapular erythematous eruption on the nose and a mild erythema on the cheeks.

Patients with pompholyx do not necessarily show hyperhidrosis.

Hidrocystomas are discussed in Chapter 24.

Bromhidrosis is foul- or abnormal-smelling sweat usually arising from the feet or axilla. It is often associated with hyperhidrosis and the odor may be overwhelming or may be largely imagined by the patient. Occasionally, generalized bromhidrosis may occur from eating garlic or onions or following the topical application of dimethylsulphoxide. Bromhidrosis smells more foul and less sweet than the odor of patients with erythroderma or extensive pemphigus vulgaris. Acrid or rancid odor may arise from the skin in areas of apocrine secretion, such as the axilla or groin.

Poral closure eruption of children is basically a type of miliaria in which the lesions are prominent at the sweat gland orifice. Occasionally, secondary suppuration occurs. Note that the eruption is not follicular, neither is it an erythema such as erythema toxicum neonatorum.

Chromhidrosis is the term used for colored sweat from the apocrine glands, commonly on the face, usually symmetrical and usually in women. The color is black or very dark and is seen in small minute (1 mm) droplets.

Recurrent palmoplantar hidradenitis in children consists of numerous small, tender erythematous papules on the palms and soles. The lesions are self-healing. Histologically, they show a dense neutrophilic infiltrate around eccrine sweat glands and extend into the hypoderm.

Apocrine gland retention cysts (see Chapter 24) and Fox-Fordyce disease (see Chapter 11) and hidradenitis suppurative (see "Acne conglobata" in Chapter 20) are also hidroses.

CHAPTER 24

Cysts

| *Encapsulated retention cavity filled with fluid, cells, and cell products.* |

Overview

A cyst is an encapsulated cavity filled with fluid, cells, and cell products.[1,2] Cysts are retention tumors. The cyst is not inflammatory though occasionally it may become secondarily inflamed. The capsule of a cyst is compressed connective tissue lined with epithelium or endothelium. The lining develops from dilated and cut-off parts of glands, glandular ducts, blood and lymph vessels, or layers of epidermis (Table 52). The contents of a cyst consist of products of the lining such as serum, lymph, sweat, sebum, epithelial cells, keratin or hairs. According to the nature and pressure of its contents, the cyst may be rubbery, doughy, or even fluctuant. In contrast to an abscess, redness and tenderness are absent. Because of the tendency of the liquid or pulpy contents to spread equally in all directions and because of regular growth, cysts are usually spherical or egg-shaped. They may be as small as a mustard seed (e.g. a milium, containing a horny pearl) or a pea (e.g. a hidrocystoma, containing sweat) or may be as large as or larger than a goose egg (e.g. an epidermal cyst, filled with lamellated keratin). If the skin covering a cyst is much stretched, the follicular openings are enlarged and form shallow pits. In some cases, the central one-third of the overlying skin may be brown, thickened, and attached to the underlying cyst. In contrast to traumatic epidermal cysts, which originate from epidermal cells displaced into the cutis, or subcutis, true epidermal cysts may show the obstructed follicle opening as a point or a small elevation. Even if the point cannot be readily seen, it frequently can be demonstrated by extrusion of a thin thread of thick keratinous material if the cyst is squeezed. Some cysts are located so superficially and have so thin a capsule that, clinically, they seem to be unilocular vesicles (miliaria crystallina, hidrocystoma, lymphangioma).

Table 52: **Cysts and Their Lining**	
Lining	**Type of Cyst**
Epidermis	Epidermoid, milia, traumatic
Epidermis	Vellus hair is present in central cyst often with a rudimentary telogen hair follicle
Outer Hair Root Sheath	Pilar Cyst
Sebaceous	Steatocystoma multiplex, eruptive vellus hair cyst
Apocrine	Hidrocystoma, cyst of gland of Moll
Eccrine	Hidrocystoma, miliaria crystallina (duct)
Synovia	Myxomatous cyst, ganglion
Vascular	Capillary and cavernous angioma, venous lake, varicosities
Lymphatics	Lymphangioma circumscriptum, cyst hygroma
Stratified Columnar	Thyroglossal or bronchial sinus or cyst
Minor Salivary Gland	Mucocele

Milium

These lesions (plural of milium is milia) are white or whitish yellow beady granules, 1 to 3 mm in size, small intraepidermic or intradermic cysts. The upper

Portions of the Overview have been taken and modified from Siemens[1] (pp. 55–58).

two-thirds of the face or the genital organs are the main locations. Milia are common along the eyelid margins and on the eyelids, especially in persons over 40 years of age. They may occur as part of the eruption in polymorphous acne or they may occur independently, especially in individuals over 50 year of age. Occasionally, these lesions can be eruptive. Milia may be present in neonates. A favorite location is the lower portion of the postauricular crease where they are often associated with true epidermal cysts. Milia also occur in the scars of porphyria and epidermolysis bullosa, in poison ivy, as part of keratosis pilaris, following dermabrasion of the face for removal of acne scars, and in the acne lesions present in dermatoheliosis.

DIFFERENTIAL DIAGNOSIS

On the eyelids, milia must be distinguished from xanthomas (which are more corn-colored, larger, dermal, and form irregular shapes); from large blackheads (which have a central black opening beneath and about which there is a yellowish white cheesy material); and from certain adnexal tumors such as syringoma and trichoepithelioma.

Epidermal Cysts

The general description of epidermal cysts is given in the Overview.

Traumatic epidermal cysts are more common on the palms and soles, particularly following trauma, as on an amputation stump, or following some surgical procedure. They are usually solitary and have no central punctum.

True epidermal cysts, on the other hand, tend to occur in areas where there are large sebaceous glands, e.g. face, neck, ear lobes, chest, back, and scrotum. To the touch, they have a degree of elasticity. True epidermal cysts usually have a central punctum. A nauseous rancid smell may be present. Commonly, more than one is present although each lesion may be of a different size. If they become inflamed and/or infected, they may resolve. Otherwise, they may stay unchanged in size, or slightly increase in size.

I doubt that inflammatory acne granulomas can develop in true epidermal cysts. If it happens it must be rare—think of the millions of acne granuloma that disappear with treatment or by themselves. Remember too, the fact that these granulomas recur at the same site does not mean they are cysts. An acne lesion recurring at the same site is not a rare phenomenon.

Pilar cysts occur mainly on the scalp, are usually multiple, and are frequently familial. No central pore is visible.

Vellus hair cysts are two to three millimeter smooth, skin-colored or pale, upper dermal papules located on the anterior chest, abdomen, and flexural aspects of the extremities.

Hundreds of cysts and/or yellowish deep dermal papules on the scalp, face, torso, and genitals occur in older patients with steatocystoma multiplex. Such patients may also have acne. Like the vellus hair cysts, steatoma multiplex lesions also are present on the flexor aspects of the extremities. Histologically, these are the only true sebaceous cysts.

Epidermal cysts should be distinguished from lipomas, which occur on the loins, buttocks, scapulas, arms, and thighs and which have a pillowy feel.

Dermoids and Teratomas

Dermoids and teratomas are relatively rare skin cysts. The dermoids occur most frequently in the brachial cleft area. Teratomas may be seen in the genital area, and may contain ectodermal and appendageal structures such as hair, sebaceous glands, teeth, and nonectodermal structures such as bone and cartilage.

Hidrocystoma

Apocrine hidrocystomas are numerous or solitary, 2 to 4 mm, firm, tense, translucent, bluish, dome-shaped elevations from which a sticky fluid is discharged on puncture. They are usually located on the head, neck, or prepuce. Rarely, a large pea-sized lesion may be seen on the trunk.

Like apocrine hidrocystomas, eccrine hidrocystomas also appear on the face and have a similar morphological picture. The difference between eccrine and apocrine nature is determined by histological examination. Contrary to current textbooks, these lesions do not occur exclusively in women exposed to a hot moist environment.

Cysts of the Gland of Moll

These are 2 to 5 mm cystic lesions occurring in the elderly on the eyelid margin or in the skin adjacent to it. The cyst has a bluish tinge, is turgid and may be composed of several microlobules or may be unilobular. Frequently, they are multiple. They are more common in the lower eyelid. They persist and slowly enlarge. They do not scar. Some have the histological picture of hidrocystoma.

DIFFERENTIAL DIAGNOSIS

An occasional basal cell carcinoma on the eyelid margin has a bluish gray, translucent aspect. However, a firmer border can usually be seen, the carcinoma will be seen to destroy or eat into the tissues, and on puncture, no or very little fluid will be obtained. The carcinoma lesions will not disappear. Also, multiple lesions of basal cell carcinoma are extremely rare on the eyelid margin.

Lymphangioma Circumscriptum and Lymphangiectases

Lymphangioma circumscriptum is a condition that consists of sago grain-sized, tense, clear, rose-colored or deep red cysts occurring in a palm-sized cluster usually on the torso or in the axilla. There are areas of normal skin between the lesions. Some of the small cystic papules are full of blood and may appear angiomatous. Occasionally, tufts of dilated capillaries are present. Sometimes, the lesions develop a verrucous keratotic surface, particularly in areas where they are continuously rubbed (e.g. between the breasts in women), closely resembling angiokeratomas. The lesions are not compressible. When punctured, a clear or blood-tinged fluid is released. One or two of the lesions are often crusted. On the anterior one-half of the tongue, these lesions may be present and cause macroglossia. Cystic hygroma is the name given to a similar lesion with larger cavities located in the subcutaneous tissue, usually on the sides and lower portions of the face and neck of infants and young children. Strictly speaking, they are not cysts, they are dilated lymphatus and small blood vessels.

Lymphangiectases (or lymphatic varicosities) are acquired dilations of the lymph channels of the skin and mucosa. They are 1 to 2mm, shiny, firm, clear, superficial, cystic papules, usually intermingled with blood and hence dark red cysts. I have seen them following surgery and radiotherapy for breast cancer, in the axilla and on the upper extremity. Lymphangiectases occur in disease states causing high lymphatic pressure. Puncture of the cystic lesions causes a persistent flow of lymph (lymphorrhea).

Miliaria Crystallina

The basic lesions of miliaria crystallina are clear, tense microcysts, usually smaller than 1mm in diameter, located in an evenly dotted fashion over the flanks and abdomen. Each cyst is made by a minute elevation of the horny layer, containing a clear watery fluid and without a congested base. The lesions look like minute drops of water. (Strictly speaking, they are not cysts but dilated sweat glands.)

Mucocele

The basic lesion is a semitranslucent cystic swelling extending upwards from the surface of the epithelium. The base of the lesion is in the superficial layers of the submucosa. There is no involvement into the tunica propria. The borders are sharply demarcated. The surface is moderately irregular, forming a lobular surface. One or two of the lobules may have a telangiectatic or hemorrhagic aspect. The lesions have a gelatinous consistency. On puncturing, clear sticky mucous fluid can be expressed. Mucoceles are located on the mucosal aspect of the lips (particularly the lower). They are multiple and are of varying size, from 2 to 8 mm.

Ranula is a cyst of the anterior portion of the floor of the mouth, usually from a blocked major salivary gland duct.

Synovial Cysts

These are subcutaneous cysts (ganglions, cutaneous myxiod cysts) occurring most commonly about the joints or on tendons on the fingers and wrists and ankles (Fig. 24.1). They are more common in elderly. At times they are invisible and can only be felt as deep, cystic, well-demarcated structures. At other times they protrude and can

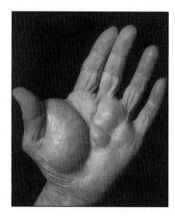

Figure 24.1 Huge multiple ganglions.

be seen as cystic structures, especially at the base of the nail. They can produce a slotted depression in the nail plate similar to that caused by periungual fibromas.

Some ganglions are true joint cysts which, on surgical exploration, can be traced into a joint. Cutaneous myxoid cyst, which occur mainly about the nails, do not communicate into the joint. Cutaneous myxoid cysts probably are best considered as pseudocysts.

DIFFERENTIAL DIAGNOSIS

The differential diagnosis includes most of the causes of juxta-articular nodes, such as gouty tophi, rheumatic nodules, Heberden's nodes, tendinous xanthomas, knuckle pads, nodules of reticulohistiocytosis, epidermal inclusion cysts, glomus tumors, and giant cell tumors of tendon sheath.

Chalazion

This is a firm elastic inflammatory or cystic enlargement of one or more meibomian glands on the eyelids usually near the tarsal plates. Most of these lesions are not true cysts, but foreign body granulomas akin to acneform granulomas.

Seroma of the auricle is not a cyst, but an accumulation of a clear, straw-colored fluid in the upper portion of the lateral side of the external ear.[3]

References

1. Siemens HW. General diagnosis and therapy of skin diseases. Weiner K, trans. Chicago:University of Chicago Press, 1958.
2. Anderson NP. Cysts, sinuses and fistulas of dermatologic interest. JAMA 1947; 135:607–612.
3. Lapins LTC, Odom RB. Seroma of the auricle. Arch Dermatol 1982; 118:503–505.

Heinrich Meibom, 1638–1700, German Anatomist

CHAPTER 25
Sinuses and Fistulae

> *Discharging tracts that are often granulomatous, sclerotic and midline, sometimes congenital.*

Overview

I make no distinction between the meanings of the terms sinus and fistula.*[1] These openings may occur as a by-product of many skin disorders and of many conditions of general medical interest. This chapter is limited to the most common and most obvious ones of dermatological interest.

To detect these lesions, pressure often must be applied, thus providing a reminder that palpation is part of the physical examination of the skin.

Congenital

Thyroglossal Sinus

In congenital thyroglossal sinuses and fistulae, on the skin over the suprasternal notch, a little to one side, is a 4 mm soft, thin, lined, translucent sac or cyst. From this lesion may be squeezed one or two drops of a clear sticky mucous fluid. All thyroglossal cysts or fistulae are located in the midline: on the chin, just above or below the hyoid bone, or lower in the midline to the suprasternal notch (Fig. 25.1).[2] Sometimes only a dimple is present. Various degrees of underlying sclerosis may be present.

Branchial Sinus

These openings may be located in the preauricular area, on the neck just at the angle of the jaw, or on a line just anterior to the sternomastoid muscle down to the clavicle

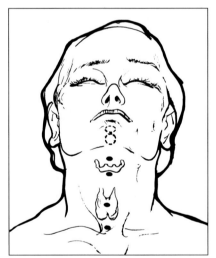

Figure 25.1 Locations of openings of thyroglossal sinuses. The broken circles indicate an intraoral location. Redrawn from Conway.[2]

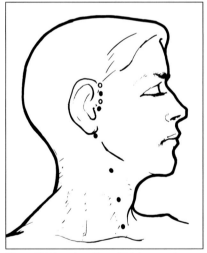

Figure 25.2 Location of branchial sinus openings (*Solid circles*) and preauricular sinus openings (*Open circles*). Redrawn from Conway.[2]

*Strictly speaking, a fistula is an abnormal communication between two cavities, e.g. from rectum to vagina, or between a cavity and the outside, e.g. from the rectum to the skin. A sinus is a blind tract and opening from a local diseased area, e.g. a discharging hidradentis suppurativa lesion. A very useful book in explaining the anatomical basis and location of many congenitally determined cysts, sinuses, and fistulae is Reference 1.

(Fig. 25.2). They are solitary and like all sinuses and fistulae may have varying degrees of inflammation, fibrosis, discharge, or pyogenic granuloma formatum. Occasionally the openings may be over the sterno-mastoid muscle.

Preauricular Sinus

This is manifest by a small dimple, pit, or orifice located usually in the preauricular area (see Fig. 25.2) The most common location is just anterior to the mid-portion of the ascending heli.Other lesions may be present in the preauricular area at the tragus and more superior areas. Rarely, multiple lesions may be present. One lesion may present on each side. Sometimes an inflamed tract or sinus, or cyst may be present. Rarely, when multiple, these tracts may communicate with each other. The tract may be felt to run superficially or may go deeply into underlying structures. Clinically, if the examiner is not alert to the possibility of preauricular fistulae, these inflamed cysts may be mistaken for acneform granulomas.

Miscellaneous Sinuses

On the lips, two pits in the center of the lower vermilion area may signify the presence of other embryological defects. Occasionally, a sinus tract may be present.

Other congenitally determined sinuses and fistulae are umbilical sinus, urachal sinus, perineal sinus, imperforate anus, blocked lactiferous duct of breast, congenital medial fistula of the nose, median raphe cysts of the penis and other sequestration dermoids in the line of embryonal concrescence and a congenital dorsal dermal sinus over the lumbosacral area sometimes associated with an overlying capillary nevus or hypertrichoses. Dermoid tumors may break down and discharge, especially if they are incompletely removed by surgery. Dermoid cysts may be present on the outer eyebrow area. Occasionally, meningoceles can cause discharging midline sinuses. Congenital midline nasal cysts, sinuses and tumors are most likely dermoids, gliomas or encephaloceles.[3]

Acquired

Dental Sinus

These present as solitary fixed openings into the skin of the cheeks, chin, and uncommonly, the neck. At the orifice a 0.5 cm, eroded, angiomatous or semicystic, inflamed structure is often present. Scarring and puckering about the orifice is common. The amount of discharge is usually minimal. A sclerotic sinus tract can often be felt by combined external and intraoral palpation. Dental sinuses can occur from buried tooth roots in patients who are seemingly edentulous.

Hair Granuloma Sinuses

The basic lesion in patients with this condition is that of multiple sinuses associated with varying degrees of inflammation, tenderness, scarring, and boggy inflammatory dermal and subdermal swellings. Pressure on one side frequently produces a watery or seropurulent discharge from one or many orifices. Occasionally, a portion of hair may be extruded, and if pulled on, a large number of long terminal hairs may be found. These sinuses are more common in patients with a dark-skinned, swarthy complexion. Much hair is frequently seen on the torso and buttocks of these patients. The most common area is in the upper portion of the natal cleft or lower sacral area. In this area, these lesions are called pilonidal sinuses. They may also be present in the umbilicus, on the face, and on the soles. In barbers, these sinuses may be located in the finger webs and the inflammatory process may cause severe pain, scarring, and infection in the palmar tissues. (See also "Foreign Body Granuloma" in Chapter 12.)

Acne Sinuses

Severe, granulomatous, inflamed, scarring acne on the face may develop sinus and fistulous tracts extending from one soft fluctuant area to another. Sometimes the tracts extend for a long distance and may, on pressure, exude foul-smelling sebaceous or keratinous material. These findings are most extensively seen in patients with acne conglobata and/or hidradenitis suppurativa and in cases of suppurating and cicatrizing folliculitis of the scalp.

Sinuses from Underlying Disease

Nodal granulomas (or gummas) may track through the hypoderm and discharge abscess material from a sinus, e.g. orofacial actinomycosis (see also Chapter 13). Also, diseased lymph nodes may break down and form sinus tracts, e.g. scrofuloderma. Sometimes the opening may be a long way from the original source, e.g. psoas abscess. Occasionally, specific organs may develop fistulous tracts, e.g. salivary gland fistulae following trauma or surgery. Multiple periparotid sinuses can develop from a draining odontogenic keratocyst in the ramus or mandible.

Crohn's disease may produce all sorts of sinuses and fistulae, usually in the genital or perianal areas. Occasionally it is associated with hidradenitis suppurativa. Bladder and bowel cancers may produce fistulae and sinuses. Fistula in ano is rarely seen in dermatological practice.

References

1. McGregor AL. du Plessis DJ. Synopsis of surgical anatomy. 10th Ed. Bristol:John Wright and Sons Ltd., 1975.
2. Conway H. Tumours of the skin. Springfield:Thomas, 1956.
3. Paller AS, Pensler JM, Tomita T. Nasal midline masses in infants and children. Arch Dermatol 1991; 427:362–366.

CHAPTER 26

Burrows

> *A tunnel in the superficial portion of the epidermis of variable size and shape made by a parasite.*

Overview

A burrow is a tunnel of variable size and shape in the stratum corneum that is made by a metazoal parasite. Creeping eruption is a classic example. Another example is scabies, in which the location of the mite-containing burrows is almost diagnostic. Other lesions as well as burrows are present in scabies and these along with the burrows are discussed in the description of scabies.

Scabies

The basic lesion in scabies is a tunnel or burrow in the stratum corneum and upper malpighian layer.[1] These are narrow, grayish tracts taking curved or sinuous courses, which do not correspond to the folds of the epidermis. A tiny deep vesicle at the head of the burrow contains the acarus. These burrows are best seen on the sides of the fingers, the fingerwebs, the thenar eminences, the penis, and the wrists. In the neonate, they are best seen on the soles. Elsewhere, the other lesions appear as small, sometimes twin, pointed papules. These are located on the axillary walls, elbows, breasts (in females), umbilicus, pubic area, buttocks, and penis. Most of these other lesions are secondary. The neck, head, and center back are not involved. Bilateral breast eczema in women is frequently scabies.

There are often many other secondary lesions: excoriated papules and linear scratch marks; the various stages of pyoderma (pustules, follicular pustules, infected ulcers, and patches of ecthyma), a blotchy eruption, scaly, slightly lichenified, in places eczematous, located mainly on the torso; in some areas, definite vesicles are present, which on the hands and wrists resemble pompholyx. Bilateral symmetry is a feature. These lesions without mites could be considered a scabid. In infants and children, the eruption is more widely spread and often involves the palmar and plantar surfaces. These surfaces are only occasionally involved in the adult. Bullous lesions may also be present.

Persistent papulonodular lesions resembling prurigo nodularis occasionally persist on the abdomen, penis, scrotum, and axilla in individuals who have had scabies. Widespread, juicy, brownish-red papules are common on the torso of infants with scabies. In these infants, the differential diagnosis includes acute parapsoriasis and histiocytosis X. These prurigo nodularis-like lesions may persist for some months after the scabies mite has been destroyed.

Rarely, patients present with nondescript excoriated papules on the sites of predilection of scabies, but no burrows can be found. This may be associated with acarophobia. Scabies is a disease that can be diagnosed by location alone. Complete examination of the skin is mandatory in any suspected case, or a correct diagnosis may be missed. The mites are easily found on the hands and wrists, or in infants and neonates, on the soles. To look for them elsewhere is usually nonrewarding, although there will be the secondary lesion of scabies elsewhere. In various members of the same family, scabies may present in different forms; for example, some may have many burrows, others, few; some, much secondary eczematous change, others, little.

Norwegian scabies is a generalized scaling process in the elderly and infirm, mentally retarded, or immunosuppressed patient. Really, it is a type of erythroderma, with varying degrees of scaling, erythema, lichenification, and excoriation. Total body involvement is the rule, including the scalp, face, neck, palmar skin, and the periungual tissues and the nail plates. In Norwegian scabies, there are innumerable mites easily found anywhere. Compare this to the average case of scabies with 11 mites located mainly on the wrists and fingers (and soles in neonates).

Differential diagnosis of scabies is provided in Table 53.

Remember that the five truly pruritic dermatoses are scabies, dermatitis herpetiformis, atopic dermatitis, insect bites, and urticaria.

Table 53: Differential Diagnoses of Scabies

Dermatitis Herpetiformis: Grouped symmetrical excoriated rather deep seated papules on lower back, scalp, elbows and knees; never on hands, rarely on genitalia; more common in adults; not contagious.

Atopic Dermatitis: Rather poorly demarcated, lichenified, scaly areas especially in flexures; may have "dyshidrosiform" pattern on sides of hands and feet; may have nummular eczematous lesions; often hypopigmentation, often involvement of head and neck.

Neurotic Excoriations: No lesions except stages of excoriation and ulceration; upper back, outer arms are favorite locations; rare on hands and genitalia; white scars may show follicular accentuation, particularly on upper back.

Insect Bites: Cat or Dog Fleas – Constellation pattern, ankles and legs
Mosquitoes – Immediate weal after insect bite
Bed Bug – Single lesion, sometimes bullous or hemorrhagic
Cheyletiella – Small dotted urticarial papules, particularly on chest

---

Creeping Eruption or Larva Migrans

This affliction presents as an irregular red line with inconsistent turns of varying size. The line is 1mm wide and is just palpable. Rarely, a small papulovesicle may be seen at the advancing head. Sometimes, the line itself has a beaded papular or papulovesicular appearance. The tract may extend as much as 3 to 4cm in a day. Sites of predilection are the ankles, feet (soles), thighs, and lower abdomen. Multiple lesions may be present.

Loa-loa may cause a burrow in the conjunctiva as it crawls across the eye.

Reference
1. Mellanby, KEW. Scabies. 2nd Ed. Faringdon, England:Classy Ltd., 1972.

Appendices

NOTE: *References for Appendices A to E inclusive are found on page 482.*

Appendix A: Method of Examination
Set Up

1. A good light is required. A 60-watt blue incandescent bulb on a wall-mounted architect-type extension lamp is a satisfactory alternative to daylight. Illuminate the lesion from several different angles.
2. You need a magnifying glass or binocular loupe 6x to 10x .[*1] A diagnosis made from a distance of greater than 20cm is, dermatologically speaking, unsound.

   If you apply a substance like oil or water to the exterior surface of the skin, you will find that the epidermis is made less obvious and it is easier to see underlying pigment and small blood vessels. Hence its desirability in looking at red, brown, and black colored skin lesions. Also, when looking at pared keratotic plantar lesions, it is easier to see where the print lines go if you use a clearing agent such as oil. This will help determine whether there is an expanding lesion (e.g. a verruca) pushing aside the print lines.

   A variation of this technique using a light source built into a magnifying glass is called epiluminescent microscopy.[2]
3. You need to make yourself and the patient comfortable, e.g. for examination of the soles of the feet the patient should be lying prone on a high (42-inch) examining table.
4. In diagnostic and long-standing problems, always look at both sides of the body, and always look all over. Many more mistakes are made by not looking than by not knowing.

Morphological Signs

Morphological signs are listed in Tables 54 and 55.[3–7]

The most indispensable historical information is what medications have been taken systemically and applied topically. Harvey's law states that when what you see does not easily resemble or remind you of a clinical diagnosis, be sure to ask yourself, "has something been done or applied to the lesion?"

I do not believe that the distinction between primary and secondary lesions is either valid or useful. A lesion is a lesion and should be seen and described and diagnosed as a part of the living gross pathology. You do not have primary and secondary aspects of other subjective medical findings, such as heart sounds, abdominal masses, or odor of certain bacterial infections. Some skin lesions may be of more significance from a diagnostic point of view, e.g. the pearly rolled border is more important than the ulcer in basal cell carcinoma, but to try to assign priority to each grossly visible change seems pointless.

---

[*]An interesting method for photographic examination of the surface of the skin indicating the polyangular units demarcated by the skin furrows has been described and illustrated by Wagner and Goltz.[1]

Table 54: Morphological Signs of the First Order
1. **Color** – The colors described in the book are those seen primarily in Caucasians.
2. **Lesion** – Remember to include the response to scratching, stroking, diascopy, pricking with a needle, and paring; in most cases, crusts should be removed so that you can see what is underneath.
3. **Consistency and Extension** – Use the ball of the third finger of the right hand for palpitation, as it is surprisingly sensitive.

Table 55: Other Morphological Signs	
Extent	Localized, disseminated, universal
Distribution	Region or regions involved
Arrangement	Grouped, linear, circular, bomb-explosion pattern
Odor[8]	
Hair, Nails, and Mucosae	
Lymph Nodes	Especially for solitary tumors and infections
Subjective Skin Symptoms	Itch, pain, burning
Systemic Signs and Symptoms	Obvious abnormalities, functional inquiry, operations
History	What applied, what drugs taken

Additional information can be obtained in References 3 to 7.

After the above examination has been done, you should be able to state, among other findings, the location of the lesion in the skin and its nature, i.e. is it above the skin, the same level as the skin, or below the skin, and is it cellular, fluid, pigment, and so on.

At our weekly teaching rounds at the Ottawa Civic Hospital, the resident is asked to sum up each case as follows: (a) a brief, one- or two-line statement on the patient's apparent age, sex, general health, and obvious abnormalities; (b) the location of the lesion; (c) the morphology; and (d) the relevant history. Then the resident is asked to give a differential diagnosis indicating reasons for excluding some and including others, and finally reasons for the most likely diagnosis.

Appendix B: Dermatological Topography

Because I have trouble remembering the details of certain anatomical areas such as the pinna, it occurs to me that others may have similar trouble, so I have included schematic drawings indicating names for the various regions of the body (Figs. B.1 to B.9).[9-11] Some of these names are quite arbitrary, but I have tried to be consistent in their use. I have also included general overall terms so that, for example, one will not call the thigh the leg. I have not used the usual Basle Nomina Anatomica (BNA) nomenclature because it is illogical to use divisions based solely on the names of underlying structures. Skin diseases do not often occur in this pattern. Also, it is impractical because there are at once too many and too few anatomical regions in the BNA nomenclature, e.g. eight areas from the tip of the chin to the suprasternal notch, and I can find no BNA name for some areas, e.g. columella of the nose, interfinger webs, and lip-cheek fold. It seems that some nomenclature scheme such as I have suggested will help accuracy in description and ease of communication. For convenience, the dermatomes and the distribution of the trigeminal nerve are also shown.

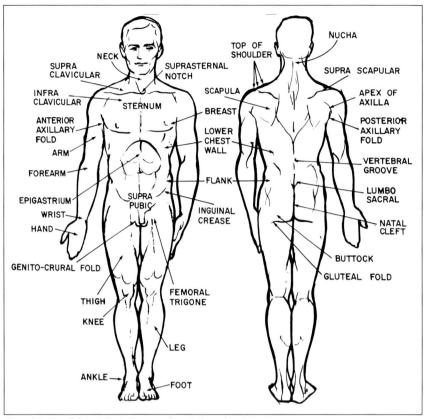

Figure B.1 Overall dermatological topography, anterior and posterior views.

Figure B.2 Dermatological topography of head and neck, side and frontal view. The synonym for the crown is the vertex; for the lip-cheek fold, the meso- or melo-labial fold; for the temple, the frontal area; and for the alar groove, the alar crease.

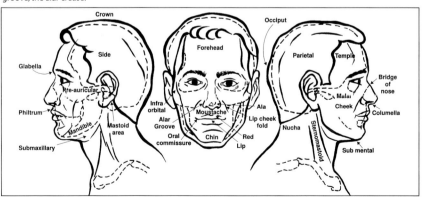

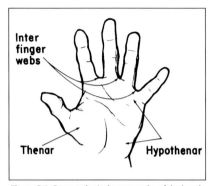

Figure B.3 Dermatological topography of the hand. Thumb, index, middle, ring, and little finger are the preferred terms.

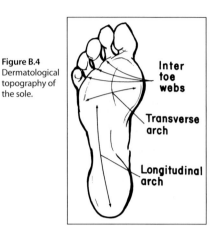

Figure B.4 Dermatological topography of the sole.

Figure B.5 Dermatological topography of the external female genitalia.

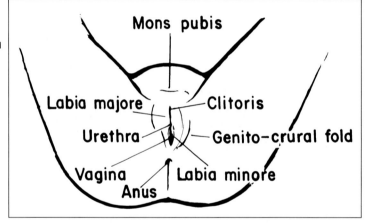

Figure B.6 Dermatological topography of the lateral portion of the pinna.

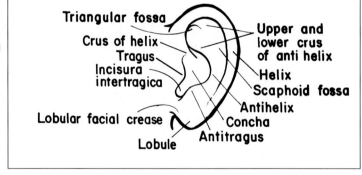

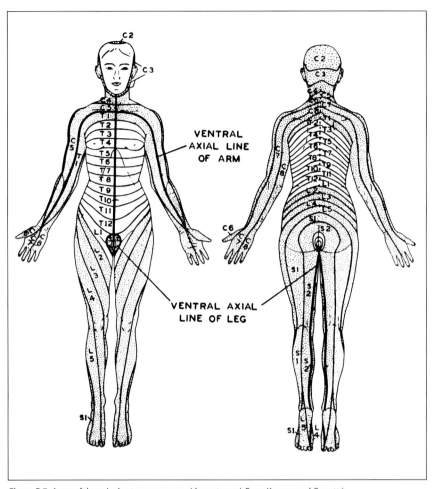

Figure B.7 Areas of the spinal cutaneous nerves (dermatomes). From Keegan and Garrett.[2]

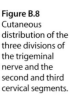

Figure B.8
Cutaneous
distribution of the
three divisions of
the trigeminal
nerve and the
second and third
cervical segments.

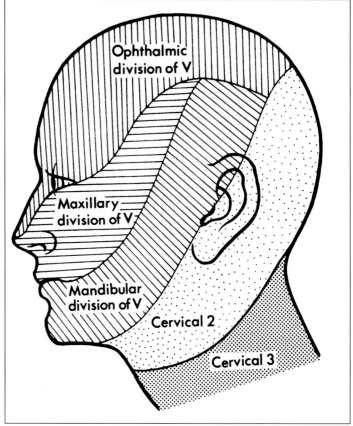

Figure B.9
The surface
anatomy of the
eyelids. Redrawn
from Wolf.[3]
X----X = Lid
closure line,
palpebral fissure.

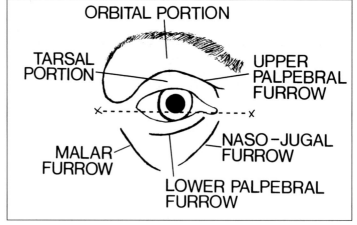

Appendix C: Color in Dermatology

The desirability of using scientifically exact names to describe the colors of skin lesions has long been advocated.[12-14] Using charts of tables as depicted in the Munsell Book of Color (Munsell Color Co. Inc., Baltimore, 1929) or by the charts of the Royal Horticultural Society (U.K.), it has been suggested that the exact value of lightness, degree of saturation, and color should be selected and used to describe, for example, the red of psoriasis.

The practicability of following such a system is very limited because the numbers of variations are so large. In the Munsell Book of Color there are 10 red colors. For each of the 10 red colors there may be 10 degrees of lightness and 10 degrees of saturation. This makes a total of 1,000 reds. Even if one had a portable set of color charts, it can be easily seen how impractical this "scientific" approach would be.

What can be done is to try and use the 24 traditional color names as proposed by the Munsell Book of Color with the explanation of color, lightness, and saturation as outlined in Table 56.

Appel[12] gives some examples of the use of this terminology as follows:

for salmon colored say weak reddish-orange or moderate orange-pink

for coral colored say pinkish-white or light red or vivid red

for fawn colored say pale brown or light yellowish-brown

I have tried to incorporate these colors into the text without reducing clarity and readability.

Many colors and hues are present in skin lesions and some are of great diagnostic import. Scattered throughout this text are several small portions about the various colors that are used to describe skin lesions. For example, the reds are discussed and classified under the erythemas and the browns under the dyschromias.

Use of the word "pigmented" as a description of a lesion without a color defining adjective is not acceptable. Is the lesion pigmented brown? black? blue? yellow? red? and so on. Almost no skin lesions are truly white—as a sheet of paper or as a lab coat. Many nonpigmented lesions are skin-colored, i.e. they have normal skin pigmentation. If one uses the term "skin- colored", one should perhaps tell the race of the patient and the location of the skin (e.g. palmar, abdominal, or scalp). In most cases, one refers to the skin adjacent to the lesion.

The biggest problem is distinguishing and describing the various red colors. What color is cooked salmon? Does it not depend on the type of salmon—and/or how it is cooked. The deep red palmar and plantar macules of secondary syphilis are of great significance in white patients. Of course, they are not a "cooked ham color" in black patients. The juvenile xanthogranuloma tends to have a yellowish or orange-brown color, the juvenile Spitz nevus has a bright angiomatous red or red-brown color, and urticaria pigmentosa has a more solid medium brown color.

Table 56: Traditional Color Names (Munsell)

| Group | Traditional Color Notation | Designation According to the Munsell System of Color Notation | | |
		Color	Lightness	Saturation
1	Pink Light Pink Pale Pink	Red pink-to red	Light	Weak to moderate
2	Rose Briar Rose Old Rose Wild Rose	Red	Middle	Moderate
3	Maroon Bordeaux Claret Red Garnet Wine Red	Red	Dark	Moderate
4	Scarlet	Red	Middle	Very Strong
5	Orange	Yellow-red	Middle	Strong
6	Tan Buff Sand	Yellow-red	Middle to light	Weak to Moderate
7	Brown Amber Auburn Chestnut Chocolate Cocoa Golden Brown Hazel Russet Seal Brown Tobacco	Yellow-red	Dark to middle	Weak to moderate
8	Ivory Buff Old Ivory Straw	Yellow	Light	Weak
9	Lemon Yellow	Yellow	Light	Strong
10	Olive Olive Drab	Yellow to green-yellow	Dark to middle	Weak to Moderate
11	Nile Green Apple Green	Green-yellow	Light	Weak to moderate

Group	Traditional Color Notation	Designation According to the Munsell System of Color Notation		
		Color	Lightness	Saturation
12	Emerald Green Jade	Green	Dark to Middle	Strong
13	Turquoise Blue Turquoise	Blue-green to blue	Middle to light	Moderate
14	Sky Blue Baby Blue Light Blue	Blue	Light	Weak to moderate
15	Royal Blue National Blue	Purple-blue	Dark	Strong
16	Navy Blue Gendarme Midnight Blue Navy Sailor Blue	Purple-blue	Dark	Weak to moderate
17	Violet	Purple	Dark	Moderate to strong
18	Lavender Lilac Mauve	Purple	Middle to light	Weak to Moderate
19	Plum Prune	Purple to red-purple	Dark	Weak to moderate
20	Orchid	Purple to red-purple	Middle to light	Weak to moderate
21	Magenta	Red-purple	Dark	Moderate to strong
22	Black Coal black	—	Very dark	None to very weak
23	Gray Battleship Gray Gunmetal Iron Gray Lead Pearl Gray Silver Slate Smoke Gray Steel Gray Taupe	—	Dark to light	None to very Weak
24	White	—	Very light	None to very weak

Various forms of the poikilodermas have various mixtures of colors—the red of telangiectasia, the brown of melanin (rarely hemosiderin), and the white of atrophy and sclerosis. In these conditions, there may be times when one or other color is predominant and this should be mentioned. For example, some radiation sequelae are pale, others are quite red, and still others are quite brown.

Atrophic lesions can have various colors. Sometimes they truly are white, more often than not they are off-white or light brown, occasionally they are more brown than the normal skin.

The color of the keratotic material must be described. For example, the solar keratoses on the dorsa of the hands often have a whitish color, those on the upper back may be reddish, and those on the face may be brownish. In pityriasis rubra pilaris, the keratoderma has the most helpful orange-brown color. A purplish-red is often present at the borders of other keratodermas.

One should never forget that agents applied to the skin (e.g. AgNO3, picric acid) or taken internally (minocycline, amiodarone) may cause a color change. Harvey's law applies to colors as to other skin morphology.

Crusts are another lesion having many colors. The honey colored crust of impetigo is not specific for impetigo; the crusts of weeping eczema may also be honey colored. Other factors such as the degree of erythema, shape of lesion, border of lesion, etc., have to be taken into account. Do not confuse a hemorrhagic crust with the black eschar of dead tissue.

Another area where color can help is in the differential between lesions having other similar morphological features. For example, the difference in the red colors between pityriasis rosea (a warm pink), psoriasis (a deep red) and tinea (a faint brown erythema) on the torso. Another example is the difference in color between papules of lichen simplex chronicus (brownish to skin colored) and those of lichen planus (violaceaus).

Table 57 lists some conditions where color is of great diagnostic significance. I am sure you could add some of your own.

Table 57: **Useful Diagnostic Colors**	
Color, Morphology, or Location	**Disease**
Streaky slate gray	Incontinentia pigmenti
Faint bluish- or greenish-brown papules	Blue nevus or "blue and true nevus"
Purply eyelid erythema	Dermatomyositis
Corn Yellow	Some xanthomas
Canary Yellow	Bile in skin
Carmine Erythema	Facial lupus erythematosus
Gray muddy–over cartilage	Argyria, ochronosis
Purplish-red in photodistribution on face	Chlorpromazine pigmentation
Pink-salmon colored palms and soles	Pityriasis rubra pilaris
Lenticular slate-blue spots on torso	Maculae caeruleae
Light gray-brown following skin lines on neck and clavicular areas	Lack of vigorous washing; build-up of stratum corneum, which gets a dirty grey color

There is a group of conditions in which both color and consistency seem to be implied (the whitish grey and firm pearly border of some basal cell carcinomas come to mind as do the apple-jelly color and consistency of some granulomas such as sarcoidosis). In these descriptions, one should remember to say apple-jelly color (dusky amber), apple-jelly consistency, or both, if that is what one means.

Appendix D: Study Aids

The purpose of the questions is to make sure that some of the more important differential diagnostic features of various kinds of eruption are being learnt. By asking for differential diagnoses of eruptions that do not have the same lesion, you can determine whether or not the student is absorbing the material.

For example, in discussing the significant differential diagnosis of annular eruptions of the chin one would expect at least some of the following to be presented:

Papular Lesions: secondary lues, sarcoidosis, lichen planus

Erythematosquame: tinea faciei

Vesiculopustular: impetigo

Follicular: kerion

Another way of doing this is to ask the student to give a classification of linear lesions (of all types—papules, blisters, dyschromias, and so on) and to explain the determinant of the pattern, e.g.:

- Blood vessels
- Lymphatics
- Dermatomes
- Nerve trunks
- Infestations
- Blaschko's lines
- Other developmental lines
- External: plants
  - collagens
  - chemical
  - thermal
  - physical
  - others

Table 58 provides a listing of lesions for discussion of differential diagnoses. Table 59 provides a listing of gross and microscopic anatomy for discussion. Study areas of embryology are listed in Table 60.

Other areas of study that have not been specifically covered are the location of the superficial lymph nodes and which areas of skin and mucosa are drained by which lymph nodes: in particular, the lymph nodes of the head and neck including the mouth; the lymph nodes of the upper and lower extremity including the axilla and groin; and finally some study of the drainage of the breast tissue.

Special attention should be paid to the tissues in the skin that provide a reason for the shape or location of many skin lesions. This should include an appreciation of dermatomal patterns, lymphatics in the skin, Blaschko's lines, blood vessels in the skin, and how their anatomy can produce certain patterns in certain diseases.

Another area to be addressed is an understanding of the anatomical bases of the ophthalmological terms used to describe eye-skin diseases.

Many of the above-mentioned study areas have been covered already in the text, especially where I have thought it directly appropriate to morphology. It is not my purpose in this text to deal with such items as lymph node location patterns and eye anatomy, but this should be part of the resident teaching programme. If it is not formally covered, the resident should see that he studies it on his own.

I suggest, as a resident exercise, that at some time they make notes on those items dealing with distribution of lesions in this text and put them all together in a "cheat sheet" format.

Table 58: Discuss the Significant Differential Diagnoses of the Following Lesions

Follicular keratoses of the loins
Erythematosquames of the inguinal crease
Purplish plaques of the left side of the neck
Scaly purplish-red plaques on the cheeks
Ulcers on the finger tips
Red lesions on the glans penis:　plaques, patches, papules
　　　　　　　　　　　　　　　　erosions
　　　　　　　　　　　　　　　　nodules
Facial erythemas
Linear keratodermas
White lesions on the tongue
Scaly lesions on the nucha
Papules on the pinna
Nodules on the nose
Patterns of eczema on the hands
Painful papules and nodules
What are the five really itchy skin eruptions?
Leonine facies
Papular and nodular tumors of the scalp
Nonblistering scaly eruptions of the sole
Papular eruptions of the flexor forearms
Distinction between pityriasis rosea and secondary lues
Brown-red facial papulonodules in children
Papules on the eyelids
Solitary keratoses on the soles
Scaly eruptions of the outer portion of the external auditory meatus
White lesions of the toe-web spaces
Multiple persistent erythematosquames on the torso
Nonpermanent swelling of the eyelids
Lichenification of the semimucosa of the anus
Scaly periungual lesions
Purpura on the dorsa of the feet and ankles
Solitary 1.0cm blister on mid-sole
Papules on the eyelid margins
Solitary hole up to 1.0cm on the face
Persistent presternal eruptions
Plaque of telangiectatic sclerosis on the sacral area
Disorders of the hair shaft of the axillae
Suprapubic papules and nodules
Lesions of the triangular fossa of the pinna
Color changes of the nail plate
A linear lesion of the upper extremity

Table 58: *continued*

Diffuse loss of eyebrows: non-scarring
                           scarring
Eyelid edema   with skin lesions
              without skin lesions
Penile edema   with skin lesions
              without skin lesions
Nodular plaques of the shins
Follicular keratoses of outer and anterior thighs
Follicular pustules on thighs and buttocks in a young male
Collarettes
Diseases with in-toeing scale
Localized poikiloderma
List 10 exophytic nodules
Acneform lesions of the hairy torso
Solitary cystic lesion on the eyelid margin
Pigmented axillary lines
Distinction between pigmented basal cell carcinoma and malignant melanoma
What are the angiomatous papulonodular tumours?
Solar cheilitis versus discoid lupus erythematosus versus lichen planus on vermilion area
   of lower lip
Fissure in natal cleft
Solitary dotted brown papule on the nose
Itchy white area on the labium majus (labia majora)
Annular eruptions on the chin
Patterns of facial eczema
Patterns of red pustular facial eruptions
Define and discuss the diagnostic significance of the semimucosae
Macroglossia
List pseudosclerodermatous (sclerodermoid?) conditions
Differential diagnosis of scaly axillary lesions
Differential diagnosis of scarring lesions of the palm
Patterns of facial melanosis
Persistent red scaly areas on sun-damaged torso
Persistent red scaly areas on sun-damaged face
Persistent red scaly areas on covered areas
Circular lesions on the torso
Inward pointing scaly patches
Orolingual paresthesias
Paresthesias of the extremities
Juxta-articular nodes
Lesions of the lobule of the ear

Table 59: **Discuss the Gross and Microscopic Anatomy**

The eyelids
Nose and nasal vestibule
Vulvar skin and semimucosae
External auditory meatus and pinna
Glans and shaft of penis
Lips and mouth
Axilla
Nails
Lymph nodes

Table 60: **Study Areas in Practical Dermatological Embryology**

Overview of Embryology of Human Skin[15]
    Various layers
    When do certain structures arise — eccrine glands, pilosebaceous units, apocrine glands, melanocytes
    Location of melanocytes in fetal epidermis, concept of their migration from the neural crest

Specific Items
    Central lower lip pit or fissure
    Congenital pre-auricular sinus
    Thyroglossal and brachial sinuses and cysts
    Lower sacral area defects
    The significance of embryological planes of the face
    Paranasal embryological defects
    Genital and peri-anal embryological defects and sinuses
    Accessory fingers versus digital fibromas
    Occipital scalp defects (aplasia cutis)
    Blaschko's lines
    Congenital cutaneous umbilical abnormalities

Concept of Multiple Congenital Defects
    Clouston's syndrome
    Epidermal nevus syndrome
    Nevoid basal cell carcinoma syndrome

Concept of Genetic Embryological Abnormality Not Present at Birth
    Possible factors determining age of onset
    Possible factors determining progression up to adulthood
    Examples: sebaceous nevus, Becker's nevus, linearepidermal nevus, nevoid basal cell carcinoma
        syndrome, the whole story of the natural progression of nevi

Appendix E: Glossary

It is surprising that standard definitions of many lesions have never been agreed upon by dermatologists.[16,17] Physicians working in the same institution may disagree on the meaning of such terms as macule, papule, nodule, node, vesicle, and bulla. What sort of science can dermatology be when the basic descriptive terms or units of measurement have no consistent meaning? Admittedly medicine, including dermatology, is not an exact science in the same sense as mathematics or physics. However, should not an attempt be made at least to standardize the basic terminology so that, for example, a nodule means the same thing in Moscow as in San Francisco? When I look at various textbooks for clarification, none can be found. This glossary is offered with humility, so that even if you do not agree with my definitions, at least you know what I am talking about.

A detailed description of many of the terms, including some basic morphological concepts, e.g. the distinction between a bulla and a vesicle, is to be found in the "Overview" in the appropriate chapter.

A useful reference book is *A Dictionary of Dermatologic Terms.*[18]

No excuse is offered for measuring lesions by the size of common fruits or vegetables.[19] Just as there is a natural variation in the size of peas, so there is natural variation in the size of vesicles, bullae, or other lesions. An eruption is classified by the size of the majority of the lesions.

- *Abscess:* A relatively large (over 2 to 3 cm in diameter) accumulation of pus forming a cavity in the dermis and subdermis. Usually pus cannot be seen from the surface, unless the lesion is draining. May be from pyogenic organisms, from nodal gran-ulomas, and from the discharging panniculitis.
- *Agminate:* Gathered together in a group.
- Ainhum: A slowly progressive, fibrous, band-like constriction, usually of the proximal phalanges of the small toes, eventually ending in withering or amputation of the digits.
- *Alopecia:* Loss of hair in any amount up to complete baldness.
- *Anetoderma:* Local atrophy of the dermis, involving mainly the elastica. The lesions may bulge or look depressed. On palpation, a sensation of herniation is felt. A type of atrophy (means slack skin).
- *Annular:* Ring-shaped with an implication of a clear, clearing, or cleared center.
- *Aphthae:* Mucosal erosions, cankers.
- *Arciform:* Bent like a bow, bow-shaped, arcuate.
- *Atrophoderma:* A very specific name for atrophies due to a defect in development, hence the name should be restricted to congenital atrophies.
- *Atrophy:* Diminution in the number or volume of constituents of the skin, in particular the elastic tissue; it is often associated with sclerosis.
- *Autosensitization:* See Id.

- *Beau's Lines:* Transverse furrows that run across all nails and grow out with the nails.
- *Blaschko's Lines:* Lines that have been arrived at as an empirical average from a large number of systematized epidermal verrucous nevi and other inflammatory linear lesions, e.g. psoriasis or lichen striatus.[20]
- *Blistering:* Can be either composed of vesicles or bullae.
- *Bomb-explosion pattern:* Large central lesion surrounded by many smaller lesions which decrease in size and number toward the periperhy, e.g. verrucae and secondary syphilis, or tinea corporis.
- *Bulla:* A liquid-filled cavity, usually unilocular, larger than a pea, i.e. larger than 1.0 cm. Bullae may be subcorneal, inter-epidermal, or subepidermal. For distinction from vesicle, see "Overview" in Chapter 8.
- *Burrow:* A tunnel in the superficial portion of the epidermis of variable size and shape made by a parasite. In scabies at one end there is a tiny deep vesicle which forms in the vicinity of the *Sarcoptes*. In creeping eruption, the metazoal parasite forms long linear red streaks in the upper epidermis (up to 10 cm).

- *Callus:* Localized horny mass of scale due to trauma.
- *Carbuncle:* Coalescence of several adjoining furuncles.
- *Circinate:* Circle-shaped, a series of curved lesions each arch of which is part of a circle. The concept of an empty circle is useful here.
- *Cockade:* From cocarde (Fr.), a rosette worn as a badge of office or a military decoration. Cockade lesions are commonly seen in linear IgA disease and in the cockade nevus.
- *Collarette:* A ring of scales, often occurring after a vesicle has subsided, e.g. eczema or flexural *Candida*.
- *Comedo:* A small horny mass with a brown or black top, the size of a pinhead to that of a millet-seed, imbedded in a dilated follicular orifice.
- *Confluent:* Refers to lesions of any type and severity when they merge to cover wide areas.
- *Corn:* A local funnel-shaped traumatic hyperkeratosis with a central light brown translucent core. In large corns, there is a central whitish core.
- *Crusts:* Deposits of dried secretions or dead tissue. May be composed of serum, pus, blood, or dead tissue. Differentiate crust from necrosis of tissue. For detailed discussion see "Overview" in Chapter 14.
- *Cutis Marmorata:* A net-like pattern of livid discoloration due to hyperemia.
- *Cyst:* Encapsulated retention cavity of any size filled with fluid, cells, and cell products. If full of pus, it is usually called an abscess. Not of inflammatory nature, but may be secondarily inflamed.

- *Deposits:* Substances, which are usually alien to the skin, laid down in the skin, mucosa, and appendages. Examples are amyloid, urates, calcium salts, and cholesterol. An accumulation of endogenous compounds in abnormal amounts or location.
- *Dermatitis:* An inflammatory condition of the skin. Meaningless unless qualified, e.g. eczematous dermatitis.

- *Dermatosis:* A pathological condition of the skin. I have used this term in the chapters on papules, nodules and nodes to encompass diseases not covered by the designation tumors and deposits. Dermatoses are usually not permanent.
- *Diascopy:* Glass or clear plastic pressure momentarily dehematizing a lesion for purposes of clearer examination. Hemorrhages, pigmentations, and cellular infiltrates persist.
- *Digitate:* Lesion assuming the shape of a finger-like mark.
- *Discoid:* Solid, round and moderately raised (cf. nummular).
- *Disseminated:* Lesions scattered over many areas. Implies concept of seeding. Widespread. Not universal, not generalized.
- *Dyschromia:* Abnormal color of skin, hair, nails, or mucosa.
- *Dyshidrosis:* A blistering, usually recurrent, eruption of the thick-skinned areas of the hands and feet. Implies an abnormality in sweating, which is not true, so I use the older, but noncommittal, term pompholyx.
- *Dystrophy:* (Literally fault of nutrition) is a variety of atrophy that may have certain combinations of finding making diagnosis clear.

- *Eczema:* A clinical process that is clearly superficial in form and that, early, is erythematous, papulovesicular, oozing and crusting and later, is red purple, scaly, lichenified, and then, brown or hypopigmented. Clinically vesiculation and histologically spongiosis must be present at some stage. For a detailed outline see "Overview" in Chapter 5.
- *Edema:* A swelling caused by retention of abnormal amounts of fluid in the tissue, usually with a connotation of diffuseness. On finger pressure, pitting occurs.
- *Enanthem:* A systemic, often febrile disease accompanied by a quickly or suddenly eruptive lesion or lesions of mucous membranes. The basic lesion may be an erythema (measles) or blister (varicella). Literally means a bursting-forth of flowers within.
- *Erosion:* Defect from loss of a portion of the epidermis, commonly following vesicles or bullae; usually nonscarring.
- *Erythema:* A reaction in the skin characterized by an active or passive redness of the skin, more or less sharply marginated, usually temporary, and which disappears upon finger pressure; may be widespread or localized. Caused by vasodilation.
- *Erythematosquamous:* Erythematosquamous eruptions are equally scaly and red.
- *Erythroderma:* A persistent inflammatory reddening of all the skin, with lichenification and scaling.
- *Exanthem:* A systemic, often febrile disease accompanied by a quickly or suddenly eruptive lesion on the skin. The basic lesion may be an erythema (scarlet fever), a blister (smallpox), or a papule (secondary syphilis). Literally means a bursting-forth of flowers to the outside.
- *Excoriation:* A defect involving damage to epidermis and upper dermis, having a linear, circular, or other geometric shape and being caused by scratching or rubbing. Usually not scarring.

- *Figurate:* Referring to a lesion in the form of a shape, such as circular, arcuate. Commonly used as an adjective to an erythema.
- *Fissure:* A linear crack involving no loss of tissue, but a loss of continuity of the epidermis and the upper dermis. Except for syphilitic fissures or rhagades, it does not scar.
- *Fistulae:* Discharging tracts that are often granulomatous, sclerotic and midline, sometimes congenital.
- *Folliculoses:* Suppurative, acneform, and keratotic eruptions that primarily involve the pilosebaceous unit.
- *Furuncle:* A deep pus-forming necrotizing folliculitis.

- *Generalized:* Term used to describe the lesions of a cutaneous disease when they are widespread and exempt no important region of the body (cf. disseminated, universal, confluent, and widespread).
- *Glabrous:* Literally smooth, usually means glabrous skin without terminal hair such as torso or face.
- *Granulations:* The vegetations on the base of ulcerative or erosive conditions.
- *Granuloma:* A microscopic pathological term having no real connotation in living gross pathology despite attempts to give it a clinical meaning. How, for example, can you compare granuloma annulare (an annular papular eruption), granuloma pyogenicum (a papular erosive angiomatous tumor), and granuloma fungoides (a nodular ulcerative tumor)? The definition really means a chronic inflammatory dermal proliferative process. But what does this look like? Does it have a "specific" gross morphological picture? Clinically, I have defined a granuloma as a deeply seated dermal or hypodermal papulonodular lesion, round, solid, well circumscribed, forming annular or arcuate borders, skin-colored or reddish-brown, and showing ulceration, scarring, and sinus formation. Be clear in your own mind when you call something a granuloma whether you are making a microscopic or living gross pathologic diagnosis.
- *Grouped:* Multiple discrete lesions occurring in a localized area.
- *Gumma:* Granulomatous abscess forming nodes of infectious origin, usually with sinus formation and scarring. By tradition, this is the nodal granuloma of tertiary syphilis.

- *Harvey's Law:* When what you see does not easily resemble or remind you of a clinical diagnosis, be sure to ask yourself… "has something been done or applied to the lesion?" (After Harvey Finkelstein, MD, resident class of 1984–1985.)
- *Hidroses:* Functional or organic disturbances of the apocrine or eccrine sweat glands.
- *Hypertrichosis:* Excessive hairiness.
- *Hypertrophies:* Persistent localized, extensive thickening of all or many layers of the skin.

- *Id:* Means in this text autosensitization dermatitis or absorptive phenomenon. These are symmetrical sterile secondary lesions occurring in other bodily areas in a patient who has an acute primary focus. This secondary lesion mimics the primary. (See Chapter 5.)

- *Intertrigo:* The congestive redness that results from mutual friction of two contiguous surfaces.
- *Iris lesions:* Multiple concentric ringed eruptions of different colors and sometimes different lesions.

- *Keratoderma:* Palmar and plantar keratoses. May be diffuse or localized, confluent or punctate.
- *Keratosis:* A localized moderate thickening of the horny layer.
- *Koebner Phenomenon:* Provocation by irritation.

- *Leukoderma:* Secondary post-inflammatory decrease in melanin.
- *Leukonychia:* White nails.
- *Leukoplakia:* Macerated mucosal or semimucosal horny thickenings that appear white. By definition, leukoplakia cannot occur on the hairy skin.
- *Lichenification:* Papules placed so close together that they no longer form separate prominences but instead a common plateau. This results in thickening of the living layers of the skin. The finer furrows of the skin surface are smoothed out by the infiltrate; this causes the few remaining ones to become deeper and more accentuated. May be fine or coarse, sharply or poorly demarcated. May be hyperpigmented with varying shades of brown (cf. plaque).
- *Livedo:* From Latin, blueness from contusion. We use the word to describe the blueness of venous congestion—racemosa (grape-shaped), reticularis (net-like).
- *Localized:* Occurring in some particular part or area of the skin; changes limited or confined to a region; regional; e.g. palms and soles, face, intertriginous areas; opposite of disseminated. In some groups of diseases, it is not possible to make a clear-cut distinction between disseminated and localized (see e.g. the keratoses).
- *Locus Minoris Resistentiae:* A place of less resistance, any part or organ more susceptible than the others to the attack of a morbific agent. A more specific definition is a site of lessened resistance; an area, structure, or organ offering little resistance to invasion by micro-organisms and/or their toxins. In his classic text on syphilis, Stokes et al.[21] used this term basically to refer to the development of syphilitic lesions at sites of physical trauma. The term has also been used to describe the location and pattern of Blaschko's lines, scar sarcoid and scar eczema.
- *Macule:* A circumscribed deviation from normal skin color without other changes. The borders may be distinct or vague. Their shapes are extremely variable. A spot. A small amount of scale can be accepted as a feature of some macules. If equally red and scaly it is an erythematosquame.
- Maculopapular

> Papuloerosive
> Papulopustular
> Papulovesicular
> Tuberoulcerative
> Vesiculobullous
> Vesiculopustular

These conjoint terms are to be used to indicate that the eruption evolves from the first type of lesion to the second, not that both types of lesion are present independently, so they are both historical and physical terms.

- *Mamillated:* Having rounded protuberances.
- *Melanoderma:* Secondary postinflammatory increase in melanin.
- *Melanosis:* Endogenous or primary melanin hyperpigmentation without preceding skin disease.
- *Multiforme:* This refers to the presence of several different types of lesions in the same disease, e.g. erythemas, bullae, and urticoid plaques in erythema multiforme. It also can have the connotation of the same disease in different patients who have different morphological lesions.
- *Mutilation:* Destruction of structures including those deeper than the skin.

- *Nevus:* This is a word with a complex meaning. Most dictionaries interpret it to mean a birthmark of red or brown color. Leider and Rosenblum[22] have this to say: "The widest implication of nevus, then, is anything, especially anything odd, abnormal or faulty, that is related to conception, gestation and post-natal development and stems from hereditary or embryogenic fault, abnormality or oddity." Those who use the word should do so carefully. Hamartoma (abnormal accumulations of normal cells and tissue) has been proposed as an alternative term.
- *Node:* A large (over 2.0 cm) solid lesion mainly or entirely subcutaneous. Distinguish from lymph node. See also gumma.
- *Nodule:* A persistent large (over 1.0 cm) epidermal-dermal, dermal, or dermal-hypodermal papule with well-defined borders. It is a solid lesion with a prominent vertical dimension. See also tuber and tubercle.
- *Nummular:* Sharply marginated, coin-sized and coin-shaped (circular and quarter-sized or larger). An implication is that the abnormality exists through the total lesion, i.e. a filled circle (see discoid).

- *Onychogryphosis:* Long, horn-shaped excrescenses of the nail plate, implying thickening and hardness.
- *Onycholysis:* Detachment of the nail plate from the nail bed.
- *Onychoses:* Diseases that affect the nail plate and surrounding structures.
- *Pachyonychia:* Columnar hyperkeratosis of finger- and toe-nails with thickened, wax-colored, opaque, and yellowish horny substance, usually beneath the distal end of the nail plate.
- *Papule:* A small (less than 1.0cm), solid persistent elevation above skin level and caused by an increase in number and size of cells and cell products rather than an accumulation of liquid. It has a solid center. It may be flattened by pressure, may be sessile (broad based), pedunculated, (constricted at the base), agminated (gathered together in groups), filiform (thread-like), acuminate (sharp or pointed); may have a central depression (dell, umbilication). They are of varying color. Shape depends in part upon the level of underlying cellular infiltration and whether papule is follicular or not.
  Darier[23] and Willan[24] have arbitrarily decided to define papular eruptions as eruptive conditions, i.e. conditions that usually eventually disappear (after perhaps

much coming and going) without scarring. Lesions of papular size that persist, e.g. xanthoma, nevi, basal cell carcinoma, are classified by them under tumors of the skin. This is very arbitrary, and Siemens[25] objects, claiming that you are basing your diagnosis on the prognosis and not vice versa. I have decided to follow exact morphology and call a papule a papule whether it is eruptive or not.

For a detailed discussion on the shape of the various types of papules, see the "Overview" in Chapter 11.

- *Papuloerosive:* See *Maculopapular.*
- *Papulopustular:* See *Maculopapular.*
- *Papulovesicular:* See *Maculopapular.*
- *Patch:* A macule larger than 1.0 cm in diameter. To be distinguished from plaque.
- *Petaloid:* Interlocking filled circles form shapes resembling flowers. Used particularly for seborrheic lesions on center chest and back.
- *Phyma:* Nodular hypertrophy of sebaceous glands and connective tissue of the nose (rhinophyma) and ear (otophyma). Implies a rounded or bullous component.
- *Plaque:* A slightly usually elevated lesion, over 1.0 cm in diameter and commonly palm-sized or larger, consisting of an area of confluent papules or occurring de novo. Plaques may or may not be lichenified. The concept of a superficial horizontal infiltration of the skin is a useful one. Two changes common in a plaque are atrophy and tumor formation. An infiltrated erythema may also be a plaque, e.g. Sweet's syndrome. A dermal plaque may have little epidermal change.
- *Poikiloderma:* Atrophy of the epidermis, brown of hyperpigmentation, white of depigmentation, red of telangiectasia. Poikiloderma may or may not be sclerotic.
- *Polycyclic:* The figure resulting from merging of peripherally extending lesions; convexities are always directed outward in the direction of growth. If the original lesions and the resulting polycyclic areas are very small, the edges may be called microcyclic (as in herpes simplex). Usually unfilled circles are present.
- *Pompholyx:* A blistering, usually recurrent eruption of the thick-skinned areas of the hands (cheiropompholyx) or feet (pedopompholyx) or both (cheiropedopompholyx).
- *Purpura:* Extravasation of red blood cells into the skin (minute = petechiae; extensive = ecchymoses; massive = hematoma).
- *Pustule:* An epidermal elevation containing a purulent liquid. These may develop from vesicles (vesiculopustules) or bullae (purulent bullae). They may be primarily epidermal, which causes no scarring, or dermal, which usually causes scarring. They may be about eccrine sweat gland openings in children or adults. They may be follicular or nonfollicular. Follicular acne pustule: a conical papule about a pilose-baceous unit with a small pustule at the top.

- *Retiform:* Net-like. Reticulate.
- *Rhagades:* These are fissures at the angles of the mouth, at commissures like the canthi and around pursed openings like the anus. If they are deep and scarring in the peri-oral area, one should think of late radiation sequelae and congenital syphilis.

- *Scale:* Independently exfoliated platelets consisting of groups of coherent horny scales. For a detailed discussion on the details of the various types of scales, see the Overview in Chapter 6.
- *Scar:* An atrophic scar has a rarefied, thinned epidermis over damaged dermis without papillae, follicles, or glands. Sclerotic scar is a condition of epidermal atrophy and cutaneous fibrosis. Hypertrophic scar may be indistinguishable from a keloid.
- *Scattered:* Widespread lesions with a pattern less uniform than disseminated.
- *Sclerosis:* A condensation and/or overproduction of connective tissue with or without other morphological changes such as atrophy and telangiectasia.
- *Semimucosae:* The transition zone between the skin and mucous membrane, partly keratinized and with no normal appendages.
- *Serpiginous:* The shape or spread of lesions in the fashion of a creep or crawl of a snake.
- *Sinuses:* Discharging tracts that are often granulomatous, sclerotic and midline, sometimes congenital.
- *Stellate:* Star-shaped, pointed outward projections. Used to described lentigines produced by the use of psoralens together with ultra violet light (PUVA).
- *Striae:* Long bands or diamond-shaped areas of epidermal and dermal atrophy.

- *Target:* Formed of rings as an archery target (cf. iris).
- *Telangiectasia:* A permanent enlargement in caliber, coiling, and sometimes increase in number of small superficial blood vessels of the skin. Macular.
- *Toxic erythema:* A symmetrical, rapidly appearing disseminated, usually febrile eruption composed of erythema, urticaria, and purpura, alone or in combination. Drugs, viruses, and certain collagen diseases are frequent causes.
- *Trichoclasis:* Irregular transverse fracture (greenstalk) of hair shaft.
- *Trichonodosis:* Individual hairs knotted.
- *Trichoptilosis:* Longitudinal splitting of distal end of hair shaft.
- *Trichoschisis:* Clean transverse fracture of hair shaft.
- *Trichoses:* Conditions where the abnormality is primarily of the hair itself.
- *Tuber or Tubercle:* A nodule of varying size in the epidermal-dermal, dermal or dermal-subdermal area. Slowly progressive, scarring, frequently ulcerative, and often arcuate. Histologically, usually a granuloma.
- *Tumor:* A swelling. I do not recommend unqualified use of this word. It has so many meanings that it has no meaning. In Chapters 11, 12, and 13, I have used it to mean benign and malignant cellular new growths, usually having a connotation of permanence.
- *Tylosis:* A condition of heavy callus formation on the palms and/or soles.

- *Ulcer:* Loss of the covering epidermis or epithelium and underlying tissue so that scars are left after healing. If externally caused, they are called wounds. Phagedenic ulcer: an ulcer that progressively increases in size by eating away or consuming adjacent tissue.

- *Universal:* A cutaneous disease or condition that is everywhere on the skin surface (cf. generalized).
- *Urticaria:* A specific type of weal, with many lesions of varying size, frequently round or oval, and of a transitory or ephemeral nature. There is no epidermal change.

- *Vegetations:* Eruptions of many small closely-packed, round, pointed, or thread-like projections.
- *Verrucosities:* Wave-like proliferations of the malpighian layer with or without a thickened stratum corneum. Other features, such as pustules, crusting, dermal granuloma, and blisters may be present. This term seems more accurate and descriptive than other terms such as papillomatous (which is not correct: there is not tumor of the papillae) and proliferating and vegetating (terms that are too general and have no specific anatomical meaning).
- *Vesicle:* A macroscopic cavity filled with clear liquid, pinhead to pea-sized (up to 1.0 cm), spherical in shape, forming little ring-shaped collars of scales (collarettes) when emptied, almost always multilocular, and possibly umbilicated.[26] For distinction from bullae, see "Overview" in Chapter 8.
- *Vesiculobullous:* See *Maculopapular.*
- *Vesiculopustular:* See *Maculopapular.*

- *Waxy:* May refer to the color (and translucency) or the consistency or both.
- *Weal (Wheal):* A transient, varying sized swelling of the skin due to diffuse dermal fluid accumulation. They are usually red at the periphery from vasodilatation, the central area may be pale, as may be the peripheral noninvolved skin. It is usually nonpitting.
- *Whitlow:* An infection or growth (acral lentiginous melanoma), (candidal, staphylococcal, herpetic) around and in the area of the cuticle. Also known as felon, run around.
- *Wound:* A loss of continuity in the skin, extending into the dermis. Usually larger and deeper than a scratch, and frequently heals with a scar. External in origin.

References — Appendices A to E

APPENDIX A

1. Wagner G, Goltz RW. Human cutaneous topography. Cutis 1979; 23:830–842.
2. Menzies SW, Crotty KA, Ingvar WH. An Atlas of Surface Microscopy of Pigmented Skin Lesions. New York, NY:McGraw-Hill Book Co., 1996.
3. Jackson R. The shapes of infectious disease lesions in the integument of plants, animals and humans. Can Med Assoc J 1967; 97:573–579.
4. Jackson R. Observations on the site, size, shape and arrangement of lesions in the human skin. Int J. Dermatol 1984; 23:370–375.
5. Jackson R. On a clear day you can see forever. Arch Dermatol 1991; 127:1151–1153.
6. Jackson R. Morphology revised. Int J Dermatol 1993; 32:77–81.
7. Jackson R. Circles: concerning circles in nature, circles produced by man and circles in dermatology. Int J Dermatol 1994; 33:818–825.
8. Smith M, Levinson B, Smith LG. The use of smell in diagnosis. Lancet 1982; ii:1452.

APPENDIX B

9. Sabourand R. Elementary manual of regional topographical dermatology. Marshall, CF trans. New York: Rebman,1906.
10. Keegan JJ, Garrett FD. The segmental distribution of the cutaneous nerves in the limbs of man. Anat Rec 1948; 102:409.
11. Wolf E. Anatomy of the eye and orbit. Warwick R, rev. 7th Ed. Philadelphia:W.B. Saunders, 1976.

APPENDIX C

12. Appel B. Decadent descriptions in dermatology. Arch Dermatol Syph 1950; 62:370-379.
13. Vertue H St H. Correspondence. Br J Dermatol 1948; 60:386.
14. Edwards C. Measurement of skin color. Retinoids today and tomorrow. 1995; Issue 38:22-25.

APPENDIX D

15. Holbrook KA, Wolff K, The structure and development of skin in dermatology in general medicine. Textbook and atlas. 3rd edition. Fitzpatrick TB, Elson AZ, Wolff K, Freedberg IM, Austen KF. McGraw Hill. New York 1987. 120–128.

APPENDIX E

16. Jackson R. Definitions in dermatology: a dissertation on some of the terms used to describe the living gross pathology of the human skin. Clin and Exp Derm 1978: 3:241–247.
17. Winkelmann, RK, Chairman, International League of Dermatological Societies, Committee on Nomenclature. Glossary of basic dermatology lesions. Acta Derm Venereol Suppl 1987; 130:1–16.
18. Carter RL. ed. A dictionary of dermatologic terms. 4th Ed. Baltimore:Williams & Wilkins, 1992.
19. Bernhardt MS. Metrology a century ago. Arch Dermatol 1991; 127:503.
20. Jackson R. The lines of Blaschko: a review and reconsideration; observations of the cause of certain unusual linear conditions of the skin. Br J Dermatol 1976; 95:349–360.
21. Stokes JH, Beerman H, Ingraham NR Jr. Modern clinical syphilology. Philadelphia:Saunders, 1944.
22. Leider M, Rosenblum M. A dictionary of dermatological words terms and phrases. West Haven CT:Dome Laboratories, 1976; 297.
23. Darier J. Textbook of dermatology. Pollitzer S, trans. Philadelphia:Lea & Febriger, 1920.
24. Willan R. On cutaneous diseases. Philadelphia:Kimber & Conrad, 1809.
25. Siemens HW. General diagnosis and therapy of skin diseases. Weiner K, trans. Chicago:University of Chicago Press, 1958.
26. Pinkus H, Mehregan AH. A guide to dermatopathology. New York:Appleton-Century-Crofts, 1969; 75–78.

Indices

In looking up something in this text there, in the main, are two possible scenarios. The first is that you have a skin disease and do not know what it is. So you analyze the basic lesion and then look up that lesion to see the possibilities. The second scenario is that you are pretty certain of your diagnosis, but wish to check the possible differential diagnoses. Using the *Table of Contents* you find your disease under the appropriate morphology and then consider the diseases described under that morphology.

So, when you look up something in this text you will usually be looking for the differential diagnosis of a basic gross morphological sign. Therefore, in general, I have planned this book and the indices, so that they are oriented towards basic signs and not disease entities.

To accomplish this I have set up an extensive *Table of Contents* at the beginning of the book and at the beginning of each chapter. As well, there is a separate *Index of Overviews* (where a sign is indexed in some detail), a separate *Index of Tables* (listing mainly differential diagnoses), and an *Index of Illustrative Material*.

Because eponyms are so widely used in dermatological terminology, I have included a separate *Index of Eponyms* with the dates, speciality, location and pagination of each entry.

There is also a separate *General Index*. One large index would not be practical because it would be so large and detailed that it would be almost impossible to use.

General Index

Index of Overviews

Index of Tables

Index of Illustrative Material

Index of Eponyms

Schamberg, Jay Frank, 1870–1934, U.S. Dermatologist, Philadelphia, PA 60
Schönlein, Johann Lukas, 1793–1864, German Physician 45, 58
Schuller, Artur, 1874–1958, Austrian Neurologist, Vienna 247, 248
Schweninger, Ernst, 1851–1924, German Dermatologist, Berlin 361
Senear, Francis Eugene, 1889–1958, U.S. Dermatologist, Chicago 143, 146, 148
Sézary, Albert, 1880–1956, French Dermatologist 130
Shulman, Lawrence, 1919–   , U.S. Rheumatologist, Baltimore 366
Sivestre 38
Siwe, Sture August, 1897–1966, German Physician 221, 226
Sjögren, Henrick Samuel Conrad, 1899–1986, Swedish Ophthalmologist 301
Sneddon, I. B., 1915–1987, English Dermatologist 83, 162, 170
Spangler, Arthur, 1916–1975, U.S. Dermatologist, Boston 152
Spence, James, 1812–1882, Scottish Surgeon, Edinburgh 333
Spiegler, Eduard, 1860–1908, Austrian Dermatologist, Vienna 246
Spitz, Sophie, 1910–56, U.S. Pathologist 205, 211, 213, 248
Stevens, Albert Mason, 1884–1945, U.S. Pediatrician 30, 286
Stewart, F.W., 1894–   , U.S. Pathologist 246
Sturge, William Allen, 1850–1919, British Physician, London 65
Sweet, Robert Douglas, English Dermatologist 23, 35, 478

Terry 433
Thomson, Mathew Sidney, 1894–1969, English Dermatologist 69, 359, 367
Tiéche, Max, Swiss Dermatologist, Zurich 212
Trélat, Ulysse Jr., 1828–1890, French Surgeon,Bordeaux 308
Trenaunay, P., 1875–   , French Physician 136
Treves, N., 1894–1964, U.S. Surgeon 246

Usher, Barney, 1899–1978, Canadian Dermatologist, Montreal, Quebec 146, 148

Vidal, Emile, 1825–1893, French Dermatologist, l'hôpital St. Louis, Paris 173, 194
Vilanova, Xavier, 1902–65, Spanish Dermatologist 257
Vincent, Henri, 1862–1950, French Physician 287
Vogt, A., 1879–1943, Swiss Ophthalmologist 345
Voigt, Christian August, 1809–90, Austrian Anatomist, Vienna 194
Von Gierke, Edgar Otto Conrad, 1877–1945, German Pathologist 343
Von Recklinghausen, Friedrich Daniel, 1833–1910, German Pathologist 219
Von Rittershain, Gottfried Ritter, 1820–83, Austrian Pediatrician 130, 157, 164

Waardenburg, Petrus Johannes, 1886–1979, Dutch Ophthalmologist 345
Weber, Frederick Parkes, 1863–1962, British Physician, London 65, 153, 257
Wegener, F., 1907–90, German Pathologist 58, 230
Werner, C. W. O., 1879–1936, German Physician 362, 367
Wickham, Louis-Frédérick, 1861–1913, French Dermatologist, Paris 77, 176, 179, 182, 183, 223, 351
Wilkinson, Darrell Sheldon, 1919–   , English Dermatologist 170
Wilson, William James Erasmus, 1809–1884, English Dermatologist 343, 352, 434
Wood, Robert Williams, 1868–1955, American Physicist 120, 219, 416
Woronoff, D. L., Moscow 25, 103

Zoon, Johannes Jacobus, 1902–1958, Dutch Dermatologist, Utrecht 187

If you can fill in any of the empty spaces, please let me know for future editions.
Many people have helped me compile this list and special mention should go to Drs. Larry Parish, Thomas Schnalke, Bob Champion, David Grinspan, Bernard Ackerman, Wolfgang Weyers and Darrel Wilkinson. I thank them very much.

Other references consulted:

Dorlands Illustrated Medical Dictionary. 28th Ed. Philadelphia, PA:Saunders, 1994.
Goodman H. Notable contributions to the knowledge of dermatology. New York, NY:Medical Lay Press, 1951.
Norman JM, ed. Morton's medical bibliography. 5th Ed. Aldershot, Hants, England:Scolar Press, 1991.
Pusey WA. The history of dermatology. Springfield, IL: Thomas, 1933.
Shelley WB, Crissey JT. Classics in clinical dermatology. Springfield, Il:Thomas, 1953.